T0321082

Innovation in Upper Extremity Fracture Treatment

Editors

ROBIN N. KAMAL
LAUREN M. SHAPIRO

HAND CLINICS

www.hand.theclinics.com

Consulting Editor
KEVIN C. CHUNG

November 2023 • Volume 39 • Number 4

ELSEVIER

1600 John F. Kennedy Boulevard • Suite 1800 • Philadelphia, Pennsylvania, 19103-2899

http://www.theclinics.com

HAND CLINICS Volume 39, Number 4
November 2023 ISSN 0749-0712, ISBN-13: 978-0-443-18189-4

Editor: Megan Ashdown
Developmental Editor: Hannah Almira Lopez

Hand Clinics (ISSN 0749-0712) is published quarterly by Elsevier Inc., 360 Park Avenue South, New York, NY 10010-1710. Months of publication are February, May, August, and November. Business and Editorial Offices: 1600 John F. Kennedy Blvd., Ste. 1800, Philadelphia, PA 19103-2899. Customer Service Office: 3251 Riverport Lane, Maryland Heights, MO 63043. Periodicals postage paid at New York, NY and at additional mailing offices. Subscription price is $444.00 per year (domestic individuals), $878.00 per year (domestic institutions), $100.00 per year (domestic students/residents), $506.00 per year (Canadian individuals), $1023.00 per year (Canadian institutions), $568.00 per year (international individuals), $1023.00 per year (international institutions), $256.00 (international students/residents), and $100.00 (Canadian students/residents). Foreign air speed delivery is included in all *Clinics* subscription prices. All prices are subject to change without notice. **POSTMASTER:** Send address changes to *Hand Clinics*, Elsevier Health Sciences Division, Subscription Customer Service, 3251 Riverport Lane, Maryland Heights, MO 63043. Customer Service (orders, claims, online, change of address): Elsevier Health Sciences Division, Subscription **Customer Service, 3251 Riverport Lane, Maryland Heights, MO 63043. Tel: 1-800-654-2452 (U.S. and Canada); 314-447-8871 (outside U.S. and Canada). Fax: 314-447-8029. E-mail: journalscustomerservice-usa@elsevier.com (for print support); journalsonlinesupport-usa@elsevier.com (for online support)**.

Reprints. For copies of 100 or more of articles in this publication, please contact the Commercial Reprints Department, Elsevier Inc., 360 Park Avenue South, New York, New York 10010-1710. Tel.: 212-633-3874; Fax: 212-633-3820; E-mail: reprints@elsevier.com.

Hand Clinics is covered in *MEDLINE/PubMed (Index Medicus)*, *Current Contents/Clinical Medicine*, *EMBASE/Excerpta Medica*, and *ISI/BIOMED*.

Contributors

CONSULTING EDITOR

KEVIN C. CHUNG, MD, MS
Charles B.G. de Nancrede Professor of
Surgery, Professor of Plastic Surgery and
Orthopaedic Surgery, Chief of Hand Surgery,
Department of Surgery, Section of Plastic
Surgery, Michigan Medicine, Assistant Dean
for Faculty Affairs, Associate Director of Global
REACH, University of Michigan Medical
School, Comprehensive Hand Center,
University of Michigan, The University of
Michigan Health System, Ann Arbor, Michigan,
USA

EDITORS

ROBIN N. KAMAL, MD, MBA, MS
Associate Professor, Medical Director, Value
Based Care and Orthopaedic Surgery, VOICES
Health Policy Research Center, Department of
Orthopaedic Surgery, Stanford University,
Redwood City, California, USA

LAUREN M. SHAPIRO, MD, MS
Assistant Professor, Department of
Orthopaedic Surgery, University of California,
San Francisco, San Francisco, California, USA

AUTHORS

ABHIRAM R. BHASHYAM, MD, PhD
Surgeon, Department of Orthopaedic Surgery,
Hand and Arm Center, Massachusetts General
Hospital, Boston, Massachusetts, USA

GABRIELLE ANNE BUI, BA, MD
Department of Orthopedics and Sports
Medicine, University of Washington Medical
Center, Seattle, Washington, USA

MARION BURNIER, MD
Surgeon, Medipole, Villeurbanne, France

NEAL CHEN, MD
Chief, Department of Orthopaedic Surgery,
Hand and Arm Center, Massachusetts General
Hospital, Boston, Massachusetts, USA

NATHANIEL FOGEL, MD
Fellow, Department of Orthopaedic Surgery,
Duke University, Durham, North Carolina, USA

EDGAR GARCIA-LOPEZ MD, MS
Physician, Department of Orthopaedics,
University of California, San Francisco, San
Francisco, California, USA

RAYMOND GLENN GASTON, MD
Fellowship Director, OrthoCarolina Hand and
Upper Extremity Fellowship, Chief of Hand
Surgery Atrium Health, The Hand Center,
OrthoCarolina, Charlotte, North Carolina,
USA

WILLIAM BARRITT GILBERT JR. MD
Physician, Department of Orthopedic Surgery,
Vanderbilt University, PGY-3, Nashville,
Tennessee, USA

RYAN HALVORSON MD
Resident Physician, Department of
Orthopaedics, University of California, San
Francisco, San Francisco, California, USA

GUILLAUME HERZBERG, MD, PhD
Surgeon, Clinique Parc Lyon, Val Ouest Lyon,
France

ANDREW W. HOLLINS, MD
Division of Plastic Surgery, Department of
Surgery, Duke University Medical Center,
Durham, North Carolina, USA

JERRY I. HUANG, MD
Professor and Program Director, Combined Hand Fellowship, Department of Orthopedics and Sports Medicine, University of Washington Medical Center, Seattle, Washington, USA

MIHIR JITENDRA DESAI, MD, MS
Associate Professor, Hand and Upper Extremity, Department of Orthopedic Surgery, Vanderbilt University, Nashville, Tennessee, USA

SANJEEV KAKAR, MD
Professor of Orthopedics, Department of Orthopedic Surgery, Mayo Clinic, Rochester, Minnesota, USA

ROBIN N. KAMAL, MD, MBA, MS
Associate Professor, Medical Director, Value Based Care and Orthopaedic Surgery, VOICES Health Policy Research Center, Department of Orthopaedic Surgery, Stanford University, Redwood City, California, USA

LYLIANE LY, MD
Hospices Civils, Lyon, France

JOSHUA J. MEAIKE, MD
Resident, Orthopedic Surgery Resident, Department of Orthopedic Surgery, Mayo Clinic, Rochester, Minnesota, USA

SUHAIL K. MITHANI, MD
Associate Professor, Division of Plastic Surgery, Department of Surgery, Duke University Medical Center, Durham, North Carolina, USA

DEVAN PATEL, MD
Fellow, Stanford University, VOICES Health Policy Research Center, Department of Orthopaedic Surgery, Redwood City, California, USA

GREGORY F. PEREIRA, MD
Physician, Department of Orthopaedics, Duke University Medical Center, Durham, North Carolina, USA

TYLER S. PIDGEON, MD, FAAOS
Associate Professor, Hand, Upper Extremity and Microvascular Surgery, Department of Orthopaedic Surgery, Duke University Medical Center, Durham, North Carolina, USA

SAMUEL L. POSEY, MD
Resident, Department of Orthopaedic Surgery, Atrium Health, Charlotte, North Carolina, USA

JILL PUTNAM, MD
The Hand and Upper Extremity Center, The Ohio State University, Columbus, Ohio, USA

JEREMY E. RADUCHA, MD
Fellow, Hand, Upper Extremity and Microvascular Surgery, Department of Orthopaedic Surgery, Duke University Medical Center, Durham, North Carolina, USA

SNEHA R. RAO, MD
Resident, Department of Orthopaedics, Duke University Medical Center, Durham, North Carolina, USA

MARC J. RICHARD, MD
Surgeon, Department of Orthopaedics, Duke University Medical Center, Durham, North Carolina, USA

LAUREN M. SHAPIRO, MD, MS
Assistant Professor, Department of Orthopaedic Surgery, University of California, San Francisco, San Francisco, California, USA

ARNOLD-PETER C. WEISS, MD
Scot Sellers Scholar of Hand Surgery, Chief, Hand, Upper Extremity and Microvascular Surgery, Vice Chairman and Professor of Orthopaedics, Alpert Medical School of Brown University, University Orthopedics, East Providence, Rhode Island, USA; Professor of Orthopaedics, Medical University of South Carolina, Charleston, South Carolina, USA

JEFFREY YAO, MD
Professor, Department of Orthopaedic Surgery, Stanford University Medical Center, Stanford, California, USA

THOMPSON ZHUANG, MD, MBA
Department of Orthopaedic Surgery, VOICES Health Policy Research Center, Stanford University, Redwood City, California, USA

Contents

Preface: Innovation in Upper Extremity Fracture Treatment—Implementation of Advanced Techniques to Improve Outcomes xi

Robin N. Kamal and Lauren M. Shapiro

Intramedullary Screw Fixation of Metacarpal and Phalangeal Fractures 475

Gabrielle Anne Bui and Jerry I. Huang

> Metacarpal and phalangeal fractures are the second and third most common hand and wrist fractures seen in the emergency department. There are a multitude of operative fixation methods for metacarpal and phalangeal fractures, including closed reduction percutaneous pinning, open reduction internal fixation, external fixation, and intramedullary screw fixation. Although intramedullary fixation is a relatively new surgical technique, it is gaining in popularity as it allows patients to resume range of motion early in the postoperative period with excellent clinical outcomes.

The Use of Patient-Specific Implants for the Treatment of Upper Extremity Fractures 489

Sneha R. Rao, Gregory F. Pereira, and Marc J. Richard

> In this article, we discuss the use of three-dimensional (3-D) printed patient-specific implants in the management of upper extremity fractures. Traditional fracture fixation methods involve the use of standard-sized implants, which may not adequately address the needs of every patient, particularly those who have complications related to fracture nonunion or malunion and those who have significant bone loss. The benefits and limitations of this technology are also discussed, along with considerations for implementation in clinical practice. Overall, the use of 3-D printed patient-specific implants holds promise for improving the accuracy and efficacy of upper extremity fracture management.

Staple Technology for Fracture Fixation and Joint Arthrodesis 505

Samuel L. Posey and Raymond Glenn Gaston

> The use of staple technology in the upper extremity has continued to evolve with the development of shape-memory alloys (SMAs) such as Nitinol that display superelastic properties that can be exploited for persistent compression. Clinical and biomechanical studies support the use of SMA staples for upper extremity fracture fixation and joint arthrodesis. To optimize biomechanical strength and clinical outcomes, it is recommended to place two staples, if possible, at the site of interest as well as to trough the staples to prevent hardware prominence.

Enhanced Approaches to the Treatment of Distal Radius Fractures 515

Devan Patel and Robin Kamal

> Distal radius fractures are among the most common fractures treated by orthopedic surgeons. Various classification systems have been described which can help in deciding the approach for fixation. In some cases, a computed tomography scan can provide better understanding of the fracture fragments and displacement for surgical planning. Plating through the volar approach is the most common approach for fractures meeting operative criteria. Several additional approaches can be used for

specific fracture patterns. These approaches can be used in isolation or in conjunction with other approaches to aid in visualization and fixation.

Innovations in Small Joint Arthroscopy

523

Joshua J. Meaike and Sanjeev Kakar

With advancements in surgical instrumentation and techniques, the role of arthroscopic and arthroscopic-assisted surgical procedures is ever-growing. Arthroscopy offers direct, magnified visualization of pathology and reductions and is more accurate than relying on intraoperative fluoroscopy alone. It also minimizes soft tissue stripping, which is of particular importance to smaller fracture fragments whose vascularity is precarious and can be injured through open approaches.

Arthroscopic-Assisted Fracture Treatment in the Wrist

533

Jeffrey Yao and Nathaniel Fogel

Wrist arthroscopy in the setting of wrist fracture affords direct visualization of reduction and identification of associated cartilage and soft tissue injuries. Further, mitigating soft tissue insult in the setting of perilunate injuries may decrease postoperative pain and stiffness while attaining outcomes equivalent to open techniques in appropriately selected patients. Technical proficiency of the surgeon continues to be a limitation of the technique. Randomized controlled studies are needed to better understand outcomes.

Role for Wrist Hemiarthroplasty in Acute Irreparable Distal Radius Fracture in the Elderly

545

Guillaume Herzberg, Marion Burnier, and Lyliane Ly

Volar locking plates for distal radius fracture (DRF) in the elderly may show complications in the most comminuted osteoporotic cases. The authors provide criteria for DRF in elderly that may not be amenable to volar plating ("irreparable DRF") and review the current results of a preliminary series of wrist hemiarthroplasty for these injuries. Between 2011 and 2019, 28 wrists with acute irreparable intra-articular DRF were treated with wrist hemiarthroplasty (96% female, mean age 79 years). A total of 17 wrists with a mean follow-up of 32 months were reviewed. At follow-up, mean visual analog scale (VAS) pain was 1/10, mean forearm rotation arc was 148°.

Intramedullary Nailing of Forearm Fractures

551

William Barritt Gilbert Jr. and Mihir Jitendra Desai

The primary goal in operative fixation of forearm fractures is to restore length, rotational stability, and maintenance of the radial bow. Plate osteosynthesis is well regarded as the gold standard of treatment though often necessitates soft tissue injury, periosteal stripping, and risk of refracture after hardware removal. While intramedullary nails have been utilized for forearm fixation since the early 1900s, technological advancements including locked intramedullary nails have lead to improved outcomes in intramedullary nail forearm fixation. In select patients, intramedullary nail fixation is an appropriate treatment option. For example, patients with mangled extremities, comminuted or segmental fractures, or soft tissue injury may benefit from this approach as it allows for smaller incisions and limits further soft tissue compromise.

Proximal Interphalangeal Joint Fractures: Various Approaches to Fixation   561

Jeremy E. Raducha and Tyler S. Pidgeon

There are numerous operative and nonoperative options for the management of proximal interphalangeal joint fractures and fracture dislocations. The treatment of choice should be guided by the fracture pattern and joint stability. The authors highlight a contemporary option for open reduction and internal fixation techniques, but all the techniques presented are viable options under the right circumstances. It is also important to set patient expectations as most of these patients will note post-injury stiffness and potential functional limitations.

Proximal Interphalangeal Joint Arthroplasty for Fracture   575

Jeremy E. Raducha and Arnold-Peter C. Weiss

Proximal interphalangeal joint arthroplasties can be performed in the setting of acute comminuted fracture, chronic fracture presentations, and posttraumatic arthritis. These surgeries provide excellent pain relief and patient satisfaction but patients should be cautioned not to expect an improvement in motion postoperatively. Despite high rates of minor complications and radiographic loosening, these implants have good rates of long-term survival with most revisions occurring in the early postoperative period. They provide viable alternatives to arthrodesis, osteotomy and amputation in the appropriate patient.

Arthroscopic-Assisted Fracture Fixation About the Elbow   587

Abhiram R. Bhashyam and Neal Chen

Arthroscopic-assisted fracture fixation can be used for some adult elbow fractures. In particular, for articular fractures of the anterior elbow (coronoid/capitellum), elbow arthroscopy can provide excellent visualization of fracture fragments using a less invasive surgical exposure. Meticulous adherence to safe techniques and utilization of specialized equipment can help maximize safety and facilitate reproducible surgical results.

Rethinking Scaphoid Fixation   597

Jill Putnam

Scaphoid fixation, whether for acute injuries or nonunion, is made challenging by the small and intra-articular nature of the most commonly fractured carpal bone. The purpose of this article is to review the techniques to simplify scaphoid fixation and to optimize healing and early return to activity.

Advances in Soft Tissue Injuries Associated with Open Fractures   605

Andrew W. Hollins and Suhail K. Mithani

Management of soft tissue injury is a key component in the overall treatment of upper extremity fractures. Hand surgeons must rely on their armamentarium for treating soft tissue deficits for functional outcomes. Understanding the role of fracture fixation and wound adjuncts, including negative pressure wound therapy and dermal regenerative templates, is the keys to success. In addition, detailed knowledge of local and free tissue options is essential for hand reconstruction.

Strategies for Perioperative Optimization in Upper Extremity Fracture Care   617

Thompson Zhuang and Robin N. Kamal

> Perioperative optimization in upper extremity fracture care must balance the need for timely treatment with the benefits of medical optimization. Care pathways directed at optimizing glycemic control, chronic anticoagulation, smoking history, nutrition, and frailty can reduce surgical risk in upper extremity fracture care. The development of multidisciplinary approaches that tie risk modification with risk stratification is needed.

Novel Tools to Approach and Measure Outcomes in Patients with Fractures   627

Edgar Garcia-Lopez, Ryan Halvorson, and Lauren Shapiro

> Upper extremity fractures are prevalent and pose a great burden to patients and society. In the US alone, the annual incidence of upper extremity fractures is 67.6 fractures per 10,000 persons. While the majority of patients with upper extremity fractures demonstrate satisfactory outcomes when treated appropriately (the details of which are discussed in prior articles), the importance of follow-up and outcome measurement cannot be understated. Outcome measurement allows for accountability and improvement in clinical outcomes and research. The purpose of this article is to describe recent advances in methods and tools for assessing clinical and research outcomes in hand and upper extremity care. Three specific advances that are broadly changing the landscape of follow-up care of our patients include: 1) telemedicine, 2) patient-reported outcome measurement, and 3) wearables/remote patient monitoring.

HAND CLINICS

FORTHCOMING ISSUES

February 2024
Malunions and Nonunions in the Forearm, Wrist, and Hand
Jerry I. Huang and Erin A. Miller, *Editors*

May 2024
Advances in Microsurgical Reconstruction in the Upper Extremity
Harvey Chim and Kevin C. Chung, *Editors*

August 2024
Peripheral Nerve Reconstruction
Sami H. Tuffaha and Kevin C. Chung, *Editors*

RECENT ISSUES

August 2023
Managing Difficult Problems in Hand Surgery: Challenges, Complications and Revisions
Sonu Jain, *Editor*

May 2023
Current Concepts in Flexor Tendon Repair and Rehabilitation
Rowena McBeath and Kevin C. Chung, *Editors*

February 2023
Diversity, Equity, and Inclusion in Hand Surgery
Michael Galvez and Kevin C. Chung, *Editors*

Preface

Innovation in Upper Extremity Fracture Treatment—Implementation of Advanced Techniques to Improve Outcomes

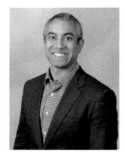 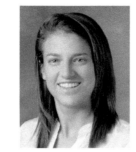

Robin N. Kamal, MD, MBA, MS   Lauren M. Shapiro, MD, MS

Editors

Does newer technology lead to improved patient outcomes and higher value care? Hand and upper extremity fractures are common, and their incidence is on the rise. These injuries impact patients and are treated by surgeons across the world. While these injuries themselves are not necessarily changing, our improved understanding of injury characteristics and parallel innovations in perioperative optimization, surgical approaches, surgical fixation, and outcome measurement continues to advance our ability to provide high-value care.

In this issue of *Hand Clinics*, thought-leaders in the field of hand and upper extremity surgery share their perspectives on innovations in the treatment of hand and upper extremity fractures and how they are advancing our ability to improve patient outcomes. These range from novel approaches (eg, arthroscopy and minimally invasive techniques) to innovative fixation methods (eg, patient-specific implants, intramedullary forearm nailing, scaphoid plates). Given the growing importance of value and quality in orthopedic surgery, this issue also includes newer perspectives on perioperative optimization and outcome measurement.

We are grateful to the authors of this issue for not only sharing their expertise in the treatment of these injuries but also being leaders in the field and sharing their experiences, pearls, and pitfalls for when innovation may lead to better patient outcomes.

Robin N. Kamal, MD, MBA, MS
Associate Professor
Department of Orthopaedic Surgery
Stanford University
450 Broadway Street
Redwood City, CA 94063, USA

Lauren M. Shapiro, MD, MS
Assistant Professor
Department of Orthopaedic Surgery
University of California–San Francisco
1500 Owens Street
San Francisco, CA 94158, USA

E-mail addresses:
rnkamal@stanford.edu (R.N. Kamal)
lauren.shapiro@ucsf.edu (L.M. Shapiro)

Hand Clin 39 (2023) xi
https://doi.org/10.1016/j.hcl.2023.07.002
0749-0712/23/© 2023 Published by Elsevier Inc.

Intramedullary Screw Fixation of Metacarpal and Phalangeal Fractures

Gabrielle Anne Bui, BA, MD[a], Jerry I. Huang, MD[b],*

KEYWORDS

- Metacarpal fracture • Phalangeal fracture • Intramedullary screw fixation • Operative fixation

KEY POINTS

- Intramedullary screw fixation is an effective, minimally invasive techniqe for fixation of metacarpal and phalangeal fractures.
- Preoperative planning and selection of appropriate screw sizes and lengths is critical.
- Antegrade and retrograde screw fixation techniques are effective for both metacarpal and phalangeal shaft fractures.
- High union rates with excellent range of motion can be expected for intramedullary screw fixation of metacarpal and phalangeal fractures.

INTRODUCTION

Metacarpal and phalangeal fractures are the second and third most common hand fractures, accounting for 18% and 23% of all forearm and hand fractures treated in the emergency department.[1,2] Previous epidemiologic studies have found that there are 13.6 metacarpal fractures per 100,000 person years.[1] Not only do metacarpal and phalangeal fractures lead to physical limitations for patients but also they have a significant economic cost as they tend to occur in young healthy laborers.[3] Given the significant opportunity costs associated with time off work, it is reasonable to consider operative fixation techniques in patients that would benefit from faster return to work/play. Although stable metacarpal and phalangeal fractures can often be managed nonoperatively, surgery may be indicated for unstable metacarpal and phalangeal fractures. Historically, operative fixation techniques have ranged from closed reduction percutaneous pinning to open reduction internal fixation and external fixation techniques. Intramedullary screw fixation is a relatively new technique that is gaining traction and popularity for its accelerated rehabilitation protocol. This article reviews the indications, biomechanics, and techniques of intramedullary screw fixation for metacarpal and phalangeal fractures.

METACARPAL FRACTURES AND INTRAMEDULLARY SCREW FIXATION
Background Information

Surgical indications for operative fixation of metacarpal factures include open fractures with bone loss, multiple adjacent metacarpal fractures, unstable fractures, multiple hand/wrist fractures, and malalignment (rotation and angulation).[4] After determining that a metacarpal fracture is indicated for operative fixation, it is critical to determine which fixation method is most appropriate given the fracture characteristics, soft tissue injury, and patient characteristics such as functional demands.

[a] Department of Orthopedics and Sports Medicine, University of Washington Medical Center, 908 Jefferson Street, Ninth Floor, Seattle, WA 98104, USA; [b] Department of Orthopedics and Sports Medicine, University of Washington Medical Center, 4245 Roosevelt Way Northeast, Box 354740, Seattle, WA 98105, USA
* Corresponding author.
E-mail address: jihuang@uw.edu

Hand Clin 39 (2023) 475–488
https://doi.org/10.1016/j.hcl.2023.05.014

Metacarpal Neck Fractures

Operative indications for metacarpal neck fractures vary by displacement and digit. Displacement is typically due to the intrinsic muscles of the hand causing an apex dorsal deformity. Malrotation with scissoring is an indication for surgery regardless of digit. There are also guidelines for acceptable degree of angulation which varies by digit. For the small finger metacarpal neck, surgery is indicated for angulation greater than 70°.[5] For the index and middle finger metacarpals, reduction and stabilization are generally recommended for angulation more than 20 to 30°. Surgical options include closed reduction with percutaneous pinning and open reduction and internal fixation with plate and screw constructs (**Fig. 1**). Most commonly, closed reduction and percutaneous pinning is performed with crossed pin constructs placed in a retrograde fashion from the metacarpal head across the neck or transverse intermetacarpal K-wires. Although K-wire constructs come with the benefit of minimal soft tissue disruption, they require additional external immobilization. In contrast, "bouquet pinning" with multiple pre-bent K-wires placed in an anterograde fashion inside the medullary canal allows for minimally invasive fixation and early mobilization.[6] In cases of inadequate stabilization with K-wires due to comminution or poor bone quality, open reduction with plate and screw fixation may be necessary.

Metacarpal Shaft Fractures

Most of the metacarpal shaft fractures can be treated nonoperatively. Indications for operative treatment include malrotation and shortening more than 5 to 7 mm. For the index and middle finger metacarpals, angulation up to 20° is well tolerated. Angulation up to 30° is acceptable for ring and small finger metacarpal fractures as the 4th and 5th carpometacarpal (CMC) joints are mobile. Interfragmentary screw fixation is indicated for long oblique or spiral fractures where the length of the fracture is more than twice the size of the diameter of the bone. Transverse patterns and comminuted fractures are usually treated with plate and screw fixation. Plate and screw constructs are excellent for restoring length but result in a significant amount of soft tissue disruption with the risk of extensor tendon adhesions as well as metacarpophalangeal (MCP) joint extension contractures.

Intramedullary Screw Fixation

Intramedullary screw fixation is a contemporary approach to metacarpal shaft fractures that offers the advantage of stable fixation through a minimally invasive approach that limits soft tissue stripping. Intramedullary screw fixation has been described for treatment of transverse, short oblique, and non-comminuted metacarpal fractures.[4] Long oblique fractures and fracture comminution are generally a contraindication for screw fixation, as displacement and shortening can occur. Intramedullary screw fixation of metacarpal neck fractures was first described by Boulton and colleagues. In that landmark article, the investigators described retrograde intramedullary fixation of a small finger metacarpal neck fracture.[7] Later, Ruschelsman and colleagues published a series of 39 metacarpal neck and shaft fractures with 100% radiographic union and excellent range of motion.[8] Then, del Pinal presented a case series of 69 fractures (48 metacarpal and 21 phalangeal) treated with intramedullary screw fixation.[9] More

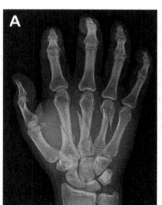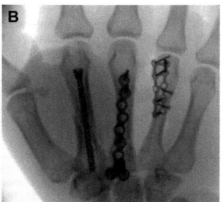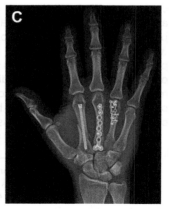

Fig. 1. (*A*) Injury films of short oblique index finger metacarpal fracture, comminuted middle finger metacarpal shaft, and ring finger metacarpal head fracture. (*B*) Managed with intramedullary fixation and plate/screw constructs and (*C*) 4-week postoperative films.

recently, Eisenberg and colleagues published a retrospective review of 91 consecutive patients treated with intramedullary (IM) screw fixation of metacarpal neck (56) and shaft (35) fractures. In this series, patients began active range of motion at 5 days postoperatively. They reported full MCP joint extension in all patients and a mean flexion–extension arc of 88°.[10]

Preoperative Assessment

Preoperative planning is a critical component of intramedullary screw fixation for metacarpal fractures. In addition to determining feasibility of IM screw fixation for the metacarpal neck or shaft fracture, implant selection is important. Hoang and colleagues performed computed tomography scan (CT) analysis on 100 hands and detailed the width of the medullary canal in the index, middle, ring, and small fingers as well as the cortical thickness.[11] Overall, they found that the ring finger tended to have the narrowest medullary canal with a mean width of 2.8 mm in the coronal plane. Excluding the thumb, the small finger had the widest midshaft medullary width at 4.1 mm in the coronal plane. Based on the data, 3.5 mm screw is generally recommended for the ring finger metacarpal, whereas 4.0 or 4.5 mm screws are recommended for the other digits. However, it is important to obtain preoperative measurements of the isthmic canal width on an anterior-posterior (AP) film.[11] The general recommended diameter and lengths for intramedullary fixation of metacarpal fractures are listed in **Table 1**.[12] It is also paramount for the surgeon to have knowledge of screw diameter options and screw lengths of various headless compression screw options as many implants have limited lengths, especially in smaller headless compression screw sizes.[13]

Table 1
Recommended screw diameter based on characteristic metacarpal widths

Headless Compression Screw (HCS) Diameter General Recommendations		
Metacarpal	Appropriate Screw Width (mm)	Appropriate Screw Length (mm)
Index and middle metacarpal	3.5–4.0 mm	45–55 mm
Ring metacarpal	3.0–3.5 mm	35–50 mm
Small metacarpal	4.0–4.5 mm	35–45 mm

Operative Technique

Intramedullary fixation of metacarpal fractures is generally performed in a retrograde fashion. However, previous studies have investigated the anatomy and efficacy of anterograde intramedullary fixation in cadaver models.[14,15] The authors first discuss the more traditional retrograde intramedullary fixation and then discuss antegrade intramedullary fixation techniques and lastly ongoing research.

Retrograde Intramedullary Fixation

A 1.5-cm transverse or longitudinal incision is made along the dorsal aspect of the metacarpal head and neck, and dissection is carried down to the extensor mechanism. The extensor tendon is split longitudinally adjacent to the sagittal band, and then an arthrotomy is performed along the dorsal joint capsule until the metacarpal head is adequately exposed. Fluoroscopy can be used to guide a closed or open reduction of the metacarpal fracture. Then, a guide pin should be placed along the dorsal one-third of the metacarpal and advanced under fluoroscopy at the level of the fracture and then across the fracture site into the proximal metacarpal shaft. Alternatively, the guide pin can be placed percutaneously without an open incision. The surgeon must then assess the quality of the reduction with a particular focus on the rotation and cascade. If the surgeon finds the reduction to be adequate, the appropriate implant should be selected based on the length of the guide pin as well as the width of the isthmus. The guide pin is then advanced to the level of the CMC joint. The pin is then over-drilled. The headless compression screw is then inserted over the guide pin with the fingers held in a fist position to ensure appropriate rotation of the fracture.

The operative technique of retrograde intramedullary fixation poses a risk to the extensor mechanism as well as an articular defect in the metacarpal head with possible involvement of its articulation with the base of the proximal phalanx.[16] However, cadaver and biomechanical studies have demonstrated that the risk to the structures above is likely acceptable with minimal damage to the articulating portion of the metacarpal head. In a study by ten Berg and colleagues using CT scans of 16 hands and ranging through an arc of MCP joint motion from 30° of hyperextension to 90° of flexion, they found that the center of the phalangeal base did not engage the entry site in 87% of the hyperextension–flexion arc.[17] Moreover, in 64% of the specimen, there was no contact of the proximal phalanx base with the entry site of the screw. The range of motion arc relative to the entry site of the screw is depicted in **Fig. 2**.[17] Urbanschitz and colleagues performed mini open metacarpal intramedullary fixation on 16 cadaver fingers and used CT to analyze the articular surface area violated and followed by dissections to quantify the degree of extensor tendon injury.[18] Overall, they found that the average metacarpal articular surface area was 132 mm^2 and that the median disruption of the articular surface was 8 mm^2 or 6% of the articular surface area. With regard to extensor tendon injury, they found that 16/16 metacarpals had less than 25% disruption of the extensor tendon width in the mini open technique.[18]

Antegrade Intramedullary Fixation

Although intramedullary fixation of metacarpal fractures is typically performed in a retrograde fashion, there is ongoing research regarding the feasibility of performing anterograde intramedullary fixation. One of the short comings of retrograde intramedullary fixation is its inability to achieve stabilization for proximal one-third metacarpal shaft fractures with shorter implants. In addition, although smaller headless compression screws cause minimal injury to the articular cartilage of the metacarpal head, larger defects are created with placing 4.0 and 4.5 mm headless compression screws. Hoang and colleagues have previously described a technique for antegrade intramedullary fixation of metacarpal shaft fractures.[14] The group performed a subsequent study demonstrating feasibility of anterograde intramedullary fixation with minimal effect on the articular surface of the CMC joint. Following screw

placement, dissection was performed to determine the location of the guide pin entry point as well as the percent of articular surface area affected. Overall, the investigators found less than 5% of the CMC joint was violated in all digits.[15]

As in retrograde techniques, a guide pin is placed in a retrograde fashion starting from the dorsal aspect of the metacarpal head. The wire is advanced from distal, across the fracture site, and toward the dorsal aspect of the metacarpal base using fluoroscopic guidance. The guide wire should be aimed dorsally to skive off the dorsal aspect of the corresponding carpal bone or clear the carpus all together. A 5- to 10-mm skin incision is then made overlaying the area where the guide pin exits from the dorsal wrist. Dissection is performed to retract the soft tissues and the extensor mechanism from the proximal aspect of the metacarpal. The guide pin is then advanced until the distal aspect of the guidewire is buried in the MCP joint. The appropriate length and width of the intramedullary screw are selected. A soft tissue protector is used, whereas a cannulated drill is used to drill past the fracture in an antegrade fashion (**Fig. 3**). The screw can then be placed in an antegrade fashion (**Fig. 4**). Like retrograde intramedullary fixation, the fingers should be kept flexed to 90° at the MCP and proximal interphalangeal (PIP) to prevent malrotation. Further studies are needed to evaluate clinical outcomes of this technique.

Strutting

Although comminution is generally considered a contraindication for intramedullary fixation, the

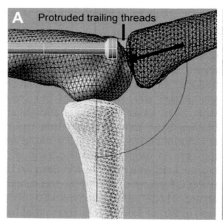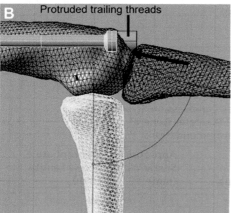

Fig. 2. (A) Arc of motion in which entry site is not engaged with center of phalangeal base (*black arrow*). (B) Arc of motion in which entry site is not engaged by the rim of the phalangeal base (*black arrow*). (*From* ten Berg PW, Mudgal CS, Leibman MI, Belsky MR, Ruchelsman DE. Quantitative 3-dimensional CT analyses of intramedullary headless screw fixation for metacarpal neck fractures. J Hand Surg Am. 2013;38(2):322-330.e2; with permission.)

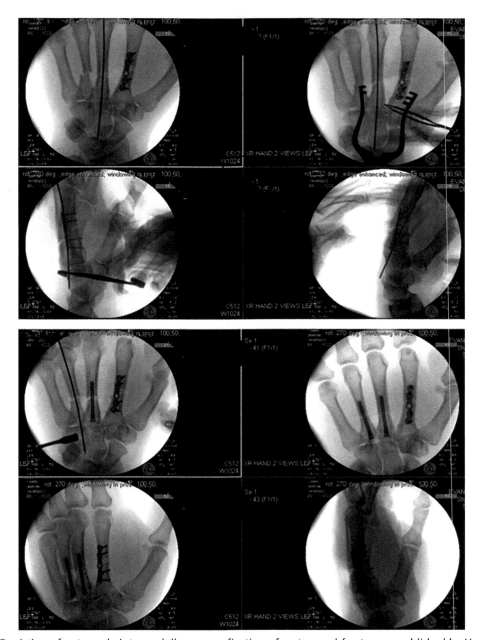

Fig. 3. Depiction of antegrade intramedullary screw fixation of metacarpal fracture as published by Hoang and colleagues. (*From* Hoang D, Huang JI. Antegrade intramedullary screw fixation: a novel approach to metacarpal fractures. J Hand Surg Global Online, 1 (4) (2019), pp. 229-235; with permission.)

previous methods have been described which use two intramedullary screws in a Y-shaped construct or "Y-strutting" (**Fig. 5**).[9] In this technique, the longitudinal screw is placed followed by the placement of an offset screw, with both screws occupying the medullary canal at their intersection. Complications associated with Y-strutting include loss of reduction, shortening, and symptomatic malunion. Further investigation is indicated to determine the efficacy of Y-strutting in complex metacarpal fractures.

Clinical Outcomes

Previous retrospective studies have demonstrated excellent outcomes after intramedullary fixation of

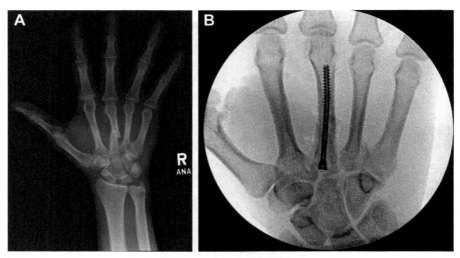

Fig. 4. (*A*) Injury films of transverse right middle finger metacarpal fracture. (*B*) Intraoperative fluoroscopy status post antegrade intramedullary screw fixation.

metacarpal fractures. In a study by Ruchelsman and colleagues, 39 patients were retrospectively followed for a minimum of 3 months after intramedullary screw fixation for metacarpal neck and shaft fractures.[8] Overall, 20 patients had sufficient follow-up for inclusion in the study and the average follow-up was 13 months. They found that 100% of patients demonstrated union 6 weeks

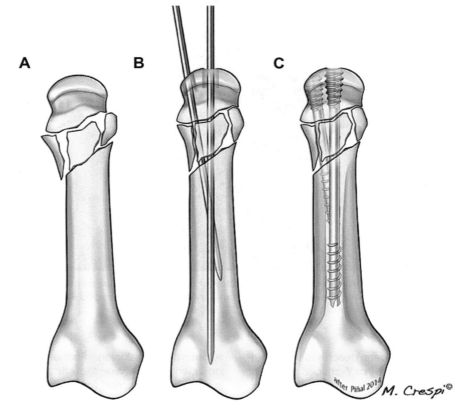

Fig. 5. Comminuted metacarpal neck fracture (*A*) reduced and followed by placement of guidepins ×2 (*B*) from the metacarpal head across the neck into the shaft, followed by placement of headless compression screws (*C*). (*From* del Piñal F, Moraleda E, Rúas JS, de Piero GH, Cerezal L. Minimally invasive fixation of fractures of the phalanges and metacarpals with intramedullary cannulated headless compression screws. J Hand Surg Am. 2015;40(4):692-700; with permission.)

postoperatively, and 100% of patients demonstrated full composite flexion with an average of 88° flexion at the MCP joint. Furthermore, mean grip strength along the operative hand was 105% compared with the contralateral hand.[8] In another retrospective study performed by del Pinal and colleagues, the investigators evaluated 48 patients with metacarpal fractures who underwent intramedullary fixation.[9] At a mean follow-up of 19 months, patients had a mean flexion of 84° at the MCP joint and total active motion (TAM; active flexion of MCP, PIP, and distal interphlanageal [DIP] joints minus extension deficits) of 249°.[9] Excellent TAM values were also found in a study performed by Poggetti and colleagues. Specifically, in this study, 173 transverse/short oblique metacarpal and phalangeal fractures underwent operative fixation with intramedullary screw. Overall, the investigators found that patients had fracture healing within 35 days and 245° TAM. They noted a 1.2% rate of malunion.[19] Another study published by Thakker and colleagues found excellent TAM after intramedullary screw fixation for metacarpal fractures. Specifically, in this retrospective study, the investigators investigated outcomes of 30 fractures in 27 patients who underwent intramedullary screw fixation. Overall, TAM at initial follow-up was 245°, and all patients returned to work over the course of 6 weeks. Despite the largely excellent range of motion, two patients required subsequent operative intervention (capsulotomy and tenolysis) 5 to 8 months postoperatively for persistent stiffness.[20] Early return to work after intramedullary fixation was also demonstrated in a systematic review published by Hug and colleagues. In this review, the mean time to return to work ranged from 3.6 to 10.9 weeks.[21]

It is worth underscoring the rehabilitation protocol in the studies. Ruchelsman and Thakker and colleagues initiated the range of motion exercises 1 week postoperatively.[8,20] In contrast, del Pinal and Poggetti and colleagues allow patients range as tolerated immediately after surgery.[9,19] Both rehabilitation protocols emphasize a critical component of intramedullary fixation being early progression of activities and possible earlier return to work.

Comparison of Outcomes

Given the multitude of methods by which to fix a metacarpal fracture, it is important to compare the clinical outcomes of intramedullary screws to those of open reduction internal fixation and those of closed reduction percutaneous pinning. In a study by Ozer and colleagues, the investigators retrospectively looked at outcomes of patients who went intramedullary screw versus open reduction with plate and screw constructs.[22] Overall, there was no significant difference in clinical outcomes as assessed by postoperative range of motion and Disability of the Shoulder and Hand (DASH) scores between the two patient groups.[22] Another study conducted by Couceiro and colleagues compared outcomes of closed reduction and percutaneous pinning to intramedullary fixation. The investigators did not note a significant difference in TAM, grip strength, pain, or patient satisfaction.[23] However, in this study, the patients who underwent intramedullary screw fixation were significantly more likely to return work earlier. Specifically, the mean time to return to work in the intramedullary screw group was 0.92 months versus 1.86 months in the closed reduction and percutaneous pinning group.[23] Furthermore, Esteban-Feliu and colleagues published a retrospective study that compared clinical outcomes and return to work for patients with metacarpal and phalangeal fractures managed with plate and screw constructs as compared with K-wire pinning and intramedullary screw fixation. The investigators reported no significant difference in groups regarding radiologic union, grip strength, TAM, or QuickDASH. Of note, however, patients who underwent intramedullary fixation were significantly more likely to return to work earlier (7.8 weeks vs 8.3 and 9.2 weeks in the plate and screw and K-wire groups, respectively).[24]

PHALANGEAL FRACTURES

Stable extra-articular phalangeal fractures can be appropriately managed nonoperatively with buddy taping and intrinsic plus splinting. However, displaced and unstable extra-articular fractures are indicated for operative fixation. Traditional minimally invasive fixation techniques include closed reduction and percutaneous pinning with crossed K-wires. However, crossed K-wires can be challenging in phalangeal shaft fractures. Belsky and colleagues described a method of K-wire fixation across the MCP joint for phalangeal shaft fractures. The proximal phalanx fracture is reduced by pulling traction, flexing the MP joint to 90° and the PIP joint to at least 45°. Followed by the placement of K-wires longitudinally through the metacarpal head, across the MCP joint, and down medullary canal of the proximal phalanx.[25] For spiral or oblique fractures, percutaneous interfragmentary screw fixation can be performed.[26] Although interfragmentary screw fixation provides more rotational stability than K-wire fixation, previous studies have not found a significant difference in the outcomes of spiral and oblique phalangeal fractures managed with K-wires as compared with interfragmentary screws.[27] Plate and screw fixation may be necessary for comminuted phalangeal fractures. Page and Stern evaluated complications following plate fixation of metacarpal and phalangeal fractures and found major complications in 36% of cases.[28] In particular, satisfactory range of motion with TAM greater than 220° was seen in only 4 of 37 (11%) of phalangeal fractures.[28]

Intramedullary fixation of phalangeal fractures was first described by del Pinal and colleagues[9] using a similar technique as that used in IM screw fixation of metacarpal fractures. Compared with K-wire fixation and plate and screw fixation, IM screw fixation offers the advantages of stable fixation and early mobilization with minimal soft tissue disruption. del Pinal described IM screw fixation of 21 transverse or short oblique phalangeal fractures. The headless screw was placed retrograde through the head of the proximal phalanx. Since this initial study, several other techniques have been described including retrograde and antegrade approaches as well as techniques using dual-screw fixation.[29–31]

Cadaveric studies have demonstrated comparable strength with cyclic loading in phalangeal fracture models treated with intramedullary screws as well as plate and screw constructs. Miles and colleagues created short oblique phalangeal fractures and compared fixation with anterograde intramedullary screws to plate and screw constructs. The cadaver hands were then loaded onto a frame and performed 2000 full flexion/extension cycle within a period of 4 seconds. The investigators noted no significant difference in the degree of fracture displacement at all time points over 2000 cyclic loading events.[32] Rausch and colleagues performed another cadaveric study which compared the torsional, distraction, bending strengths of proximal phalanx fractures managed with intramedullary screws as compared with K-wires and T-plate and screw constructs. The investigators found that the cannulated compression screws had a significantly higher cyclic load to failure in bending compared with T-plates and K-wire fixation (96N ± 29N in cannulated compression screw [CCS] vs 64 ± 22N in T-plates vs 42 ± 21N, $P<.05$). Although T-plates had greater load to failure with torsional loads, both T-plates and cannulated cortical screws had a significantly higher load to failure as compared with K-wires (0.80 ± 0.21 N in T plates vs 0.63 ± 0.61 N in CCS vs 0.16 ± 0.09 in K-wires, $P<.05$).[33]

Preoperative Assessment

Preoperative planning is a critical component of intramedullary screw fixation for phalangeal fractures. The isthmus of the fractured phalanx should be measured on a lateral film. Generally, for phalanx fractures, a screw diameter of 2.0 to 3.0 mm is recommended. IM screw fixation can be performed for extra-articular fractures of the phalangeal neck, shaft, and base.

Operative Technique

Intramedullary screw fixation can be performed using an antegrade or retrograde approach. The main disadvantage of a retrograde approach is the defect created in the articular surface of the head of the proximal phalanx as well as injury to the central slip. del Pinal used CT scans to calculate the percentage of the defect in the proximal phalanx head created by a 2.5- and 3.0-mm headless screw. The 2.5-mm screw created a defect of about 13% to 18% of the articular surface, whereas the 3.0-mm screw created a defect of about 19% to 25% of the articular surface.[9]

The investigators begin by creating a 3.0-mm incision over the MCP joint. The MCP joint is maximally flexed followed by the placement of a guide pin along the dorsal aspect of the MCP joint. The guide pin is advanced from the dorsal aspect of the base of the proximal phalanx, across the fracture site, into the phalangeal neck. We next drill over the guide pin and place a headless cannulated screw (**Fig. 6**). When satisfactory reduction cannot be obtained using this intra-articular approach, one may use a trans-articular approach through the metacarpal head. In the trans-articular approach, the K-wire is placed through the distal aspect of the metacarpal head and advanced through the MCP joint to the base of the proximal phalanx. The trans-articular approach should be avoided when possible as it causes iatrogenic damage to the articular surface of both the distal metacarpal head and the proximal phalanx.

Although intramedullary fixation of proximal phalanx fractures is typically done in an anterograde fashion, retrograde fixation has also been described. In this technique, a 3.0-mm incision is made overlying the PIP joint. With the PIP joint flexed at 90°, a guide pin is advanced from the head of the proximal phalanx to the base of the proximal phalanx. After over-drilling the guide pin, a headless compression screw is placed, taking care to ensure the screw is 2 to 3 mm below the articular surface (**Fig. 7**).[16]

In addition to the single-screw fixation methods described above, dual-screw

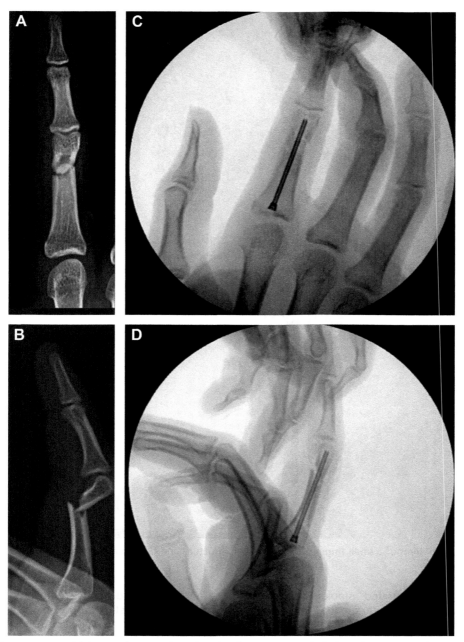

Fig. 6. (*A*) Injury AP and (*B*) injury lateral of a left index finger proximal phalanx fracture and (*C, D*) status post antegrade intramedullary screw fixation.

intramedullary techniques have also been described to achieve more stable fixation of phalangeal fractures. In the metacarpal section, we discussed the technique of Y-strutting, described by del Pinal and colleagues, in which a longitudinal screw is first placed in the standard fashion and then a smaller oblique screw is placed as a strut to provide support and prevent shortening in the setting of comminution.[9] Gaspar and colleagues published a modified Y-strutting, in which two screws were placed in an anterograde fashion for phalangeal shaft fractures.[31] Through a small 5-mm incision, a 2.4- or 3.0-mm screw was first placed followed by the placement of a second 2.4-mm screw. In this case series of 10 patients, Gaspar and

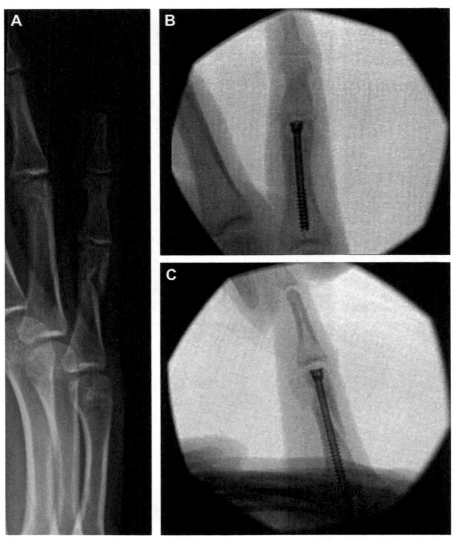

Fig. 7. (*A*) Injury films of a small finger proximal phalanx fracture and (*B, C*) managed with retrograde intramedullary fixation.

colleagues demonstrated stable fixation and excellent outcomes with mean TAM of 258° and mean grip strength of 97% of the contralateral side.[31] More recently, Gray and colleagues published a technique paper, which describes double barrel screw fixation for proximal phalanx fractures.[34] In this technique, fracture is reduced followed by provisional fixation with a single longitudinal 0.062 K-wire down the center of the proximal phalanx. Medial and lateral incisions are made along the collateral recess of the metacarpal heads. Medial and lateral guidewires are then advanced through each incision and advanced across the fracture site. Intramedullary screws are then sequentially placed over the medial and lateral guidewires.

del Pinal also described a technique termed axial strutting to stabilize proximal phalanx fractures with dorsal comminution (**Fig. 8**).[9] In this technique, reduction is obtained and a guidewire is introduced along the dorsal most aspect of the medullary canal. A headless compression screw, which is slightly shorter than the total length of the phalanx, is then inserted until its leading tip abuts the subchondral plate at the base of the phalanx. Blocking screws have also been described in conjunction with intramedullary fixation and are placed from radial to ulnar along the volar aspect of the phalanx. Blocking screws can increase stability for proximal phalanx and phalangeal shaft fractures by decreasing the width of the medullary canal (**Fig. 9**).

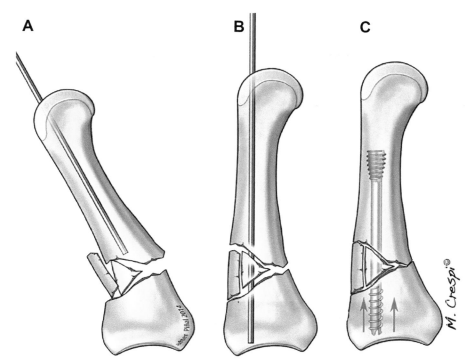

Fig. 8. Retrograde screw fixation of a comminuted proximal phalanx fracture with placement of a guidepin as a joystick through the head of the proximal phalanx (*A*). The fracture is reduced followed by advancement of the guidewire into the base of the proximal phalanx (*B*), followed by placement of a headless cannulated compression screw (*C*).. (*From* del Piñal F, Moraleda E, Rúas JS, de Piero GH, Cerezal L. Minimally invasive fixation of fractures of the phalanges and metacarpals with intramedullary cannulated headless compression screws. J Hand Surg Am. 2015;40(4):692-700; with permission.)

First, a guidewire is placed in a retrograde fashion along the intramedullary canal, and then a guidewire is placed anterior to the screw from radial to ulnar into the metaphyseal portion of the base of the proximal phalanx, followed by placement of a second headless screw. Fader and colleagues noted that blocking screws did not improve three-point bending strength of the construct.[35] However, the investigators believe that the blocking screw can provide rotational stability to the construct by decreasing the functional size of a capacious medullary canal.

Dangers and complications
Cadaver studies have been performed to assess the risk of articular and extensor tendon injury for the various methods of intramedullary fixation of phalangeal fractures. Urbanschitz and colleagues found that the median distal articular surface of the proximal phalanges was 59 mm^2, and that the median defect along the distal aspect of the proximal phalanx was 7 mm^2 or 12% of the articular surface. In the middle phalanx, they found the median proximal joint

surface area was 83 mm^2 whereas the distal middle phalanx articular surface area was 45 mm^2. The median defect of the proximal surface was 4 mm^2 or 6% of the proximal articular surface, whereas the median defect size of the distal articular surface of the middle phalanx was 4 mm^2.[18] The investigators did not find a significant difference in the degree of tendon damage between retrograde or anterograde screw insertion for middle phalanx fractures.

Clinical outcomes
Although there is a paucity of studies looking at long-term outcomes of phalangeal fractures managed with intramedullary nailing, there is a growing amount of evidence that suggests that the short-term and intermediate outcomes of intramedullary screws are acceptable. Giesen and colleagues performed a study that evaluated the clinical outcomes of patients who underwent anterograde intra-articular fixation or transarticular anterograde fixation of both proximal and middle phalangeal fractures.[30] Of the 31 fractures that met inclusion criteria, all but one

A

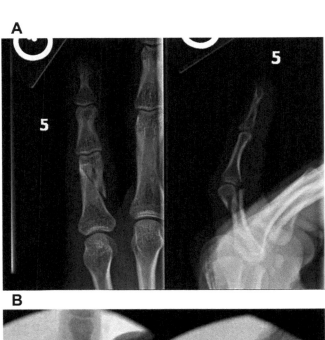

Fig. 9. (*A*) Preoperative imagines of a long oblique proximal phalangeal fracture with dorsal translation of the distal segment. (*B*) Intraoperative images (AP and lateral) demonstrating the use of a blocking screw. (*C*) Six-month postoperative films status post fixation with interval healing of the proximal phalanx fracture.

B

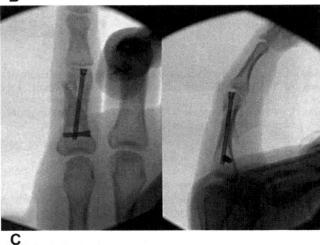

C

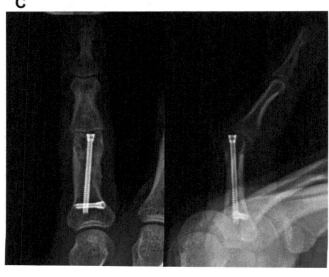

demonstrated radiographic union within 31 days. Furthermore, the mean TAM was 222° in all digits at the last follow-up appointment.[30] Aita and colleagues published a prospective study of 41 patients with 48 unstable extra-articular proximal phalanx fractures and compared the patients' range of motion and outcome scores to that of the contralateral hand.[36] Overall, they found that there was no significant difference between the ranges of motion compared with the contralateral side. Similarly, they noted improvement in DASH scores and visual analog scores (VAS) such that no differences were seen between the operative hand and the contralateral hand at a mean of 17 months.[36]

SUMMARY

The use of cannulated compression screws for intramedullary fixation of metacarpal and phalangeal fractures is a relatively new surgical fixation method. Early research studies investigating outcomes have demonstrated excellent results regarding union, range of motion, and return to work. Indications for intramedullary fixation include transverse or short oblique fractures without comminution. Although metacarpal fractures are generally fixed using retrograde screw fixation, there is ongoing research regarding the feasibility of antegrade fixation. Phalangeal fractures can be treated using numerous techniques including anterograde or retrograde and intra-articular or trans-articular approaches. Intramedullary fixation comes with inherent risk of damage to the extensor tendons as well as the articular cartilage. However, cadaver and biomechanical studies have demonstrated a minimal and thus acceptable degree of iatrogenic injury to both structures. As postoperative protocols after intramedullary fixation tend to allow for early range of motion/weight-bearing, this surgical technique may become especially important in the laboring population. This is critical as metacarpal and phalangeal fractures are predominantly seen in young laborers. Further clinical research is needed to compare the long-term clinical outcomes of intramedullary screw fixation and how it compares to plate and screw and K-wire constructs.

REFERENCES

1. Nakashian MN, Pointer L, Owens BD, et al. Incidence of metacarpal fractures in the US population. Hand (N Y) 2012;7(4):426–30.
2. Chung KC, Spilson SV. The frequency and epidemiology of hand and forearm fractures in the United States. J Hand Surg Am 2001;26(5):908–15.
3. Gardner DC, Goodwill CJ, Bridges PK. Cost of incapacity due to fractures of the wrist and hand. J Occup Med 1968;10(3):118–20.
4. Wolfe SH, Robert, Pederson William, et al. Green's operative hand surgery. 7th edition. Philadelphia: Elsevier/Churchill Livingston; 2017.
5. Statius Muller MG, Poolman RW, van Hoogstraten MJ, et al. Immediate mobilization gives good results in boxer's fractures with volar angulation up to 70 degrees: a prospective randomized trial comparing immediate mobilization with cast immobilization. Arch Orthop Trauma Surg 2003; 123(10):534–7.
6. Foucher G. "Bouquet" osteosynthesis in metacarpal neck fractures: a series of 66 patients. J Hand Surg Am 1995;20(3 Pt 2):S86–90.
7. Boulton CL, Salzler M, Mudgal CS. Intramedullary cannulated headless screw fixation of a comminuted subcapital metacarpal fracture: case report. J Hand Surg Am 2010;35(8):1260–3.
8. Ruchelsman DE, Puri S, Feinberg-Zadek N, et al. Clinical outcomes of limited-open retrograde intramedullary headless screw fixation of metacarpal fractures. J Hand Surg Am 2014;39(12):2390–5.
9. del Pinal F, Moraleda E, Rúas JS, et al. Minimally invasive fixation of fractures of the phalanges and metacarpals with intramedullary cannulated headless compression screws. J Hand Surg Am 2015; 40(4):692–700.
10. Eisenberg G, Clain JB, Feinberg-Zadek N, et al. Clinical Outcomes of Limited Open Intramedullary Headless Screw Fixation of Metacarpal Fractures in 91 Consecutive Patients. Hand (N Y) 2020;15(6): 793–7.
11. Hoang D, Vu CL, Jackson M, et al. An Anatomical Study of Metacarpal Morphology Utilizing CT Scans: Evaluating Parameters for Antegrade Intramedullary Compression Screw Fixation of Metacarpal Fractures. J Hand Surg Am 2021;46(2):149 e1–e149 e8.
12. Chao J, Patel A, Shah A. Intramedullary Screw Fixation Comprehensive Technique Guide for Metacarpal and Phalanx Fractures: Pearls and Pitfalls. Plast Reconstr Surg Glob Open 2021;9(10):e3895.
13. Okoli M, Chatterji R, Ilyas A, et al. Intramedullary Headless Screw Fixation of Metacarpal Fractures: A Radiographic Analysis for Optimal Screw Choice. Hand (N Y) 2022;17(2):245–53.
14. Hoang D, Huang JI. Antegrade Intramedullary Screw Fixation: A Novel Approach to Metacarpal Fractures. Journal of Hand Surgery Global Online 2019;1(4):229–35.
15. Hoang D, Vu CL, Huang JI. Evaluation of Antegrade Intramedullary Compression Screw Fixation of Metacarpal Shaft Fractures in a Cadaver Model. J Hand Surg Am 2021;46(5):428 e1–e428 e7.
16. Guidi M, Frueh FS, Besmens I, et al. Intramedullary compression screw fixation of metacarpal and

phalangeal fractures. EFORT Open Rev 2020;5(10): 624–9.

17. ten Berg PW, Mudgal CS, Leibman MI, et al. Quantitative 3-dimensional CT analyses of intramedullary headless screw fixation for metacarpal neck fractures. J Hand Surg Am 2013;38(2):322–330 e2.

18. Urbanschitz L, Dreu M, Wagner J, et al. Cartilage and extensor tendon defects after headless compression screw fixation of phalangeal and metacarpal fractures. J Hand Surg Eur Vol 2020;45(6): 601–7.

19. Poggetti A, Fagetti A, Lauri G, et al. Outcomes of 173 metacarpal and phalangeal fractures treated by intramedullary headless screw fixation with a 4-year follow-up. J Hand Surg Eur Vol 2021;46(5): 466–70.

20. Thakker A, Sharma SC, Gupta M. Intramedullary Headless Screw Fixation of Distal Metacarpal Fractures - the Birmingham Experience. J Hand Surg Asian Pac 2021;26(1):52–9.

21. Hug U, Fiumedinisi F, Pallaver A, et al. Intramedullary screw fixation of metacarpal and phalangeal fractures - A systematic review of 837 patients. Hand Surg Rehabil 2021;40(5):622–30.

22. Ozer K, Gillani S, Williams A, et al. Comparison of intramedullary nailing versus plate-screw fixation of extra-articular metacarpal fractures. J Hand Surg Am 2008;33(10):1724–31.

23. Couceiro J, Ayala H, Sanchez M, et al. Intramedullary Screws versus Kirschner Wires for Metacarpal Fixation, Functional, and Patient-Related Outcomes. Surg J 2018;4(1):e29–33.

24. Esteban-Feliu I, Gallardo-Calero I, Barrera-Ochoa S, et al. Analysis of 3 Different Operative Techniques for Extra-articular Fractures of the Phalanges and Metacarpals. Hand (N Y) 2021;16(5):595–603.

25. Belsky MR, Eaton RG, Lane LB. Closed reduction and internal fixation of proximal phalangeal fractures. J Hand Surg Am 1984;9(5):725–9.

26. Freeland AE, Orbay JL. Extraarticular hand fractures in adults: a review of new developments. Clin Orthop Relat Res 2006;445:133–45.

27. Horton TC, Hatton M, Davis TR. A prospective randomized controlled study of fixation of long oblique and spiral shaft fractures of the proximal phalanx: closed reduction and percutaneous Kirschner wiring versus open reduction and lag screw fixation. J Hand Surg Br 2003;28(1):5–9.

28. Page SM, Stern PJ. Complications and range of motion following plate fixation of metacarpal and phalangeal fractures. J Hand Surg Am 1998;23(5): 827–32.

29. Borbas P, Dreu M, Poggetti A, et al. Treatment of proximal phalangeal fractures with an antegrade intramedullary screw: a cadaver study. J Hand Surg Eur Vol 2016;41(7):683–7.

30. Giesen T, Gazzola R, Poggetti A, et al. Intramedullary headless screw fixation for fractures of the proximal and middle phalanges in the digits of the hand: a review of 31 consecutive fractures. J Hand Surg Eur Vol 2016;41(7):688–94.

31. Gaspar MP, Gandhi SD, Culp RW, et al. Dual Antegrade Intramedullary Headless Screw Fixation for Treatment of Unstable Proximal Phalanx Fractures. Hand (N Y) 2019;14(4):494–9.

32. Miles MR, Krul KP, Abbasi P, et al. Minimally Invasive Intramedullary Screw Versus Plate Fixation for Proximal Phalanx Fractures: A Biomechanical Study. J Hand Surg Am 2021;46(6):518 e1–e518 e8.

33. Rausch V, Harbrecht A, Kahmann SL, et al. Osteosynthesis of Phalangeal Fractures: Biomechanical Comparison of Kirschner Wires, Plates, and Compression Screws. J Hand Surg Am 2020; 45(10):987 e1–e987 e8.

34. Gray RRL, Rubio F, Heifner JJ, et al. Double Barrel Screw Fixation for Proximal Phalanx Fracture. Tech Hand Up Extrem Surg 2022;26(4):214–7.

35. Fader L, Robinson L, Voor M. Headless Compression Screw Fixation for Proximal Phalanx Fractures: A Biomechanical Study. Hand (N Y) 2022;17(2): 239–44.

36. Aita MA, Mos PAC, de Paula Cardoso Marques Leite G, et al. Minimally invasive surgical treatment for unstable fractures of the proximal phalanx: intramedullary screw. Rev Bras Ortop 2016;51(1):16–23.

The Use of Patient-Specific Implants for the Treatment of Upper Extremity Fractures

Sneha R. Rao, MD*, Gregory F. Pereira, MD, Marc J. Richard, MD

KEYWORDS

- 3-D printing • Patient-specific instrumentation • Personalized surgery • Malunion

KEY POINTS

- 3-D printing technology can improve intraoperative precision.
- Patient-specific intraoperative guides can be particularly helpful in improving accuracy during complex upper extremity deformity correction.
- The main limitations of 3-D printing technology include implant cost and manufacturing time.

INTRODUCTION

Three-dimensional (3-D) printing and patient-specific instrumentation (PSI) have become progressively more common within orthopedics during the past decade, with the creation of customized guides, implants, and models representing the dawn of personalized surgery.

Three-dimensional printing and PSI have multiple applications in preoperative planning, complex reconstruction, multiplanar cutting guides, education, and implant design.[1,2] To this end, recent literature have focused on evaluating the advantages and disadvantages of these technologies. A recent systematic review by Wong and colleagues, provided evidence that 3-D printing in orthopedics reduced operating time, blood loss, fluoroscopy times, bone union time, pain, increased accuracy and function, and did not increase the rate of complications.[3] Despite these positive findings, concerns about implant costs and time required to produce PSI still limit its widespread use.[1]

In upper extremity surgery, 3-D printed implants and PSI have been applied to a wide array of cases from complex corrective osteotomies to ligament reconstructions and segmental bone loss.[2] As this technology advances, the applications and indications in upper extremity surgery will continue to broaden. This article aims to review current experiences using 3-D printed implants and PSI in the upper extremity to assist with complex reconstruction.

RELATIVE INDICATIONS

For the purposes of this article, PSI will include 3-D printed implants that remain in the patient after surgery, as well as traditional, PSI, used only intraoperatively as guides. Although there are no agreed-upon absolute indications for PSI in the literature, we present frequent indications for which it has been used in the literature for surgery of the upper extremity.

Complex Malunion Correction

Both nonoperatively and operatively managed fractures of the upper extremity can progress to malunion. Distal radius fractures are the most common fracture of the upper extremity and malunion is the most common complication, occurring in 11% to 24% of cases.[4–6] If symptomatic, these malunions may require an osteotomy to correct the deformity, often in multiple planes. Accurate preoperative planning of complex corrective osteotomies is challenging, and the intraoperative execution of these plans is often even more difficult. Campe and colleagues demonstrated that current preoperative planning techniques enabled precise correction of distal radius malunion in only 40% of patients within their cohort.[7] Inability to

Department of Orthopaedics, Duke University Medical Center, Box 3000, Durham, NC 27710, USA
* Corresponding author.
E-mail address: sneha.rao@duke.edu

Hand Clin 39 (2023) 489–503
https://doi.org/10.1016/j.hcl.2023.05.002
0749-0712/23/© 2023 Elsevier Inc. All rights reserved.

restore radial length was associated with increased stiffness and pain; highlighting the need for more precise preoperative and intraoperative techniques to help achieve and maintain the planned deformity correction.[7]

The recent advances in additive manufacturing and PSI have implemented cost-effective production of patient-specific osteotomy guides. These guides have been shown to be effective and reliable for complex corrections of common malunions of the upper extremity including those of the metacarpals and distal radius.[8] These guides can help minimize technical errors and may yield more reproducible results.

Intercalary Segmental Defect

Large intercalary bone defects of the upper extremity pose a challenging problem to surgeons and frequently lead to discussions about salvage or palliative treatments including amputation. Traditional reconstructive approaches such as the induced membrane technique[9] and distraction osteogenesis[10] are reasonable options to manage segmental bony defects, although it frequently requires multiple sequential procedures, especially for larger defects. Similarly, free vascularized bone flaps are technically very challenging and have associated donor-site morbidity and prolonged convalescence. The use of 3-D-printed, PSI with ingrowth surfaces provides another approach to address this challenging problem. Unlike other options, this procedure may provide a solution for the intercalary defect in a single surgery.

Patient-Specific Instrumentation for Cortical Autograft Harvest

Obtaining appropriate cortical autografts to get ideal congruity with the recipient site is often a challenge to preoperatively plan and intraoperatively execute. Using 3-D modeling and computer-assisted surgical planning, donor and recipient sites can be assessed to determine optimal cuts for the intended use.[2] Subsequently, cutting guides may be printed to minimize guesswork on the intraoperative execution of these plans. Such cutting guides have been used to harvest optimally congruent iliac crest bone graft for cases of glenoid deficiency with shoulder instability and in scaphoid nonunion[11] being managed with osteoarticular medial femoral condyle vascularized grafting.

Intraoperative Patient-Specific Instrumentation Guides

Intraoperative PSI guides and virtual 3-D surgery planning technology have the potential to optimize

hardware placement and minimize articular damage for periarticular upper extremity fracture management. This technology has already been validated in shoulder arthroplasty with the implementation of preoperative 3-D planning technology and corresponding patient-specific guides for glenoid hardware placement. A randomized control trial by Iannotti and colleagues showed the precise placement of glenoid implant placement with the use of preoperative 3-D planning and use of patient-specific guides.[12] Translating this technology to the management of upper extremity fractures could have similar advantages. The use of patient-specific guides and 3-D preoperative planning can be particularly efficacious in fractures that require hardware removal followed by deformity correction because these cases may necessitate techniques that minimize bone resection while utilizing new screw paths in an area with less bone stock. Fillat-Goma and colleagues addressed this challenge in the correction of periarticular distal humerus fracture malunion by use of 3-D printed cutting guides that enabled precise removal of hardware while also providing accurate placement for new drill paths with adequate bone stock.[2] As noted in their case report, the use of headless compression screws in fracture fixation can pose a challenge during hardware removal due to the difficulty of identifying entry points for screw removal; therefore, preoperative computer-assisted surgery planning enabled them to plan surgical techniques and model potential intraoperative challenges. In conjunction with the 3-D printing technology, they were able to utilize precise intraoperative guides that helped facilitate the removal of hardware, accurate correction of deformity, and subsequent fixation.

Reported Outcomes

Given that this technology is still in its infancy in terms of clinical applications, there are relatively few reports of small series with clinical outcomes data to evaluate postoperative outcomes and clinical complications.

Currently, postoperative clinical outcomes data examining the use of patient's specific implants and upper extremity fracture management has involved the use of 3-D printed models of the fracture and preoperative planning. Yang and colleagues evaluated the use of 3-D printed models of complex elbow fractures both for physician preoperative planning and for the preoperative patient encounters.[10] In the cohort of 40 patients with elbow fractures, of which 20 received a 3-D printed model preoperatively and 20 patients received only a standard computed tomography

(CT) scan of the fracture, patients who received the personalized 3-D printed fracture models had higher patient satisfaction scores than those who obtained standard CT scanograms.[10] Patients who received the 3-D printed fracture model also had shorter surgical duration, lower blood loss, and higher functional scores. Surgeons included in the study who answered a questionnaire rated higher subjective efficacy of preoperative surgical planning for the patients who received the 3-D model preop.[10] Similar results were noted in a randomized controlled trial by Chen and colleagues who utilized 3-D printed models in AO type C fractures of the distal radius and found reduced intraoperative use of fluoroscopy, lower blood loss and operative time in patients who had a 3-D printed model of their complex distal radius fractures used in the preoperative planning stages.[11] This study also showed that patient satisfaction was higher in the 3-D printed cohort due to the patients' perceived benefit of the technology.[11] However, there was no difference in postoperative functional scores in distal radius fractures treated with or without the 3-D printed models.[11]

The use of custom 3-D printing has been well established in oral maxillofacial surgery and while this technology has not been fully integrated into orthopedic surgery, we can learn a great deal from its applications in adjacent surgical subspecialties. Martelli and colleagues conducted a systematic review of more than 158 studies utilizing 3-D printing in various applications for both maxillofacial and orthopedic surgery. Although the majority of the studies were published in oral maxillofacial literature, 25% of the studies originated from the orthopedic surgery literature. Development of 3-D anatomic models for preoperative planning was the most common application with 71.5% of studies citing this technology. The use of surgical guidance, templates, and 3-D printed implants were less common with 25.3% and 9.5% of studies in this systematic review utilizing these technologies. Across all studies, the main advantages that were reported were improved preoperative planning (48.7%), accuracy of the technology (33.5%), and decreased intraoperative time (32.9%). The main limitation cited across studies was the time required to develop and implement the 3-D printing technology in the clinical setting (19.6%) and the increased cost of this technology (19%).

CASE REPORTS
Case 1

Anatomical region: distal radius.

Case description
Complex distal radius malunion in a 28-year-old active military patient.

Patient-specific instrumentation
Custom cutting guide and 3-D-printed implant for 3-D patient-specific correction of distal radius malunion.

Brief history
A 28-year-old woman sustained a left distal radius fracture 10 years earlier while serving in the military that was treated nonoperatively and subsequently went on to malunion. She reported daily pain, reduced range of motion, functional limitation, and was unable to continue to work as a mechanic and fulfill her military training obligations.

Clinical outcome
At the patient's most recent visit, approximately 6 months postop, the patient reports 0 out of 10 pain and reports that she can perform her job as a mechanic without difficulty. On examination, the patient has 75° of wrist extension, 60° of wrist flexion, 60° of pronation, and full supination.

Preoperative radiographs (**Fig. 1**)
Preoperative CT (**Fig. 2**)
Preop 3-D reconstruction (**Fig. 3**)
Intraoperative fluoroscopy (**Figs. 4–7**)
Most recent visit (**Fig. 8**)

CASE 2
Anatomical Region

Ulna midshaft.

Case Description

Multiply revised both bone forearm fracture with previously infected nonunion.

Patient-Specific Instrumentation

Custom cutting guide and 3-D-printed custom implant to fill in an intercalary defect of the ulnar shaft.

Brief history
A 47-year-old previous smoker sustained a both bone forearm fracture from a fall downstairs that underwent open reduction and internal fixation (ORIF) and went on to nonunion requiring revision ORIF. This was complicated by compartment syndrome with subsequent infected fasciotomy sites and finally deep surgical site infection. After removal of hardware, insertion of an antibiotic spacer, and multiple courses of antibiotics guided by the Infectious Disease service, the infection was cleared, and the patient underwent a revision ORIF with a vascularized free fibular graft to the

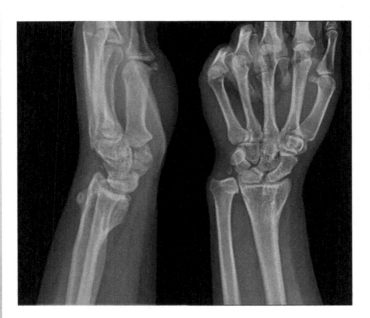

Fig. 1. Preoperative lateral (*left*) and posteroanterior (*right*) radiographs with volar translation of the carpus relative to the articular surface of the radius, decreased radial inclination, decreased radial height, and ulnar positive variance.

radius and conventional bone grafting to the ulna. The radius went on to union but the ulnar nonunion persisted. The patient continued to have symptoms related to the ulna nonunion and was offered a one-bone forearm procedure versus a 3-D-printed custom implant to preserve pronosupination, which remained similar to the contralateral, uninjured side.

Clinical outcome

At the patient's most recent visit, approximately 6 months postop, the patient reports 0 out of 10 pain and has been able to use her forearm for light activities. On examination, the patient has 45° of wrist extension, 45° of wrist flexion, 70° of pronation, and 60° of supination.

Preoperative radiographs and CT (**Fig. 9**)

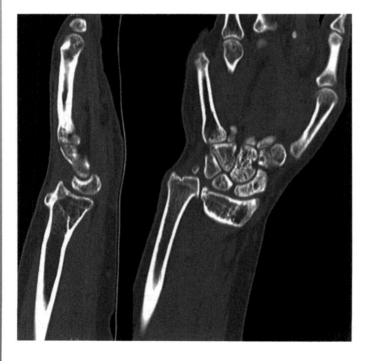

Fig. 2. Redemonstration of preoperative deformity with volar translation of the carpus relative to the articular surface of the radius, decreased radial inclination, decreased radial height, and ulnar positive variance via sagittal (*left*) and coronal (*right*) CT cuts.

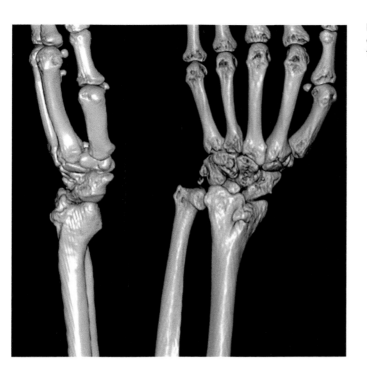

Fig. 3. Three-dimensional reconstruction of the preoperative osseous anatomy from a standard CT scan.

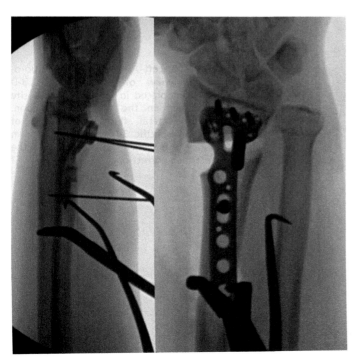

Fig. 4. Left–Lateral fluoroscopic view of the patient-specific cutting guide for the planned osteotomy held on the volar surface of the radius with Kirschner wires. Right–Anteroposterior fluoroscopic view of osteotomized distal radius with a volar locking plate based on the pretemplated cut and planned patient-specific 3-D implant.

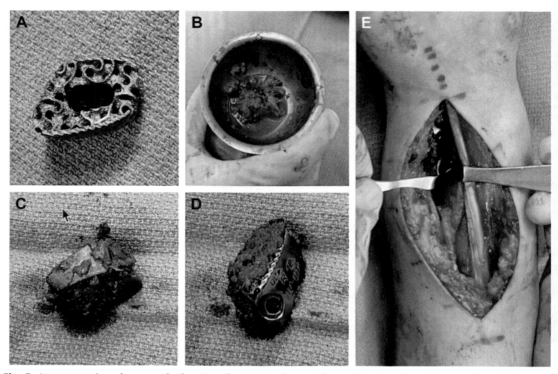

Fig. 5. Intraoperative photograph showing the 3-D implant with machined surfaces that enable adherence of bone graft (*A*). Images B–D show the harvested iliac crest autograft and application of the bone graft onto the machined surfaces of the implant. Final application of the implant with the bone graft shown in image E.

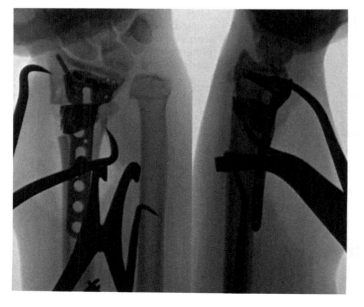

Fig. 6. Left–Anteroposterior fluoroscopic view of patient-specific 3-D implant placed in prior osteotomy site to maintain the planned correction. Right—Lateral fluoroscopic view of patient-specific 3-D implant placed in prior osteotomy site to maintain the planned correction.

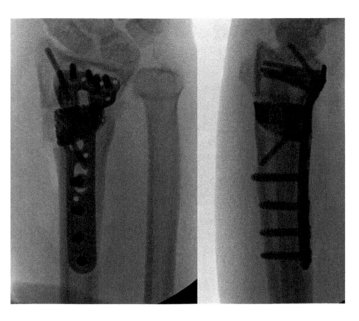

Fig. 7. Left–Anteroposterior fluoroscopic view of the patient-specific 3-D implant in its appropriate corrective position fixed to the volar locking plate. Note that cancellous iliac crest autograft has been placed in the defect adjacent to the implant. Right–Lateral fluoroscopic view of the patient-specific 3-D implant in its appropriate corrective position fixed to the volar locking plate.

Intraoperative fluoroscopy (**Figs. 10–12**)
Most recent visit (**Fig. 13**)

CASE 3
Anatomical Region

Distal radius.

Case Description

Distal radius malunion.

Patient-Specific Instrumentation

Custom 3-D-printed cutting guides for correction of malunion deformity.

Brief History

A 59-year-old woman with remote history of breast cancer and prior stroke presented as a second opinion regarding evaluation and treatment of malunion of extra-articular right distal

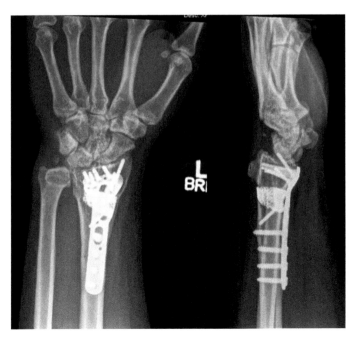

Fig. 8. Most recent posteroanterior (*left*) and lateral (*right*) radiographs from 6-month postop showing maintenance of the reduction, osseous integration, and no concern for hardware failure.

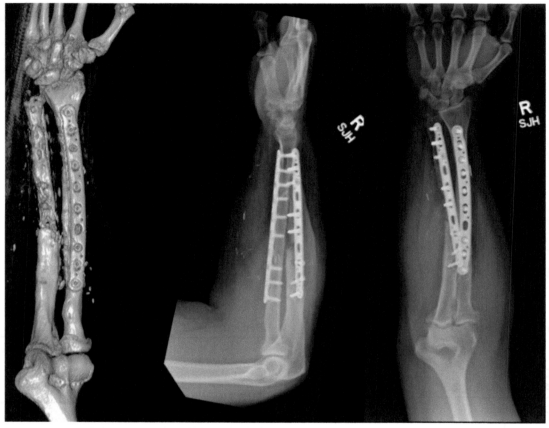

Fig. 9. Anteroposterior (*right*) and lateral (*middle*) radiographic images and 3-D CT reconstructed image (*left*) showing status after vascularized fibular bone flap with operative fixation of both radius and ulna, there is union of the radius with persistent nonunion of the ulna.

radius fracture following nonoperative treatment. She sustained the initial injury due to a fall on the right hand and was subsequently evaluated by a local orthopedic surgeon and treated with 4 weeks

of cast immobilization. The patient presented for a second opinion 2 weeks following due to persistent wrist pain and limited range of motion. At the initial clinic visit, the patient's range of motion

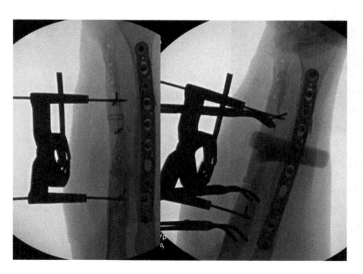

Fig. 10. Left–Anteroposterior fluoroscopic view of the patient-specific cutting guide for the planned osteotomy held on the ulna with Kirschner wires. Right–Anteroposterior fluoroscopic view of the patient-specific cutting guide with completed osteotomy.

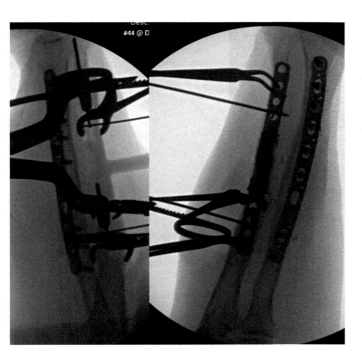

Fig. 11. Left–Anteroposterior fluoroscopic view after the osteotomized segment was removed with proximal and distal osseous segments held with serrated clamps. Right—Anteroposterior fluoroscopic view with patient-specific 3-D implant filling and spanning the ulnar defect.

was limited to 15° of wrist flexion, 20° of wrist extension, full pronation and supination limited to −10 (unable to achieve neutral wrist position), with painful motion. The patient is deaf and communicates via American Sign Language, which is adversely affected by her functional limitation at the wrist. Radiographs at the initial evaluation showed extra-articular distal radius fracture with loss of reduction and increased volar tilt measuring 27° compared with 15° following cast removal and shortening of 2.5 mm as measured by ulnar variance. CT scan obtained at 8 weeks following injury reveal a nondisplaced intra-articular fracture component and well reduced distal radial ulnar joint (DRUJ). Given the degree of her symptoms and the persistent increased volar angulation and shortening of the fracture, the decision was made to undergo corrective

Fig. 12. Anteroposterior (*left*) and lateral (*right*) fluoroscopic views with the patient-specific 3-D implant in place.

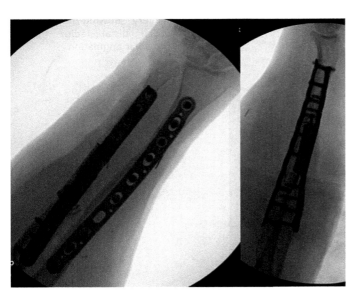

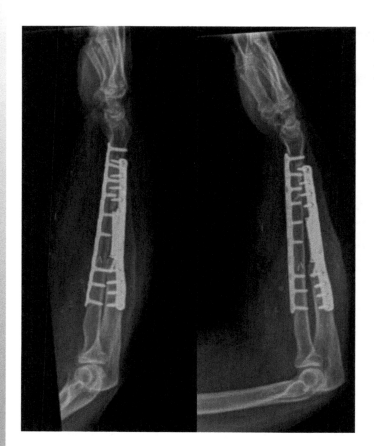

Fig. 13. Most recent lateral radiographs from 3-month postop showing maintenance of the alignment, osseous integration, and no concern for hardware failure.

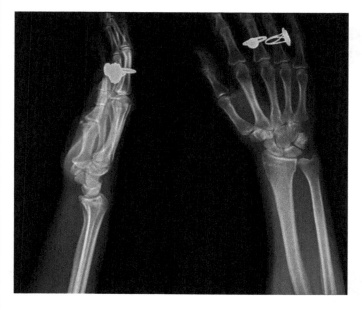

Fig. 14. Radiographs obtained at the time of injury showing nondisplaced extra-articular distal radius fracture with 15° of volar angulation.

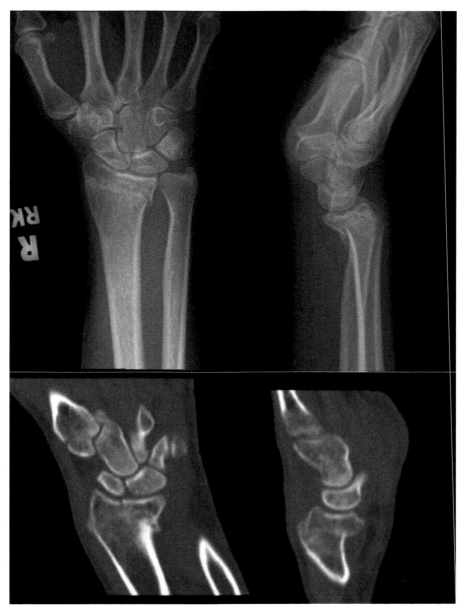

Fig. 15. Radiographs obtained following 4 weeks of cast immobilization showing displacement of extra-articular distal radius fracture with increased volar angulation to 27°. CT scan reveals a nondisplaced intra-articular component of the fracture.

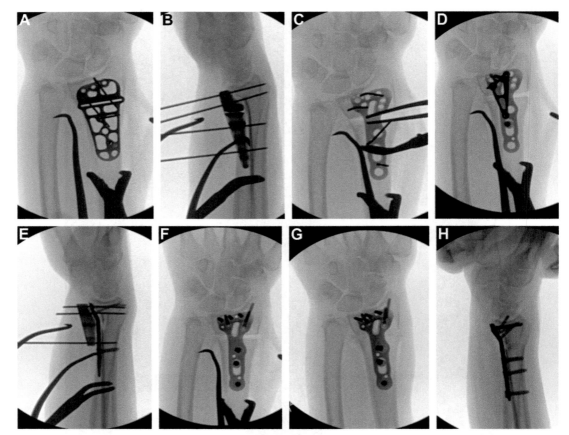

Fig. 16. Figures A through H show the application of the 3-D printed custom cutting guide (*A*, *B*), AP and lateral views following distraction osteotomy and placement of volar plate, and application of custom guide to maintain reduction of osteotomy during volar plate fixation (*C–E*) Final fluoroscopic AP and lateral images as shown in (*G* and *H*) show final volar plate construct with iliac crest autograft and anatomic alignment of the distal radius.

osteotomy with custom 3-D printed cutting guide and bone graft from ipsilateral iliac crest.

    Radiographs at the time of injury (**Fig. 14**)

    Preoperative radiographs and CT scan (**Fig. 15**)

    Intraoperative fluoroscopy and clinical images (**Figs. 16–18**)

    Postoperative radiographs (**Fig. 19**)

DISCUSSION

Three-dimensional printing technology and PSI are being rapidly integrated into many clinical settings, including preoperative and intraoperative surgical applications. Although the indications for this technology have not yet been clearly defined, there are a few common clinical scenarios in which 3-D printing and PSI have been shown to improve preoperative planning for complex surgical problems and reduce technical difficulties intraoperatively.[1] The use of 3-D printed, patient-specific intraoperative guides and 3-D printed implants have been shown to be successful in the planning and execution of complex deformity correction in the setting of malunion and nonunion of upper extremity fractures.[13] In our experience, this technology enables us to not only preoperatively plan for intraoperative challenges but also to build patient-specific 3-D printed implants and intraoperative surgical guides that would address these challenges and minimize deviation from the preoperative plan. We think that the overall benefit of this technology in improving our intraoperative precision is worth further investigation with larger case series.

Our experience mirrors that of other groups that have addressed challenging clinical problems by utilizing 3-D printing technology. In the upper extremity trauma setting, Chen and colleagues showed that 3-D printed preoperative models of complex fractures and malunions have been shown to decrease intraoperative surgical time and increase postoperative patient satisfaction

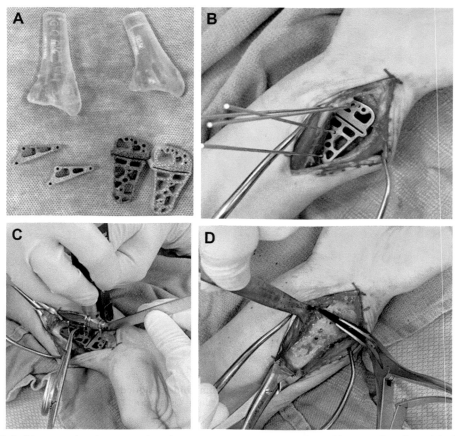

Fig. 17. Clinical images showing 3-D printed custom cutting guides along with 3-D printed model of the distal radius (A). Images (B–D) depict placement of the custom cutting guides through the standard FCR approach for distal radius fractures and planned osteotomy at the site of malunion.

because they were able to have a better understanding of their complex injury.[14] The majority of the case series currently published in the literature include preoperative planning applications of this technology; however, the few published case series investigating the use of 3-D printed custom implants and 3-D printed custom surgical guides for intraoperative use demonstrate great potential for this technology to improve our precision intraoperatively and help provide solutions for complex surgical problems.

The main limitations of using 3-D printing and PSI are the higher implant costs and preoperative planning time that is inherently associated with these newer techniques.[1] In addition, due to the lack of high-level studies in the literature and the lack of robust clinical outcomes data, the indications for this technology are not yet clearly defined. Along with exploring the clinical applications, there is a need to continue to study this technology and further our understanding of its potential and limitations. These patients often have challenging clinical problems and they represent a very heterogeneous group of patients and skeletal defects, hence the need for custom implants. These technologies are currently used in other orthopedic applications such as oncologic reconstruction, lower extremity trauma, and revision arthroplasty. These experiences can guide their use in upper extremity surgery. Future studies can address these gaps in the literature to expand the clinical applications of 3-D printing technology.

SUMMARY

Three-dimensional printing technology can help improve our intraoperative precision and preoperative planning to address challenging upper extremity trauma such as complex malunion/nonunion and fracture patterns with large intercalary bone defects. Although this new frontier of medicine is still in its infancy, the innovative solutions that are possible to achieve with this technology have the potential to improve outcomes for patients that have complex injuries and/or resulting complications from those injuries.

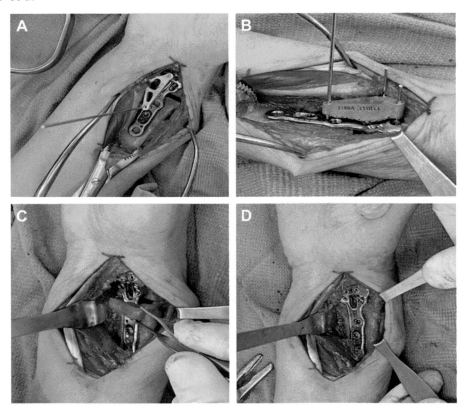

Fig. 18. Clinical images (*A, B*) show application of 3-D custom guide designed to both hold reduction of the osteotomy site and enable application of volar distal radius plate. Osteotomy site filled with ipsilateral iliac crest autograft (*C*). Final implant construct shown in image D.

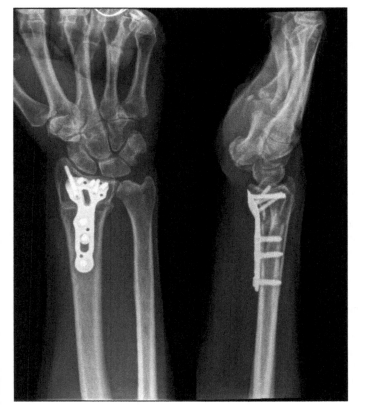

Fig. 19. Postoperative PA and lateral radiographs reveal stable hardware and healing osteotomy site with incorporation of the iliac crest autograft.

CLINICS CARE POINTS

- Intraoperative patient-specific implants can help achieve desired deformity correction for the treatment of malunited upper extremity fractures.
- The added benefit of improved accuracy when using patient spefic implants/intraoperative guides must be weighed against the increased cost of implants.
- The clinical benefit of PSI and 3D printing technology has not been clearly delineated in the literature.
- We recommend considering the use of this technology in the surgical treatment of complex upper extremity fracture malunion and nonunion.

REFERENCES

1. Martelli N, Serrano C, van den Brink H, et al. Advantages and disadvantages of 3-dimensional printing in surgery: A systematic review. Surgery 2016; 159(6):1485–500.
2. Fillat-Goma F, Marcano-Fernandez FA, Coderch-Navarro S, et al. 3-D printing innovation: New insights into upper extremity surgery planning. Injury 2021;52(Suppl 4):S117–24.
3. Wong RMY, Wong PY, Liu C, et al. 3-D printing in orthopaedic surgery: a scoping review of randomized controlled trials. Bone Joint Res 2021;10(12): 807–19.
4. Amadio PC, Botte MJ. Treatment of malunion of the distal radius. Hand Clin 1987;3(4):541–61.
5. Dobyns JH, Linscheid RL, Cooney WP 3rd. Fractures and dislocations of the wrist and hand, then and now. J Hand Surg Am 1983;8(5 Pt 2): 687–90.
6. Sharma H, Khare GN, Singh S, et al. Outcomes and complications of fractures of distal radius (AO type B and C): volar plating versus nonoperative treatment. J Orthop Sci 2014;19(4):537–44.
7. von Campe A, Nagy L, Arbab D, et al. Corrective osteotomies in malunions of the distal radius: do we get what we planned? Clin Orthop Relat Res 2006; 450:179–85.
8. Hirsiger S, Schweizer A, Miyake J, et al. Corrective Osteotomies of Phalangeal and Metacarpal Malunions Using Patient-Specific Guides: CT-Based Evaluation of the Reduction Accuracy. Hand (N Y) 2018;13(6):627–36.
9. Masquelet AC. Induced Membrane Technique: Pearls and Pitfalls. J Orthop Trauma 2017;31(Suppl 5):S36–8.
10. Ruette P, Lammens J. Humeral lengthening by distraction osteogenesis: a safe procedure? Acta Orthop Belg 2013;79(6):636–42.
11. Houdek MT, Matsumoto JM, Morris JM, et al. Technique for 3-Dimesional (3-D) Modeling of Osteoarticular Medial Femoral Condyle Vascularized Grafting to Replace the Proximal Pole of Unsalvagable Scaphoid Nonunions. Tech Hand Up Extrem Surg 2016;20(3):117–24.
12. Martin TG, Iannotti JP. Reverse total shoulder arthroplasty for acute fractures and failed management after proximal humeral fractures. Orthop Clin North Am 2008;39(4):451–7.
13. Yang L, Grottkau B, He Z, et al. Three dimensional printing technology and materials for treatment of elbow fractures. Int Orthop 2017;41(11):2381–7.
14. Chen C, Cai L, Zheng W, et al. The efficacy of using 3-D printing models in the treatment of fractures: a randomised clinical trial. BMC Musculoskelet Disord 2019;20(1):65.

Staple Technology for Fracture Fixation and Joint Arthrodesis

Samuel L. Posey, MD[a], Raymond Glenn Gaston, MD[b],*

KEYWORDS

- Nitinol staple biomechanics • Wrist arthrodesis • Scaphoid fracture fixation
- Trapeziometacarpal arthrodesis

KEY POINTS

- Memory staples provide an excellent fixation option for upper extremity joint arthrodesis and fracture fixation.
- Modern memory staple designs allow for easy application and continuous compression at the targeted site of bone healing.
- Troughing and unicortical placement of staples with the legs being within 2 mm of the far cortex maximizes the biomechanical strength of the construct while minimizing hardware prominence.
- Staple fixation alone is supported for partial wrist fusions as well as fixation of carpal fractures; applications throughout the upper extremity are increasing such as in the case of provisional fixation of an osteotomy.
- When possible, it is recommended to place two staples at a fracture or fusion site and preferably on the compression side of the fracture.

INTRODUCTION AND HISTORY

Although originally developed for military equipment such as the hydraulic lines of the F-14 fighter aircraft, shape-memory alloys (SMAs) have provided a unique area of innovation to the orthopaedic community with the development of SMA staples for fracture fixation and arthrodesis.[1,2] More traditional staples requiring external methods of compression have become obsolete with the development of SMA staples that have intrinsic properties of compression.[3,4] Nitinol (nickel–titanium; Naval Ordnance Laboratory, Nitinol Devices and Components, Inc, Fremont, CA) is a nickel–titanium alloy that exhibits temperature-sensitive deformation that allows for continuous compression across a fracture or arthrodesis site.[1,2,5] SMA staples have been used for fracture fixation since 1983 with broadening indications ranging from joint arthrodesis to intra-articular fracture fixation.[6,7]

The use of SMA staples has increased in the upper extremity literature.[8,9] With simple application and the ability to provide continuous compression, SMA staples achieve a higher union rate than the more traditional staples.[8,9] One of the more frequent complications of staples includes impingement from hardware prominence,[9,10] but current techniques of troughing or countersinking the staple have become more commonplace with no compromise in biomechanical strength of the construct.[7] Troughing is defined as removing bone between the planned staple legs to provide a recess for the staple to sit, thus making it less prominent (**Fig. 1**). Although there is a dearth of prospective literature comparing SMA staple constructs to other forms of fixation for upper extremity fractures or arthrodesis, understanding the proper technique and indications for SMA staple placement can be a helpful emerging technique for hand surgeons.

a Department of Orthopaedic Surgery, Atrium Health, 1000 Blythe Boulevard, Charlotte, NC 28203, USA; b The Hand Center, OrthoCarolina, 1915 Randolph Road, Charlotte, NC 28207, USA
* Corresponding author.
E-mail address: Glenn.Gaston@orthocarolina.com

Hand Clin 39 (2023) 505–513
https://doi.org/10.1016/j.hcl.2023.05.010

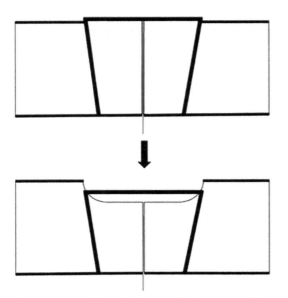

Fig. 1. No trough (top) and troughed constructs (bottom). After troughing, the staple is countersunk to avoid impinging on surrounding structures.

NATURE OF THE PROBLEM

In upper extremity surgery, the primary goal of fracture fixation or arthrodesis is to obtain a stable union that allows for pain relief as well as restoration of function. Unfortunately, nonunion rates as high as 25% to 35% have been reported for some partial wrist arthrodeses with a subsequent need for revision surgery or even salvage procedures.[8,11] In addition, the function of the hand relies on tendons that are intimately associated with the underlying skeletal structures as opposed to more proximal portions of the arm or lower extremity where the soft tissue envelope is larger. Therefore, fixation constructs should be low profile in nature to avoid tendon or soft tissue irritation. Although compression screws have led to improvements in union rates as compared with Kirschner wires (K-wires) for midcarpal arthrodesis,[12] these screws are subject to osteolysis and proximal migration that can require subsequent hardware removal in up to one-third of cases.[10,13]

To achieve stability while preserving blood supply to a fracture or fusion site, the surgeon must determine the appropriate fixation construct to allow for sufficient stability while simultaneously respecting the local biology.[14] Many of the original reports of capitolunate fusions using K-wires required a transition to a four-corner fusion for a larger surface area for fusion, but this was before the advent of more quality fixation constructs such as SMA staples or compression screws.[15,16]

Isolated intercarpal arthrodeses have more recently been shown to have high union rates and require less OR time and bone graft when used as compared with more extensive fusions. To accomplish the goal of a fusion in a low-profile manner, SMA staples offer an appealing option for various upper extremity fractures and joint arthrodesis procedures that include midcarpal fusions (four-corner, isolated capitolunate, two or three column fusions), radiocarpal fusions, carpometacarpal (CMC) joint fusions, carpal fractures, and even provisional fixation for transverse long bone fractures or osteotomies such as humerus and forearm, including ulnar shortening osteotomy.

BIOMECHANICS

Nitinol is the most common alloy used for SMA staples and it exists in two crystallographic phases depending on the local temperature: martensite and austenite.[2] At lower temperatures, Nitinol remains in its more malleable martensite phase; meanwhile, at higher temperatures near body temperature, it transforms to the stronger austenite phase with a more cubic crystalline structure.[1] In addition to this shape memory characteristic, Nitinol displays an incredible amount of superelasticity that allows it to recover a large amount of strain as it returns to its "trained" shape.[17] Many modern SMA staple designs capitalize on both Nitinol's shape memory and superelasticity characteristics that result in a staple that inherently wants to "pull" (or compress) its legs together at body temperature. Most current SMA staples are held by an external applicator with legs that are parallel to each other in a "strained" version of the austenite phase that compresses as soon as the applicator is removed from the staple (**Fig. 2**).

In clinical and biomechanical studies, the two staples applied orthogonally to each other provide increased stability.[2,18] Regardless, it is recommended to place two staples when possible to double the compressive force, stiffness, and bending strength of the fixation; moreover, a recent biomechanical study showed that the effective leg length for an SMA staple is extended 2 mm distal to the tip of the staple leg so Nitinol staples do not have to be placed bicortically to achieve compression of the far cortex.[7] The same study demonstrated that countersinking the staple to avoid implant prominence did not have a negative biomechanical effect of the construct; by contrast, troughing to recess staples actually increased the bending strength of the construct.[7] To achieve higher contact forces at the fracture or fusion site in osteoporotic bone, increasing the bridge length

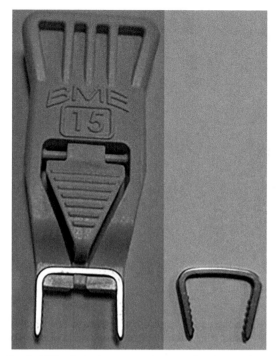

Fig. 2. Nitinol staple mounted on application tool uncompressed (left), and after deployment in compression mode (right). Once placed into bone, staple legs move together, applying compression between the legs.

was shown in one finite element analysis study to both increase compression at the osteotomy site and lower stresses in osteopenic bone.[17] The ability to increase bridge length, of course, is dictated clinically by the anatomic location of the fusion or fracture site; nonetheless, being able to apply these various biomechanical principles is paramount for proper SMA staple application in each clinical scenario.

PREOPERATIVE/PREPROCEDURE PLANNING

Preoperative planning for an upper extremity fusion or fracture fixation with SMA staples starts with quality imaging of the anatomy of interest. Although biplanar radiographs are often sufficient, advanced imaging such as a computed tomography (CT) scan, may be helpful to estimate the desired bridge length and leg length preoperatively to ensure implant availability. Moreover, understanding the surgical approach may allow for thoughtful staple placement. For example, the surgical approach may dictate a surgeon's ability to place two staples or at least one staple on the compression side of the anticipated loading to improve construct stability.[2] Although we place

most standard plate constructs on the tension side of a fracture to enhance stability, SMA staples produce the most compression on the "far" side near the ends of its effective legs that want to return to the aforementioned "trained" state; therefore, placing the staple on the compression side of anticipated loading allows its dynamic compression to work better on the tension side of a fracture or fusion site.

PREP AND PATIENT POSITIONING

The standard skin prep and positioning for upper extremity fractures or fusion procedures are followed at the authors' institution. The patient is typically supine with the operative extremity prepped and draped on a hand table.

PROCEDURAL APPROACH: USE OF BULLETED OR NUMBERED LISTS IN THESE SECTIONS IS ENCOURAGED
Capitolunate Arthrodesis

- A standard dorsal wrist approach is used between the second and fourth extensor compartments distal to the EPL.
- A capsulotomy is performed to identify the proximal and distal carpal rows.
- The scaphoid is excised and used for supplemental bone graft.
- The cartilage and subchondral/sclerotic bone of the capitolunate joint is removed using a rongeur or osteotomes until there is visible cancellous bone. We prefer to avoid using power for this step to prevent any thermal necrosis to the cancellous bone.
- Provisional reduction of the capitolunate joint is performed typically with palmar pressure on the capitate and radial translation of the lunate.
- The capitolunate reduction is then pinned with a K-wire.
- Using fluoroscopy, one must next critically assess the alignment of the capitate and lunate to ensure they are colinear on the lateral image and that a natural "scaphoid shadow" is present on the AP image.[19]
- The guide for drilling the SMA staple is then placed on the capitate and lunate such that two parallel staples can be placed across the capitolunate articulation.[9] Some systems have a cannulated drill guide option to improve accuracy of the drilling.
- The drill bit is then drilled through one cortex of the capitate but does not have to exit the second cortex; it simply needs to be within

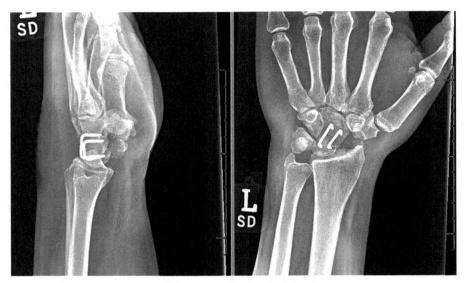

Fig. 3. Capitolunate fusion with two parallel SMA staples for final fixation.

2 mm of the second cortex for optimal compression.[7]

- A pin is placed in the drill hole through the guide to maintain the selected length of the SMA staple measured.
- The second hole is then unicortically drilled in the lunate ideally just beneath the subchondral bone distally.
- A small rongeur is used to create a trough between the two drill holes in the lunate and capitate to allow the staple to sit at or below the dorsal cartilaginous rim of the lunate to avoid impingement of the staple and the dorsal lip of the radius. This has been shown to have no significant impact on biomechanical strength of the construct and may actually improve bending strength of the construct.[7]
- Bone graft from the scaphoid is packed densely into the fusion site.
- A depth measurement is then made with the depth gauge to ensure a proper leg length of staple is chosen. The depth should be measured on the capitate as it has a smaller diameter in the sagittal plane than the lunate and volar staple prominence may be mitigated.
- The appropriately sized SMA staple is placed into the predrilled holes with its application tool in uncompressed mode (see **Fig. 2**). A mallet or tamp is then used to seat and ideally recess the staple.
- The application device is removed once the staple is fully seated and the steps are repeated for placement of the second parallel staple. The staples will move into their

compression mode once they reach physiologic body temperature and their applicator is removed (**Fig. 3**).
- The position of the staples is checked under fluoroscopy to ensure proper placement and remove the provisionally placed K-wire.
- After irrigation and incision closure, the patient is placed into a volar splint until their first appointment at 2 weeks postoperatively.
- In the setting of a Type 2 lunate, we will either use an osteotome to remove the proximal aspect of the hamate or prepare the lunate-hamate articulation and include it in the fusion mass with the second staple spanning this articulation depending on the size of this articulation.
- In certain cases, later recognition of an lunotriquetral (LT) tear resulted in persistent ulnar-sided wrist pain following capitolunate (CL) fusion (**Fig. 4**). Therefore, it is recommended to closely scrutinize the LT relationship radiographically and consider a four-corner fusion in that setting.

Four-Corner Arthrodesis

- A similar approach and exposure steps to the capitolunate arthrodesis procedure described above are used.
- The scaphoid is excised and used for later bone graft. When additional autograft is needed, we will use the distal radius at the level of Lister's tubercle.
- The lunate extension is corrected with either volar pressure applied to the capitate as

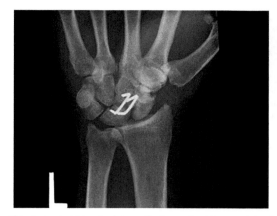

Fig. 4. Lunotriquetral tear that resulted in persistent ulnar-sided wrist pain following CL fusion.

described above or using wrist flexion and a pin across the radius and lunate. The wrist can then be extended (through the midcarpal joint) to align the capitate and lunate and the pin driven into the capitate.

- The lunate, capitate, hamate, and triquetrum are temporarily pinned with 1.14-mm (0.45-in) K-wires (**Fig. 5**).
- The articular cartilage and subchondral bone are removed from the planned fusion site with rongeurs and curettes.
- Using similar steps for staple placement as described above with planned bridge length and troughing, staples are placed in standard fashion to adjoin the lunate, capitate, hamate, and triquetrum.

First Carpometacarpal Joint Arthrodesis

- Similar to the technique described by Richards and Newington,[20] a dorsal approach is used between the abductor pollicis longus and extensor pollicis brevis tendons.
- A capsulotomy is performed, and the first CMC joint is excised with an oscillating saw or rongeur to minimize bone excision and thereby preserve thumb height.
- Once both the base of the first metacarpal and the trapezium have exposed the cancellous bone, the joint is provisionally pinned with a K-wire.
  - Ensure the pinned thumb is in 35° of radial abduction, 35° of palmar abduction, 15° of pronation, and 10° of extension.[21] We typically use a Coban roll in the palm to position the thumb during pin placement.
- Place two SMA staples in an orthogonal fashion after troughing the bone between the staple drill holes to avoid prominence (**Fig. 6**).

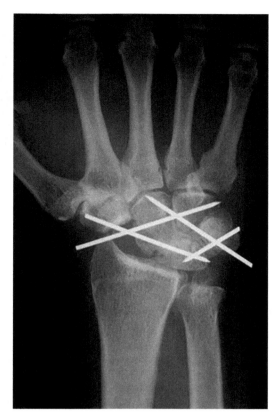

Fig. 5. Wrist posteroanterior radiograph following provisional K-wire fixation for planned four-corner fusion.

Scaphoid Waist Fracture Fixation

- Although it is the authors' preference to use cannulated screw fixation for acute scaphoid waist fractures, SMA staples remain a viable option for fixation, especially in the setting of revision surgery or nonunion.
- This technique is contraindicated in proximal third or distal third fractures as there is not enough bone surface area to place the staple in such a manner to capture the fracture fragment.
- A longitudinal incision is made overlying the flexor carpi radialis (FCR) and curved toward the base of the first metacarpal at the distal wrist crease.[22]
- The FCR tendon is retracted ulnarly, and the thenar musculature is divided in line with its fibers.
- The volar wrist capsule is incised sharply and elevated to expose the scaphoid.
- This can be extended proximally to the radioscaphocapitate ligament which can then be either retracted proximally with a small Ragnell retractor or divided and subsequently repaired.

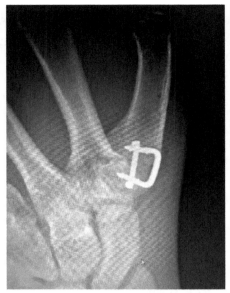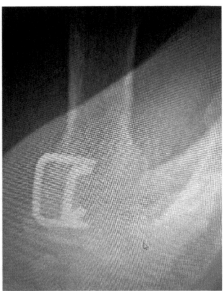

Fig. 6. Thumb CMC arthrodesis with perpendicular SMA staple construct.

- Using separate K-wires as joy sticks in the proximal and distal fragments, the scaphoid fracture is reduced and provisionally pinned with a retrograde K-wire.
- Ulnarly deviating and extending the wrist will extend the distal aspect of the scaphoid, enhance visualization, and help facilitate staple placement.
- Sample radiographs of the SMA staple construct for a scaphoid waist fracture are depicted in **Fig. 7**.

Humerus (or Radius/Ulna) Fracture Adjunct Fixation

- Diaphyseal humerus fractures are an area where SMA staples can provide excellent provisional reduction as well as compression at the fracture site, especially in the case of transverse fracture patterns.
- Another more unique case demonstrates similar use of a staple for a humeral shortening osteotomy (designed to preserve the condyles while shortening the limb for improved prosthetic fit and rotational control). An SMA staple in this case can provide similar compression and provisional fixation before neutralization plate placement (**Fig. 8**).

RECOVERY AND REHABILITATION (INCLUDING POSTPROCEDURE CARE)

After capitolunate arthrodesis or four-corner arthrodesis, sutures are removed at the patient's

first postoperative appointment, and a short-arm cast is placed. Patients are instructed to avoid weight-bearing on the operative extremity. Repeat radiographs are evaluated at 6 weeks postoperatively; if the fusion seems apparent and the patient has little or no pain, patients are transitioned to a removable Velcro wrist splint. Active and active-assisted range of motion exercises are started at the 6-week postoperative mark with passive range

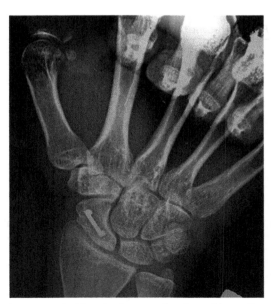

Fig. 7. Scaphoid waist fracture fixation with an SMA staple. (*Courtesy of* Miguel Cruz, MD, Gilbert, AZ).

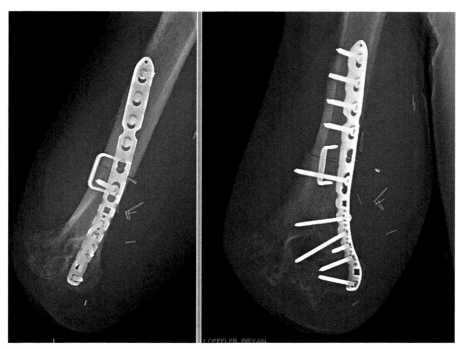

Fig. 8. Provisional fixation of a humeral shortening osteotomy with an SMA staple.

of motion and strengthening exercise beginning at 8 to 12 weeks based on radiographic and clinical healing.[10]

The first CMC arthrodesis and scaphoid waist fractures fixed with SMA staples are converted from their postoperative thumb spica splint to a thumb spica cast at their first postoperative visit when sutures are removed. They remain immobilized in a cast until their 6-week postoperative appointment, where they are then transitioned into a removable thumb spica Velcro brace to begin active range of motion exercises. In the case of SMA staples for humeral shaft fractures, the postoperative management is variable based on the situation and additional fixation that is used.

OUTCOMES

There are no prospective clinical trials currently that compare the outcomes of SMA staples to other forms of fixation for midcarpal fusions. For patients with scaphoid nonunion advanced collapse and scapholunate advanced collapse wrist, a recent retrospective study found that SMA staples had comparable union rates when evaluating staples (97%) to compression screws (89%) for a capitolunate arthrodesis.[23] Both cohorts of patients in this study had similar patient-reported outcome measures and incidences of hardware complications. Of note, the staple cohort had no incidents of hardware prominence

after the surgical technique was adjusted to include troughing so that the staple was countersunk. A more recent systematic review found similar union rates between all forms of fixation for four-corner arthrodesis when comparing K-wires alone, plate fixation, and staples.[24]

For the younger patient with first CMC arthritis, a first CMC arthrodesis has been described to have good functional outcomes but a high complication rate from hardware prominence with all techniques used.[25] At present, there are no comparative, prospective studies to evaluating fixation techniques and complication rates.[26] Although Singh and colleagues[27] noted a 20% nonunion rate in patients undergoing first CMC arthrodesis with K-wire fixation alone, the investigators reported union in all cases with SMA staple or headless compression screw fixation. A study by Richards and colleagues[20] reporting on 14 young patients undergoing first CMC arthrodesis with SMA staple constructs noted a 100% union rate and no secondary operations.

Although less common than headless compression screw fixation, scaphoid waist fractures are amenable to SMA staple fixation. A recent retrospective study of 131 patients with scaphoid waist fractures undergoing fixation with an SMA staple similar to our described method above demonstrated a greater than 97% union rate with a mean operative time of 34 minutes.[28] A more recent systematic review by Dunn and colleagues,[29] reported a 100% union rate for SMA staple fixation of acute scaphoid waist fractures with a complication rate of approximately 9%. The most common complication noted in this study was the need for hardware removal in two patients which the investigators attributed to technical error in staple placement.

SUMMARY

Staple technology use in the upper extremity has continued to evolve with the development of SMA such as Nitinol that displays superelastic properties that can be exploited for persistent compression at the fracture site. Biomechanical studies support the use of SMA staples for upper extremity fracture fixation and joint arthrodesis. To optimize biomechanical strength and clinical outcomes, it is recommended to place two staples, if possible. Countersinking the staples to prevent hardware prominence is also recommended when possible. Placing the staples perpendicular to each other and having one staple on the compression side of the fracture site increase stability of the construct. The current literature supports the use of staple technology for not only joint arthrodesis in the upper extremity but also for fracture fixation with non-inferior outcomes as compared with other methods of fixation for various clinical situations.

CLINICS CARE POINTS

- Memory staples provide an excellent option for upper extremity arthrodesis and fracture fixation.

- Modern memory staple designs allow for easy application and continuous compression at the targeted site of bone healing.

- Troughing and unicortical placement of staples with the legs within 2 mm of the far cortex allows for fewer hardware complications with no compromise in the biomechanical strength of the construct.

- Staple fixation alone is supported for both intercarpal wrist arthrodesis and fixation of scaphoid fractures; applications throughout the upper extremity continue to expand with utilization of staples for provisional fixation of fractures and osteotomies.

- When possible, it is recommended to place two staples at a fracture or arthrodesis site, preferably on the compression side of the site of interest.

DISCLOSURE

R.G. Gaston is a consultant to Biomedical Enterprises, Synthes (West Chester, PA).

REFERENCES

1. Wadood A. Brief overview on nitinol as biomaterial. Adv Mater Sci Eng 2016;2016. https://doi.org/10.1155/2016/4173138.
2. Hoon QCJ, Pelletier MH, Christou C, et al. Biomechanical evaluation of shape-memory alloy staples for internal fixation-an in vitro study. J Exp Orthop 2016;3(1). https://doi.org/10.1186/S40634-016-0055-3.
3. Shibuya N, Manning SN, Meszaros A, et al. A compression force comparison study among three staple fixation systems. J Foot Ankle Surg 2007;46(1):7–15.
4. Wu JC, Mills A, Grant KD, et al. Fracture fixation using shape-memory (Ninitol) staples. Orthop Clin North Am 2019;50(3):367–74.
5. Mahtabi MJ, Shamsaei N, Mitchell MR. Fatigue of nitinol: the state-of-the-art and ongoing challenges. J Mech Behav Biomed Mater 2015;50:228–54.
6. Dai KR, Hou XK, Sun YH, et al. Treatment of intra-articular fractures with shape memory compression staples. Injury 1993;24(10):651–5.
7. McKnight RR, Lee SK, Gaston RG. Biomechanical properties of nitinol staples: effects of troughing, effective leg length, and 2-staple constructs. J Hand Surg Am 2019;44(6):520.e1–9.
8. Bain GI, Ondimu P, Hallam P, et al. Radioscapholunate arthrodesis - a prospective study. Hand Surg 2009;14(2–3):73–82.
9. Ronchetti PJ, Topper SM. Lunocapitate fusion using the OSStaple compression staple. Tech Hand Up Extrem Surg 2006;10(4):231–4.
10. Gaston RG, Greenberg JA, Baltera RM, et al. Clinical outcomes of scaphoid and triquetral excision with capitolunate arthrodesis versus scaphoid excision and four-corner arthrodesis. J Hand Surg Am 2009;34(8):1407–12.
11. Ledgard JP, Siddiqui J, Pelletier MH, et al. Midcarpal arthrodesis biomechanics: memory staples versus cannulated screws. J hand Surg Asian-Pacific 2018;23(4):474–8.
12. Goubier JN, Teboul F. Capitolunate arthrodesis with compression screws. Tech Hand Up Extrem Surg 2007;11(1):24–8.
13. Yao YC, Wang JP, Huang TF, et al. Lunocapitate fusion with scaphoid excision for the treatment of scaphoid nonunion advanced collapse or scapholunate advanced collapse wrist. J Chin Med Assoc 2017;80(2):117–20.
14. Baker CE, Moore-Lotridge SN, Hysong AA, et al. Bone fracture acute phase response—a unifying theory of fracture repair: clinical and scientific

implications. Clin Rev Bone Miner Metab 2018;16(4): 142–58.

15. Calandruccio JH, Gelberman RH, Duncan SFM, et al. Capitolunate arthrodesis with scaphoid and triquetrum excision. J Hand Surg Am 2000;25(5): 824–32.

16. Watson HK, Goodman ML, Johnson TR. Limited wrist arthrodesis. Part II: Intercarpal and radiocarpal combinations. J Hand Surg Am 1981;6(3):223–33.

17. Curenton TL, Davis BL, Darnley JE, et al. Assessing the biomechanical properties of nitinol staples in normal, osteopenic and osteoporotic bone models: a finite element analysis. Injury 2021;52(10):2820–6.

18. Choudhary RK, Theruvil B, Taylor GR. First metatarsophalangeal joint arthrodesis: a new technique of internal fixation by using memory compression staples. J Foot Ankle Surg 2004;43(5):312–7.

19. Rizzo M. Wrist Arthrodesis and Arthroplasty. In: Wolfe S, Pederson W, Kozin S, Cohen M, editors. Green's Operative Hand Surgery. Philadelphia, PA: Elsevier; 2022. p. 439–500.

20. Richards T, Newington D. The results of carpometacarpal joint arthrodesis of the osteoarthritic thumb in younger patients using memory staples. J Hand Microsurg 2020. https://doi.org/10.1055/S-0040-1716613.

21. Li J, Li D, Tian G, et al. Comparison of arthrodesis and arthroplasty of Chinese thumb carpometacarpal osteoarthritis. J Orthop Surg Res 2019;14(1). https://doi.org/10.1186/S13018-019-1469-2.

22. Congiusta DV, Basyuk Y, Vosbikian MM, et al. The use of nitinol compression staple fixation and bone graft for scaphoid waist fractures and nonunion: a surgical technique. Tech Hand Up Extrem Surg 2020;25(1):35–40.

23. McKnight RR, Tait MA, Bracey JW, et al. Retrospective comparison of capitolunate arthrodesis using headless compression screws versus nitinol memory staples for SLAC and SNAC wrist: radiographic, functional, and patient-reported outcomes. Hand (N Y) 2021. https://doi.org/10.1177/1558944721999732.

24. Hayes E, Cheng Y, Sauder D, et al. Four-corner arthrodesis with differing methods of osteosynthesis: a systematic review. J Hand Surg Am 2022;47(5): 477.e1–9.

25. Dharamsi MS, Caudle K, Fares A, et al. Arthrodesis for carpometacarpal joint arthritis: a systematic review. Hand (N Y) 2022. https://doi.org/10.1177/15589447221105541. 155894472211055.

26. London DA, Stern PJ. Carpometacarpal arthrodesis: indications and techniques. Hand Clin 2022;38(2): 231–40.

27. Singh HP, Hoare C, Beresford-Cleary N, et al. Nonunion after trapeziometacarpal arthrodesis: comparison between K-wire and internal fixation. J Hand Surg Eur 2015;40(4):351–5.

28. Rocchi L, Merendi G, Cazzato G, et al. Scaphoid waist fractures fixation with staple. Retrospective study of a not widespread procedure. Injury 2020; 51:S2–8.

29. Dunn J, Kusnezov N, Fares A, et al. The scaphoid staple: a systematic review. Hand (N Y) 2017; 12(3):236.

Enhanced Approaches to the Treatment of Distal Radius Fractures

Devan Patel, MD, Robin Kamal, MD, MBA, MS*

KEYWORDS

• Distal radius • Fractures • Wrist • Approaches

KEY POINTS

- Distal radius fractures are common injuries and can be a sign of osteoporosis in the elderly.
- A thorough examination and patient history can help define patient goals and ultimately guide treatment.
- A variety of surgical approaches, including volar, dorsal, or radial, can be used.
- Approaches can be used in isolation or in conjunction based on the visualization needed for reduction and fixation.

INTRODUCTION

Distal radius fractures are among the most common injuries treated by orthopedic surgeons. Studies estimate the incidence of distal radius fractures accounts for 1.5% to 2.5% of all emergency room visits with a trend for increasing incidence.[1] The incidence occurs in a bimodal distribution, with peaks seen in the children or adolescence population and the elderly population. Younger age groups tend to have higher energy mechanisms of injury, and children are at risk because of skeletal immaturity of the wrist. Elderly patients, over the age of 65 years, tend to have a lower energy mechanism, with a ground-level fall being the most common mechanism.[2] The rate of distal radius fractures in the young adult population is relatively low compared to that in the other two groups but is often due to high-energy mechanisms. Due to the overall rise in patients sustaining distal radius fractures, a thorough understanding of the treatment principles for additional radius fracture is essential for surgeons.

CLASSIFICATIONS

There are a variety of classifications describing distal radius fractures. The AO, Frykman, and Fernandez classification are among the most common classification used.[3] Although classification systems are different, the primary goal is to group similar fracture patterns to help surgeons decide appropriate management. No system has been found to be perfect in determining treatment or predicting outcomes, but they may help surgeons recognize behavior of fractures and communicate with other physicians.

Because the historic distal radius classification systems do not align with contemporary understanding of distal radius fractures (eg, volar lunate facet fractures), the authors prefer an Instability-Based Distal Radius Fracture Classification system. In this system, the distal radius injury is analyzed for 4 unique patterns of instability.

1. Axial instability: fractures that involve the metaphysis of the distal radius leading to translation, loss of radial height (in reference to the ulna), radial inclination, and/or volar tilt.

[a] Stanfod University, VOICES Health Policy Research Center, Department of Orthopaedic Surgery, 450 Broadway Street, MC: 6342, Redwood City, CA 94063, USA
* Corresponding author. Department of Orthopaedic Surgery, Stanford University, 450 Broadway Street MC: 6342, Redwood City, CA 94603.
E-mail address: rnkamal@stanford.edu

Hand Clin 39 (2023) 515–521
https://doi.org/10.1016/j.hcl.2023.07.001

2. Articular joint instability: fractures that involve the articular surface of the distal radius leading to articular step off greater than 2 mm. These injuries require greater focus on obtaining anatomic articular reductions with various surgical approaches and reduction techniques.
3. Radiocarpal joint instability: fractures associated with nondissociative carpal instability patterns. These include the more severe trans-styloid perilunate and ulnocarpal translocations of the carpus, the more subtle volar lunate facet and dorsal lunate facet fragments leading to carpal subluxation. These injuries require a focus on repair of the capsular injuries along with fixation of the associated fractures (including size and bone quality).
4. Distal radioulnar joint (DRUJ) instability: fractures that are associated with injury to the triangular fibrocartilage complex (TFCC) or base of the ulnar styloid fractures leading to volar or dorsal instability between the radius and the ulna at the sigmoid notch. These injuries require either specialized splinting with later initiation of motion or additional operative treatments to stabilize the DRUJ.

RELEVANT ANATOMY

The structure of the distal radius plays a critical role in allowing the patient's hand to be placed in optimal positions for functions of the digits. The articular surface of the distal radius articulates with the carpus, specifically, the scaphoid facet and the lunate facet which articulate with the respective carpal bones. The articulation of the distal radius with the carpal bones allows for the flexion and extension, as well as radial and ulnar deviation of the wrist. Malalignment of the articular surface can limit these motions and thus limit hand function.[4]

In addition, the distal radius includes the sigmoid notch on the most ulnar aspect, which articulates with the ulnar head, known as the distal radial and ulnar joint (DRUJ). In conjunction with the proximal radial ulnar joint (PRUJ), the DRUJ allows for forearm rotation. The relative stability of this joint is primarily provided by the triangular fibrocartilage complex. The TFCC is comprised of both volar and dorsal radial ulnar ligaments which act as the primary stabilizer of the TFCC. In addition, the fibrocartilaginous disc, the ulnocarpal ligaments, and the floor of the extensor carpi ulnaris (ECU) tendon also contribute to the stability.[5] These structures are at risk of injury in the setting of distal radius fractures and may require additional repair.

INITIAL MANAGEMENT

A thorough initial evaluation of the patient is crucial in the management of patients with distal radius fractures. The history should include hand dominance, previous injuries, activity level, and medical comorbidities. These factors can play a crucial role in the management decision of these injuries.[6] In addition, distal radius fractures can be a sign of osteopenia or osteoporosis. The bone quality of older patients should be evaluated, and if concerns exist, the patient may warrant referral to an osteoporosis specialist.[7] Furthermore, it may be a sign of impaired mobility, and physicians should evaluate ambulatory status in this population.

A detailed physical examination should be performed before operative intervention to evaluate for any concomitant injuries. When treating fractures that involve significant displacement of the distal radius or a radiocarpal dislocation, a detailed examination evaluating the median nerve should be performed. If persistent paresthesias are present after the reduction, there should be consideration for emergent carpal tunnel release and fracture fixation.[8]

In most cases, initial management of nondisplaced distal radius fractures should consist of a reduction with splint or cast application followed by repeat radiographs to evaluate the residual displacement (for up to 3 weeks). If the fracture pattern is truly nondisplaced, the patient can initially be placed in a cast as a form of definitive management. A cast or splint should be accompanied by a three-point mold to maintain the position of the fracture within the cast.

Displaced fractures, however, should undergo closed reduction followed by splint application. A hematoma block using local anesthetic can help with patient analgesia and make reduction more tolerable for patients. In contrast to casts, splints allow for subsequent swelling after reduction.

The patient should be advised to elevate the extremity to mitigate swelling after reduction. Immobilization should end proximal to the metacarpal phalangeal joints to allow for full finger range of motion. After the initial management and immobilization, patients with displaced fractures should follow up to evaluate for any subsequent displacement within the splint or cast.

NONOPERATIVE MANAGEMENT

The decision for operative or nonoperative management is multifactorial based on the fracture pattern, fracture displacement, patient's functional status (typically using age as a guide), medical comorbidities amongst others. Ultimately the decision for treatment management should be made by the patient in conjunction with the surgeon. The patient should have the understanding that residual displacement of the fracture may result in decreased objective function of the wrist and hand, but subjective function may not vary based on functional demands. Recent evidence suggests there may be limited benefit of surgical treatment in geriatric patients.[9]

Generally accepted criteria for operative management are articular step off greater than 2 mm, ulnar variance greater than 4 mm, ulnar shift greater than 6 mm, and dorsal tilt greater than 10°.[10] Patients undergoing nonoperative management can be transitioned to a cast after an initial period of 2 to 3 weeks in a splint. Several factors have been established as risk factors for loss of reduction in closed management of distal radius fractures. Lafontaine proposed dorsal tilt greater than 20°, dorsal comminution, intra-articular fracture, ulnar fracture, and age greater than 60 years were all associated with an unstable pattern and subsequent loss of reduction.[11] More recent evidence has supported these risk factors and emphasized age as a primary risk factor for loss of reduction.[12–14]

IMAGING

The initial imaging of the distal radius should include the standard three views of the wrist (PA, oblique, and lateral).[15] Radiographs of the hand as well as the forearm should be performed to evaluate for concomitant injuries.

The PA view of the wrist allows for measurement of the radial inclination, which is measured by a line along the distal articular surface to a line that is 90° perpendicular to the radial shaft. The average radial inclination is approximately 23°. The ulnar variance can also be measured on the initial PA view. The ulnar variance is calculated between 2 parallel lines, which are perpendicular to the axis of the radial shaft. One line is through the distal articular margin of the ulna. The other is a line from the midpoint of the lunate facet articular margin. Ulnar variance is typically 1 to 2 mm but can vary widely, and therefore, contralateral radiographs are useful.[15]

The lateral view is useful in measuring the volar tilt, which is the angle between a line between the distal margins of the volar and dorsal lunate facets and a line perpendicular to the longitudinal axis of the radial shaft. The average volar tilt is approximately 11°. The lateral radiograph is also helpful in evaluating the lunate facet, which is a critical structure contributing stability of the radiocarpal joint. This is represented by the teardrop

seen on the lateral view which is the palmar aspect of the lunate facet.[15]

A radial inclination lateral view can help better define the articular margin of the distal radius. The beam is inclined about 10° to 20° to account for the normal radial inclination of the distal radius to allow for a lateral view down the radial carpal articular surface without overlap of the radial styloid.[15]

If there is intra-articular involvement, there should be consideration to obtain a CT scan. A CT scan allows for better characterization of the fracture fragments as well as the severity of the injury at the joint surface.[16] Three-dimensional reconstructions can help better define the relationship of the fracture fragments and aid in planning the approach for proper fixation.

PREP AND PATIENT POSITIONING

In general, patients are positioned on the operating room table in the supine position with a hand table on the operative side. Supine positioning allows for access to both the volar and dorsal aspects of the wrist with adequate baseline rotation of the forearm. Patients can undergo surgery under regional block or general anesthesia. A tourniquet should be applied on the upper arm for hemostasis throughout the case. Intraoperative fluoroscopy should be available to evaluate the fracture reduction as well as the position of the implants during the procedure.

PROCEDURAL APPROACHES
Percutaneous Pin Fixation

Percutaneous pin fixation can be an effective strategy for patients with extra-articular fractures and simple intraarticular fractures that can be reduced anatomically. A variety of pin orientations can be used to stabilize the fracture fragment. One of the most common strategies involves pins from the radial styloid aimed ulnarly into the intact radial shaft. When placing radial sided pins, care must be taken to avoid damage to the radial sensory nerves, extensor tendons, as well as the radial artery if deviating too volar. A mini open approach can be used over the distal aspect of the radial styloid just dorsal extensor pollicis brevis. After closed reduction, the initial pin from the radial styloid to the intact shaft can be placed. Additional pins can be placed from either the radial styloid or dorsal-ulnar aspect of the distal radius just radial to the sigmoid notch to the intact shaft acting as a cross pin relative to the radial styloid pin.[17] More than one pin should be placed in the fracture fragment to control rotation. Pins can be buried or left out to be removed after 4 weeks. Alternatively, a headless compression screw can be used for fixation.

External Fixation

External fixation remains a useful tool stabilizing distal radius fractures in patients with significant soft tissue injuries about the wrist. This fixation strategy can be used for both temporary and definitive fixation depending on the goals of treatment.

Begin with a 2- to 3-cm incision on the dorsoradial aspect of the index finger metacarpal. Blunt dissection can be used to dissect down to bone avoiding extensor tendons ulnarly and neurovascular bundle radially. Once dissection is carried down to visualize bone, two 2.5-mm or 3-mm half pins can be placed along the dorsoradial axis to be parallel to and bicortical in the metacarpal. Then, a 6-cm dorsoradial incision can be made proximal to the wrist joint out of the zone of injury and proximal to the fracture. Blunt dissection is used to visualize the dorsoradial aspect of the radius ulnar to brachioradialis. Sufficient retraction is necessary to avoid damage to the soft tissues and dorsal sensory branch of the radial nerve. Two pins are then placed through the radius proximal to the fracture.[18] Fluoroscopy is used to confirm that all pins are bicortical and well-spaced. After the frame is assembled, the reduction can be achieved by stabilizing the frame proximally and pulling traction on the distal pins and securing the frame. Additional bars and cross-bars can be used to strengthen the fixation construct. External fixation can also be used in addition to other forms of fixation including percutaneous pin fixation.

Dorsal Bridge Plating

Dorsal bridge plating can be used as an alternative to external fixation if the soft tissue envelope is amenable. Bridge plating mitigates the risk of pin site infection and the presence of an external device compared to external fixation. However, it requires an additional procedure to remove the plate.[19] In cases with significant axial and articular instability, bridge plating can be used to restore length and overall alignment of the distal radius articular surface.[20] Similarly, a dorsal bridge plate can also reduce radiocarpal instability as it can fix the position of the radius to the metacarpals/distal carpal row. In addition, the bridge plate can be used in conjunction with other fixation techniques including percutaneous pinning and volar plating to maintain reduction and joint stability.

A 3-cm incision is made on the dorsal aspect of the second or third metacarpal. Either metacarpal can be used for distal fixation. Blunt dissection is used to expose the dorsal aspect of the bone. A periosteal elevator can be used to dissect soft tissue off the proximal aspect of the metacarpal. Then, a retractor can be used to mobilize the extensor tendons inserting onto the metacarpal base dorsally allowing a clear path to place the plate proximately. A periosteal elevator can be used to create a path proximally across the wrist underneath the fourth dorsal compartment. The plate can be palpated approximately along the dorsal aspect of the radius. Before fixation, it is critical to ensure that the plate is in the correct path and not overlying the soft tissues of the dorsal compartment of the forearm. Once the plate is in appropriate position, the plate can be fixed distally to the metacarpal using a combination of nonlocking followed by locking screws. Fluoroscopy is used to guide the incision over the proximal aspect of the plate. Blunt dissection can be used to expose the plate proximally. Three additional screws are placed through the proximal plate.[21] Plates are generally removed in 3 to 4 months or after radiographic evidence of fracture healing.

Henry/Modified Henry

The volar approach is the most used approach for surgical treatment of distal radius fractures. The approach provides visualization of the volar articular surface for volar plating or fragment-specific fixation. The classic Henry approach uses the interval between the radial artery and flexi carpi radialis (FCR). This approach is extensile and can be used for fractures on the middle and proximal aspects of the radius as well. For the exposure of the distal radius, an 8-cm incision is made just proximal to the wrist crease medial to the brachioradialis tendon on a line from the radial styloid to a point just lateral to the insertion of the biceps tendon. After the incision is made, superficial dissection includes identification of the radial artery just ulnar to the brachioradialis. After identification of the radial artery, the dissection is carried between the radial artery and FCR tendon down to the radial edge of the pronator quadratus. The pronator quadratus is incised along its radial edge and proximal to the distal insertion, leaving a cuff for possible repair, and a periosteal elevator is used to expose the distal radius.[22] It is critical to make sure that exposure includes the volar ulnar corner as well as distally enough for adequate plate fixation. Distally, care must be taken to not remove the volar extrinsic ligaments of the wrist, which are within 5 mm of the distal insertion of pronator quadratis.[23]

An alternative to the classic Henry approach is the modified approach which uses a similar interval through the FCR subsheath. The incision is centered over the distal FCR tendon. Dissection is carried down to the FCR sheath. It is critical to stay radial to the FCR tendon as the palmar cutaneous branch of the median nerve is often just medial to the tendon. Once the sheath over the tendon is incised, the FCR is retracted ulnarly, and the subsheath of the tendon is incised along the length of the incision, and the FPL muscle belly below is exposed. The FPL muscle belly is bluntly dissected on the radial boarder and retracted ulnarly exposing the pronator quadratus. In the pronator, quadratus is incised in similar fashion to the classical Henry approach.[24] A carpal tunnel release can be performed by extending the incision distally with a Brunauer incision over the wrist crease or through a separate incision.

The volar approach can also be extended for improved exposure of marginal fragments along the articular surface. First, the distal radius is pronated, and the insertion of the brachioradialis is incised as well as the floor of the first dorsal compartment. This allows exposure of the dorsal aspect of the radial styloid for reduction and fixation. The exposure is then carried proximally, and subperiosteal dissection is carried out to expose the distal radial shaft. The distal radial shaft can then be pronated with a bone clamp, which allows visualization and reduction of the central and dorsal marginal fractures.[25]

Dorsal Approach

The dorsal approach to the distal radius is useful to address dorsal cortical fragments as well as directly visualize the articular surface. A 6- to 8-cm incision is made just ulnar to Lister's tubercle. Dissection is carried down to the extensor retinaculum. The extensor retinaculum over the extensor pollicis longus (EPL) tendon is incised in line with the path of the tendon. The tendon can then be mobilized, and the fourth dorsal compartment can then be subperiosteally elevated off the radius. The second dorsal compartment can also be elevated if needed for fracture visualization or plating.[26] The capsulotomy can be made longitudinally in line with the incision, or a ligament-sparing approach can be used to visualize articular fragments. The ligament-sparing approach involves two limbs, and proximal limb is in line with the dorsal radiocarpal ligament with the distal limb in line with the dorsal intercarpal ligament. The residual flap is then elevated from ulnar to volar off the triquetrum to expose the articular surface.[27] An alternative to this approach is the capsular window approach that uses two separate capsulotomies. One capsulotomy is along the distal margin the DRC and the other along the distal margin of the DIC, while preserving the insertion at the triquetrum.[28]

Radial Approach

Isolated fractures involving the radial styloid can be reduced and fixed through a radial-based approach. Radial column or pin plates can be placed through this approach. A 6-cm approach is made from the radial styloid proximally along the radial boarder of radius. Radial sensory nerves need to be protected within the subcutaneous tissues below the skin. The retinaculum over the first dorsal compartment is incised longitudinally, and the abductor pollicis longus (APL) and extensor pollicis brevis (EPB) tendons are retracted to expose the styloid. The brachioradialis, located volar to the first dorsal compartment, can be released for further visualization, and eliminate primary deforming force on the styloid fragment.[29] The radial styloid is then exposed and can be extended proximally along the distal radial shaft for plate fixation.

Ulnar Approach

The volar ulnar approach is a useful approach to address small volar ulnar fragments as well as fractures involving the DRUJ. A 5- to 6-cm incision is made between palmaris longus and the flexor carpi ulnaris (FCU) beginning just proximal to the wrist crease. The ulnar neurovascular bundle is then identified and retracted ulnarly. The flexor tendons are then retracted radially, which allows for visualization of the volar ulnar aspect of the distal radius after the PQ is incised and elevated. The ulnar approach can also be extended distally to facilitate a carpal tunnel release if necessary.[30]

Volar Intraarticular Extended Window Approach

Direct visualization and manipulation of articular fragments can be achieved with either the volar intraarticular extended window approach (VIEW) or an arthroscopic approach. In addition to the articular surface of the distal radius, arthroscopy allows for visualization of the TFCC, lunate, scaphoid, SLIL, and the volar radiocarpal ligaments; however, arthroscopic approaches have not been demonstrated to improve patient outcomes when used for distal radius fractures.[31] Although the dorsal approach to the articular surface is often employed, as we typically use a volar approach for fixation of distal radius fractures, we prefer the VIEW approach when the fracture pattern would benefit from direct visualization. In this approach, the modified Henry exposure is taken distally over the volar capsule. In the setting of articular instability, the sagittal split between the scaphoid and lunate is used as a guide to release the capsule in an oblique pattern toward the mid-carpal joint. Thus, an oblique capsulotomy is performed from the radius to the radial border of the lunate between the short radiolunate ligament (SRL) and long radiolunate ligament (LRL). A retractor is used to protect and mobilize the SRL ligament, which remains overlying the lunate. Care must be taken to avoid damaging the underlying SL ligament. In cases where greater visualization of the articular surface is necessary, the LRL ligament can be released radially off the distal radius. This release is performed subperiosteally from the LRL ligament insertion in the distal radius. Stay sutures are used in the volar capsule to facilitate joint visualization, and in this manner, both the scaphoid and lunate fossa can be evaluated.[32] Longitudinal traction can be used to facilitate articular visualization. A blunt joker can be used to assist in traction and improve visualization, or the wrist can also be placed into a traction tower. A dental pick and smooth K-wires can be used to perform direct reduction, and then 0.035-inch smooth or threaded K-wires can be used for provisional fixation. Once anatomic reduction is confirmed, final fixation using plate-locking screws is performed.

RECOVERY AND REHABILITATION

Postoperatively patients are splinted to immobilize the wrist and allow for postoperative swelling. At 2 weeks, sutures are removed, and repeat radiographs are performed to ensure maintenance of reduction and implant position. Patients are typically placed in removeable wrist immobilization and encouraged to begin passive and active assisted range of motion of the wrist. After 8 weeks, patients should attempt to wean out of the wrist splint and continue range-of-motion exercises. Throughout the period of immobilization, patients should be encouraged to perform range of motion of the fingers as well as elbow if no additional injuries exist.

CLINICS CARE POINTS

- The decision to proceed with surgical management of distal radius fractures is based on several factors including patient comorbidities, functional goals, and fracture pattern.

- A thorough understanding of fracture patterns and fragments are necessary when deciding on the surgical approach and can be guided by an instability classification of distal radius fractures (axial, articular, radio-carpal, and DRUJ instability).
- The distal radius can be approached through a volar, dorsal, or radial approach, which can be used in isolation or in conjunction with one another.
- If direct articular visualization is necessary, the VIEW approach may be used.

DISCLOSURE

The authors have nothing to disclose.

REFERENCES

1. Nellans KW, Kowalski E, Chung KC. The Epidemiology of Distal Radius Fractures. Hand Clin 2012. https://doi.org/10.1016/j.hcl.2012.02.001.
2. Corsino CB, Reeves RA, Sieg RN. Distal Radius Fractures. StatPearls. Published online May 1, 2022. Accessed September 4, 2022. Available at: https://www.ncbi.nlm.nih.gov/books/NBK536916/
3. Kleinlugtenbelt Y v, Groen SR, Ham J, et al. Acta Orthopaedica Classification systems for distal radius fractures Does the reliability improve using additional computed tomography? Classifi cation systems for distal radius fractures Does the reliability improve using additional computed tomography? Acta Orthop 2017;88(6):681–7.
4. Freeland AE, Luber KT. Biomechanics and Biology of Plate Fixation of Distal Radius Fractures. Hand Clin 2005. https://doi.org/10.1016/j.hcl.2005.03.002.
5. Haugstvedt JR, Langer MF, Berger RA. Distal radioulnar joint: Functional anatomy, including pathomechanics. J Hand Surg: European Volume 2017; 42(4):338–45.
6. Langerhuizen DWG, Janssen SJ, Kortlever JTP, et al. Factors Associated with a Recommendation for Operative Treatment for Fracture of the Distal Radius. Wrist Surg 2021. https://doi.org/10.1055/s-0041-1725962.
7. Freedman BA, Potter BK, Nesti LJ, et al. Missed opportunities in patients with osteoporosis and distal radius fractures. Clin Orthop Relat Res 2007;454:202–6.
8. Pope D, Tang P. Carpal Tunnel Syndrome and Distal Radius Fractures. Hand Clin 2018. https://doi.org/10.1016/j.hcl.2017.09.003.
9. Shapiro LM, Kamal RN. American Academy of Orthopaedic Surgeons Appropriate Use Criteria: Treatment of Distal Radius Fractures. J Am Acad Orthop Surg 2022;30(15). https://doi.org/10.5435/JAAOS-D-22-00139.

10. Watson NJ, Asadollahi S, Parrish F, et al. Reliability of radiographic measurements for acute distal radius fractures. BMC Med Imaging 2016. https://doi.org/10.1186/s12880-016-0147-7.

11. Lafontaine M, Hardy D, Delince P. Stability assessment of distal radius fractures. Injury 1989;20:208–10.

12. Nesbitt KS, Failla JM, Les C. Assessment of instability factors in adult distal radius fractures. J Hand Surg Am 2004;29(6):1128–38.

13. Mackenney PJ, McQueen MM, Elton R. Prediction of instability in distal radial fractures. J Bone Joint Surg Am 2006;88(9):1944–51.

14. Myderrizi N. Factors Predicting Late Collapse of Distal Radius Fractures. Malays Orthop J 2011. https://doi.org/10.5704/MOJ.1111.006.

15. Medoff RJ. Essential radiographic evaluation for distal radius fractures. Hand Clin 2005;21(3):279–88.

16. Lichtman DM, Bindra RR, Boyer MI, et al. American Academy of Orthopaedic Surgeons clinical practice guideline on: the treatment of distal radius fractures. J Bone Joint Surg Am 2011;93(8):775–8.

17. Luchini PM, Glener JE, Vaida J, et al. Percutaneous Threaded Pin Fixation of Distal Radius Fracture in the Athlete. Hand (N Y) 2020. https://doi.org/10.1177/1558944720975135. 1558944720975135.

18. Capo JT, Swan KG, Tan V. External fixation techniques for distal radius fractures. Clin Orthop Relat Res 2006;445:30–41.

19. Wang WL, Ilyas AM. Dorsal Bridge Plating versus External Fixation for Distal Radius Fractures. J Wrist Surg 2020;9(2):177–84.

20. Perlus R, Doyon J, Henry P. The use of dorsal distraction plating for severely comminuted distal radius fractures: A review and comparison to volar plate fixation. Injury 2019;50(Suppl 1):S50–5.

21. Boateng HA, Payatakes AH. Distal Radius Fractures: Dorsal Bridge Plating. Oper Tech Orthop 2015; 25(4):282–7.

22. Berdia S, Yu R. Volar Approach to Distal Radius Fractures. Oper Tech Orthop 2009;19(2):65–9.

23. Tedesco LJ, Wu CH, Strauch RJ. How Close Are the Volar Wrist Ligaments to the Distal Edge of the Pronator Quadratus? An Anatomical Study. Hand 2022; 17(1):35–7.

24. Protopsaltis TS, Ruch DS. Volar Approach to Distal Radius Fractures. J Hand Surg Am 2008;33(6): 958–65.

25. Orbay JL, Badia A, Indriago IR, et al. The Extended Flexor Carpi Radialis Approach: A New Perspective for the Distal Radius Fracture. Tech Hand Up Extrem Surg 2001;5.

26. Via GG, Roebke AJ, Julka A. Dorsal Approach for Dorsal Impaction Distal Radius Fracture-Visualization, Reduction, and Fixation Made Simple. J Orthop Trauma 2020;34:S15–6.

27. Berger RA, Bishop AT, Bettinger PC. New dorsal capsulotomy for the surgical exposure of the wrist. Ann Plast Surg 1995;35(1):54–9.

28. Loisel F, Wessel LE, Morse KW, et al. Is the Dorsal Fiber-Splitting Approach to the Wrist Safe? A Kinematic Analysis and Introduction of the "Window" Approach. J Hand Surg 2021;46(12):1079–87.

29. Pirela-Cruz MA, Scher DL. Exposure of distal radius fractures using a direct radial approach with mobilization of the superficial branch of the radial nerve. Tech Hand Up Extrem Surg 2010;14(4):218–21.

30. Tordjman D, Hinds RM, Ayalon O, et al. Volar-Ulnar Approach for Fixation of the Volar Lunate Facet Fragment in Distal Radius Fractures: A Technical Tip. J Hand Surg 2016;41:e491–500.

31. Shihab Z, Sivakumar B, Graham D, et al. Outcomes of Arthroscopic-Assisted Distal Radius Fracture Volar Plating: A Meta-Analysis. J Hand Surg 2022; 47(4):330–40.e1.

32. Kamal RN, Ostergaard PJ, Shapiro LM. The Volar Intra-Articular Extended Window Approach for Intra-Articular Distal Radius Fractures. J Hand Surg 2023. https://doi.org/10.1016/j.jhsa.2022.09.018.

Innovations in Small Joint Arthroscopy

Joshua J. Meaike, MD, Sanjeev Kakar, MD*

KEYWORDS

- Arthroscopy • Small joint • Carpometacarpal • Metacarpophalangeal • Fracture • Fixation • DRUJ
- TFCC

KEY POINTS

- Arthroscopy offers direct, magnified visualization of intra-articular pathology and structures, overcoming limitations of fluoroscopy and partial visualization with open approaches, improving intra-operative decision-making.
- With advances in technology, surgeon knowledge, and technical skill, the indications for small joint arthroscopy continue to expand.
- The introduction of smaller, flexible arthroscopes and low-profile surgical instruments enable the progression of minimally invasive surgery.

INTRODUCTION

Hand fractures including those of the carpus, metacarpals, and/or phalanges account for 20% to 30% of all fractures.[1,2] Intra-articular injuries are particularly challenging, with several fracture patterns and characteristics resulting in a complex treatment algorithm. In general, treatment goals focus on the restoration of anatomic alignment and joint congruity with stable fixation allowing for early motion in an effort to decrease degenerative changes and stiffness, respectively.[3] Some of the more frequently encountered intra-articular injuries of the hand include thumb carpometacarpal (CMC) fractures,[2] metacarpal head fractures,[4] interphalangeal joint (IPJ) fractures,[5] and scaphoid fractures.[6] Soft tissue ligament injuries to the IPJs, carpus, and distal radioulnar joints (DRUJs) can also result in joint malalignment and subsequent sequelae.[7]

Improper or inadequate treatment of these injuries can result in chronic pain, stiffness, and disability.[8–10] Of particular importance, as is the case with nearly all intra-articular fractures, is anatomic reduction and reestablishment of congruent articular surfaces.[11] Traditional surgical options include percutaneous Kirschner (K) wire fixation, open reduction and internal fixation, distraction techniques, and salvage procedures.[3]

The importance of anatomic articular reduction can be understood to some degree from our knowledge of distal radius fractures, where articular step-off greater than 2 mm can result in an increased risk and rate of post-traumatic arthritis (although this can remain clinically asymptomatic).[12,13] Typically, joint reduction is assessed with the use of fluoroscopy. Despite this, fluoroscopy can often underestimate the degree of intra-articular injury and the quality of the joint reduction. In a review of 231 consecutive intra-articular distal radius fractures treated with fluoroscopic reduction and pinning followed by arthroscopic assessment of the reduction, Abe and colleagues reported a 21.2% rate of malreduction greater than 2 mm that were identified arthroscopically.[14] In a fresh frozen cadaveric model of Bennett fractures involving one-fourth to one-third of the articular surface, Yin and colleagues noted that fluoroscopy was inaccurate at assessing both articular step-off and gap, $P < .05$.[15] With the advancements of arthroscopic-assisted techniques, our ability to obtain improved articular reduction as well as diagnose and treat concomitant pathologies may result in improved patient

Department of Orthopedic Surgery, Mayo Clinic, 200 1st Street Southwest, Rochester, MN 55905, USA
* Corresponding author.
E-mail address: kakar.sanjeev@mayo.edu

Hand Clin 39 (2023) 523–531
https://doi.org/10.1016/j.hcl.2023.05.003

outcomes.[16–20] In this article, the authors review the use of arthroscopy in the management of certain injuries within the hand and DRUJ.

Small joint arthroscopy of the hand follows general arthroscopic principles implemented elsewhere throughout the body.[21] One must first have an appreciation of the local anatomy including neurovascular and musculotendinous structures at risk and how they relate to surface and palpable landmarks. It is also important to have an understanding of the intra-articular joint anatomy for surgical efficiency and safety.[22] Gupta and colleagues highlighted the importance of appropriately sized arthroscopes, namely 2 to 3 mm for the wrist and less than 2 mm for smaller joints, and associated instrumentation.[23] Shih and colleagues noted the volume of the thumb CMC joint to be approximately 104 to 140 mm^3, in contrast to the 1240 to 1340 mm^3 of space within the radiocarpal joint.[24,25] The advent of the 1.9 mm arthroscope and corresponding surgical instruments have allowed for safe arthroscopic visualization and instrumentation of the smaller joints within the hand. With its smaller size, the 1.9-mm Nanoscope (Arthrex, Naples, Fl) and its 2.2-mm outer trocar sheath require less distraction force (5 to 7lbs) compared with the more traditional 10 to 12lbs for 4.0 mm cannulas.[26] The camera is lightweight, disposable, and flexible allowing surgeons to navigate the complex anatomy of the smaller joints without causing articular injury. Although fluid and pressure systems may be used for joint distention, we routinely use "dry arthroscopy" for debridement, fracture fixation, and reparative procedures of these small joints.[16,17,19,27] We find this beneficial as fluid extravasation into the soft tissues with wet arthroscopy may contribute to postoperative pain, edema, and stiffness. Fluid extravasation may also cause soft tissue distension, making any planned or unplanned open approaches more challenging. In addition, one can make larger portals when using dry arthroscopy allowing larger shavers and burrs to be placed within the joint, thereby increasing surgical efficiency.

CASE EXAMPLES
Triangular Fibrocartilage Complex Injuries

Ulnar-sided wrist pain following distal radius fractures has been reported at rates as high as 36%, the most frequent postoperative complaint following this injury.[28,29] Triangular fibrocartilage complex (TFCC) injuries are commonly involved. In a prospective study of 50 adult distal radius fractures, acute injury to the TFCC (peripheral, central, and combined tears) was identified in

78% of cases.[30] Furthermore, of the 11 patients with complete peripheral TFCC tears, 10 (91%) were found to have instability 1 year following treatment of their distal radius fractures, with DRUJ instability negatively impacting functional outcome measures.[7] In a prospective series of 56 arthroscopically assisted distal radius fractures, 13 cases of complete foveal TFCC disruption were identified and arthroscopically repaired. At a mean follow-up of 24 months, none of the patients had ulnar-sided wrist pain, and 12 of the 13 patients had an excellent outcome, with a mean functional disabilities of the arm, shoulder, and hand (DASH) score of 13.

In symptomatic patients with suspected TFCC injuries that are recalcitrant to nonoperative treatment, we typically perform arthroscopic-assisted TFCC repair.[16] Wrist arthroscopy is performed with the patient in the supine position with the arm suspended in a well-padded arthroscopic tower. We typically perform arthroscopy with the forearm in the vertical position, although horizontal arthroscopy has been described.[31] Finger traps are placed on the small to index fingers to allow even distraction across the hand and wrist. With the advent of smaller, flexible arthroscopic systems, we use 5 to 7 pounds of distraction.[26] We typically perform "dry" wrist arthroscopy and have found this particularly advantageous for the management of fractures and disorders of the TFCC and DRUJ.[16,17,19,27,32,33] Alternatively, arthroscopy with fluid instillation can be used. For wrist arthroscopy, we typically start with the development of radiocarpal 3-4 and 6-R portals and proceed with diagnostic wrist arthroscopy including evaluation of the articular surfaces of the distal radius and proximal row as well as the extrinsic ligaments including the radioscaphocapitate, long radiolunate, short radiolunate, and ulnocarpal ligaments. As one comes to the ulnocarpal joint, the TFCC is inspected and its integrity examined using a combination of the trampoline, hook, and suction tests.[34–36] When foveal tears are suspected, we find DRUJ arthroscopy to be a critical tool in its diagnosis and management.[37,38] With the arthroscope in the 3-4 portal looking at the TFCC, the distal DRUJ portal is located proximal and radial to the 6-R portal.[39] The distal end of the ulna is palpated, and an 18 gauge needle is inserted distal to the ulna and underneath the TFCC. This is confirmed with the arthroscope that is within the radiocarpal joint. The portal is then created and the camera placed within the distal DRUJ portal to examine the undersurface of the TFCC, the fovea, and the DRUJ. The direct foveal portal is created and acts as a working portal.[40] Given the close proximity of underlying neurovascular structures, it is critical that for each portal, the surgeon bluntly dissects down through the skin incision, soft tissues, and joint capsule. In a study of 10 fresh frozen cadaveric specimen, Munaretto and colleagues found that on average, the 3-4 portal was 18.9 mm from the superficial branch of the radial nerve, though as close as 14.3 mm.[26] The mean distance from the extensor pollicis longus (EPL) was 2.8 m (range 0.01–10 mm). The 6-R portal was on average 1.7 mm from the extensor carpi ulnaris (range 0.01–3.6 mm) and 14.7 mm from the dorsal sensory branch of the ulnar nerve (range 10.3–19.5). Volar portals are created when clinically needed.[41]

We present the case of a 15-year-old girl with a chief complaint of ulnar-sided wrist pain with associated DRUJ instability 2 years after nonoperative management of a distal radius buckle fracture with short-arm cast immobilization (**Fig. 1**A, B). On examination, her pain was localized to the fovea with DRUJ laxity in neutral, supinated, and pronated positions. Radiographs demonstrated a healed distal radius fracture with no signs of malunion when compared with her contralateral side (**Fig. 1**C, D). A non-contrast wrist MRI was read by musculoskeletal trained radiologists as normal, with no identified pathology. Given the clinical suspicion of a TFCC foveal injury, wrist arthroscopy was performed, which demonstrated a structurally intact but functionally incompetent TFCC tear with normal trampoline and hook tests but abnormal suction test. Foveal disruption was confirmed with DRUJ arthroscopy (**Fig. 1**E). An arthroscopic-assisted ulnar tunnel foveal TFCC repair was performed (**Fig. 1**F).[42] Three months postoperatively, the patient was pain free with full pronosupination, a 105° arc of wrist flexion–extension, 91% grip strength compared with her contralateral dominant hand, and a clinically stable DRUJ on examination.

Trehan and colleagues reported on 26 cases of pediatric arthroscopic TFCC repairs with mean clinical follow-up of 21 months (range 3–66).[43] The investigators noted a high rate of associated pathology including prior distal radius fractures, ulnar styloid nonunions, and intercarpal ligament injuries among others. At final follow-up, QuickDASH improved to a median of 2 which was significantly improved compared with preoperative values (P < .05). They found a high rate of return to sport and 9/10 satisfaction for both patients and parents. Injuries to the TFCC can be seen with pediatric distal radius buckle fractures as well.[46] In a retrospective review of 85 cases of DRUJ instability from pediatric wrist injuries, 79% of cases were associated with a distal radius and/or ulna fracture, including 12 distal radius buckle fractures.[47]

Thumb Carpometacarpal Bennett Fractures

Arthroscopic assistance in the management of thumb CMC fractures offers many of the same benefits, notably including direct visualization of fracture reduction, confirmation of extra-articular positioning of hardware, and preservation of the stabilizing soft tissue structures.[20,44,45] With the complex shape and multiplanar movement afforded by the first CMC joint, compressive forces are localized with grip and thumb pinch grasps, highlighting the importance of an anatomic articular reduction.[11] Fluoroscopy has been shown to have limitations when guiding the articular reduction, whereas arthroscopy provides a direct evaluation of articular surface reduction and step-off.[44,48] In a cadaveric model of simulated Bennett's fractures, when compared with open caliper measurements, fluoroscopy underappreciated fracture displacement (3.05 vs 0 mm, P < .01), step-off (2.07 vs 0.31 mm, P < .001), and gap formation (0.92 vs 0.56 mm, P = .2) following percutaneous reduction and fixation.[44] Fifty percent of simulated cases had a residual articular step-off that was greater than 2 mm.

Current indications for surgical management of these intra-articular CMC fractures include articular step-off greater than 1 mm, articular gap greater than 1 mm, articular fragment greater than 20% of the joint surface, and/or the presence of joint subluxation.[11] In treating these fractures, we use dry arthroscopy with automatic washout to guide articular reduction. For thumb CMC arthroscopy, 5 to 7 pounds of longitudinal traction is placed on the thumb with a single finger trap. Standard thumb CMC portals include the 1-R portal, immediately radial to the abductor pollicis long and the 1-U portal, immediately ulnar to the extensor pollicis brevis (EPB).[49,50] To create a wider working space, we typically create the 1-U portal followed by the trans-thenar portal.[51] Oftentimes, we will alternate between these portals to ensure a complete inspection of the joint. As with other portals, a superficial skin incision followed by blunt dissection down to and through the joint capsule is imperative with the 1-R and 1-U portals being intimately associated with both tendinous structures and branches of the superficial radial nerve.[52] The accessory thenar portal is located approximately 2 to 3 cm from the motor branch of the median nerve, however, is within 2 mm of its two main terminal branches. Using the Nanoscope (Arthrex, Naples, Fl), we start with arthroscopic mobilization of the fracture fragment and debridement of hematoma and scar tissue (**Fig. 2**A). We then obtain control of the fracture fragments with 0.045 inch K wires placed under oscillate mode using fluoroscopy

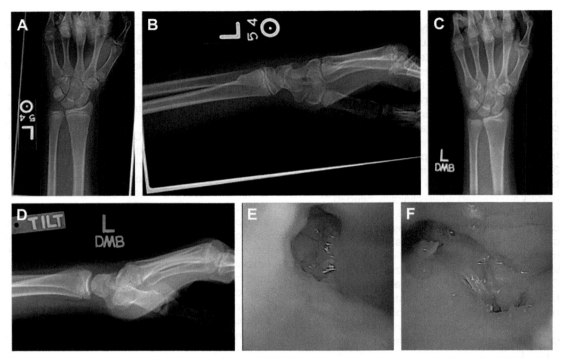

Fig. 1. Injury posterior-anterior (PA) (*A*) and lateral (*B*) left wrist radiographs demonstrating a buckle fracture. Two-years post-injury PA (*C*) and lateral tilt (*D*) left wrist radiographs demonstrating healing and acceptable alignment. Intraoperative arthroscopy demonstrating TFCC foveal disruption (*E*) and subsequent repair (*F*).

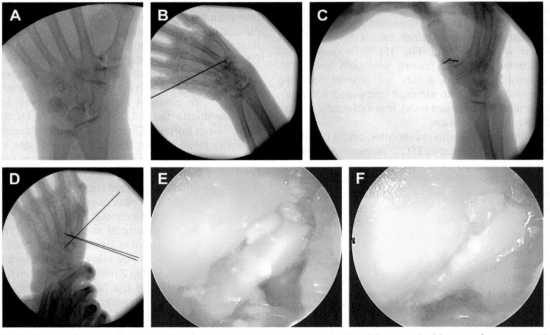

Fig. 2. Bennett fracture demonstrating fracture displacement prereduction (*A*), control of fracture fragment with percutaneous Kirschner wire (*B*), final arthroscopic-assisted reduction on fluoroscopy (*C, D*), arthroscopic visualization of fracture prereduction (*E*), and arthroscopic visualization of fracture postreduction (*F*).

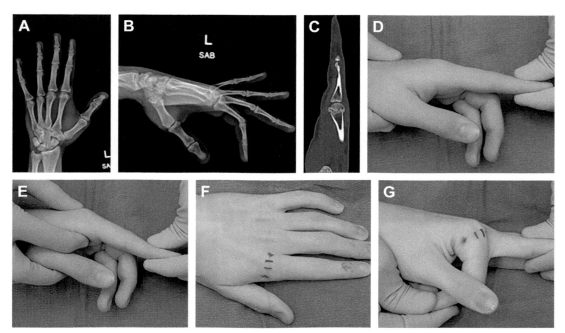

Fig. 3. Oblique (*A*) and lateral (*B*) hand radiographs demonstrating an index finger metacarpal head fracture with intra-articular step-off. Sagittal computed tomography (CT) (*C*) demonstrating articular step-off of approximately 1.7 mm. Preoperative MCPJ motion of 10° to 25°(*D*, *E*). Portal placement in reference to the extensor mechanism with final passive range of motion noted after arthroscopic treatment (*F*, *G*).

(**Fig. 2**B). The articular surface is reduced first using K wires as joysticks. Once the articular surface is reduced (**Fig. 2**C–F), additional K wires are placed from the thumb metacarpal into the trapezium for added stability (see **Fig. 2**D) and into the second metacarpal (as needed). We typically bury the K wires under the skin in an effort to minimize possible pin site complications.[53] Alternatively, if the fragments are large enough, once the articular reduction has been obtained under arthroscopic control, the surgeon can definitely stabilize the fracture with rigid internal fixation.

Pomares and colleagues retrospectively reported on 21 patients with Bennett fractures, 11 treated with arthroscopically assisted reduction and percutaneous fixation and the remaining 10 treated with open reduction and internal fixation (ORIF).[48] The arthroscopy group achieved 100% union without any encountered malunions or hardware complications, whereas the ORIF group had two cases of malreduction and four cases of intra-articular hardware. Both groups had similar Quick-DASH scores, strength, and motion at final follow-up, though the arthroscopy cohort had significantly shorter tourniquet times and shorter duration of postoperative immobilization in addition to a lower complication rate (9.1% vs 60%) and a higher rate of return to pre-injury work/activities (91% vs 70%).

Metacarpal Head Fractures

Metacarpal fractures occur at an incidence of 13.6 per 100,00 person years and approaches 70 per 100,000 person years in males 10 to 19 years of age, with approximately 5% being intra-articular metacarpal head fractures.[54,55] Open approaches are either volar through the A1 pulley or dorsal through the extensor mechanism and may provide limited access to the articular surface.[11] More extensile approaches can lead to damage of the tenuous blood supply of the fracture fragments resulting in avascular necrosis of the metacarpal head fragments.[56]

With the advent of smaller arthroscopes, arthroscopy of the metacarpophalangeal joints (MCPJs) has become much more feasible.[57] The MCPJs are accessed through dorsoradial and dorsoulnar portals, immediately adjacent to the extensor tendon at the level of the joint line.[18] During portal creation, the incision should occur through the skin only, followed by blunt dissection to access the joint given the close proximity of the extensor mechanism complex and neurovascular structures.[18,58] The neurovascular bundles are located at the volar recess and one must be careful with instrumentation in this area.[18]

Fig. 3A–C shows the radiographic studies demonstrating an intra-articular metacarpal head

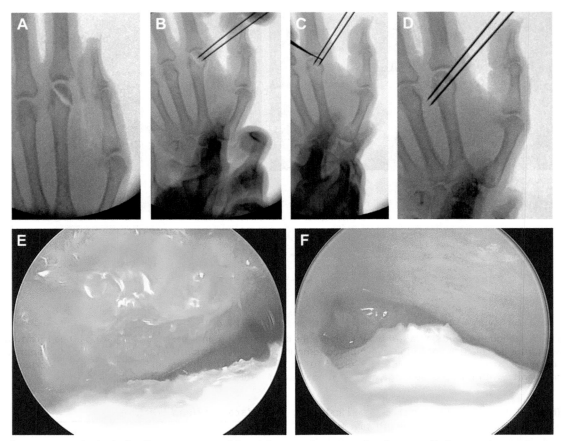

Fig. 4. Intra-articular index finger metacarpal head fracture demonstrating fracture displacement prereduction (*A*), control of fracture fragment with percutaneous Kirschner wires (*B*), arthroscopic-assisted fracture reduction (*C*), final arthroscopic-assisted reduction on fluoroscopy (*D*), arthroscopic visualization of fracture prereduction (*E*), and arthroscopic visualization of fracture postreduction (*F*).

fracture malunion of a patient following an injury to the left index finger treated nonoperatively and was referred to see us several months later with a 15°arc of motion (flexion to 10° and extension to 25°, **Fig. 3**D, E) with pain. After failing nonoperative treatment, he underwent arthroscopic synovectomy (**Fig. 3**F, G), debridement, and loose body removal and at final follow-up had MCPJ range of motion of 0° to 80° of active and passive motion.

Using the principles of ligamentotaxis and arthroscopic reduction, small joint arthroscopy can be used to manage metacarpal head fractures. As can be seen in **Fig. 4**, following arthroscopic debridement, 2 K wires are placed within the fracture fragment under fluoroscopic control. With the fracture reduction confirmed with arthroscopically, the K wires are advanced across the fracture for bicortical fixation (**Fig. 4**B–F). Alternatively, screw fixation can be used for definitive stabilization.

Slade and Gutow reported on 14 cases (included 6 thumbs) of arthroscopically assisted percutaneous fixation of metacarpal head fractures, with non-thumb digits on average achieving 81° of MCPJ flexion and 99° of proximal interphalangeal joint (PIPJ) flexion at final follow-up.[59] Compared with a matched open cohort, the investigators reported earlier return of motion and greater arc of motion at final follow-up. There was one loss of reduction treated with revision arthroscopic reduction, percutaneous fixation. The average return to unrestricted activity was 8 weeks.

Thumb Ulnar Collateral Ligament Injuries

Injuries to the thumb ulnar collateral ligament (UCL) are common, with up to 20,000 cases occurring annually in the United States.[60] These injuries can be classified as acute, often termed skiers thumb, or chronic as gamekeepers thumb. If at any time the distal insertion of the UCL becomes trapped superficial to the adductor aponeurosis, a Stener lesion is created, thereby impairing the thumb UCL injury to heal with resultant chronic pain, instability, and functional limitations.[11,61] Traditionally, repair is performed through an open approach, taking care to protect superficial sensory nerves.[11] Both the adductor aponeurosis and joint capsule are taken down with this technique and must be repaired.

Thumb MCPJ arthroscopy follows similar principles and steps previously outlined for finger MCPJ arthroscopy, however, noting the presence of both the EPB and EPL tendons coursing dorsally across the thumb MCPJ. Both dorsal radial and dorsal ulnar portals are created first with a transverse incision through the skin only followed by blunt dissection and joint penetration.[18] Ryu and Fagan described their experience with arthroscopic reduction of thumb UCL Stener lesions in eight consecutive cases.[62] Suspension was isolated through the thumb with a single finger trap, relying on the weight of the arm for traction with no added weight. Their first portal was created dorsal to the radial collateral ligament and radial to the EPL, using a 20-gauge needle and 2 mL of saline to confirm their location within the joint. This was followed by a radiopalmar portal, created under direct visualization, just palmar to the radial collateral ligament. Debridement was required to visualize the key structures, at which point a probe from the radiopalmar portal was passed along the metacarpal head and underneath the adductor aponeurosis to hook the origin of the UCL and pull its distal insertion inside the joint. The MCPJ was then pinned in 20° to 30° of flexion and immobilized in a thumb spica short-arm cast. Their average surgical time was 47 minutes (range 28–64). At final follow-up, mean tip pinch, key pinch, and grip strengths were 109%, 108%, and 116% of the contralateral side. Seven of eight (87.5%) patients were pain free at final follow-up with the remaining patient having mild pain when opening jars. They attributed their successes to the minimally invasive, soft tissue sparing technique afforded by arthroscopy when compared with an open approach, which they associated with stiffness, hyperesthesia of sensory nerves, and painful scar formation. Others have been able to reproduce good clinical outcomes without complications in small case series.[18,59]

SUMMARY

With advancements in surgical instrumentation and techniques, the role of arthroscopic and arthroscopic-assisted surgical procedures is ever-growing. Although arthroscopy offers direct,

magnified visualization of pathology, reductions, and structures of interest and is more accurate than relying on intraoperative fluoroscopy alone, the impact of arthroscopic techniques on clinical outcomes as compared with open techniques is an area of active investigation. Arthroscopic techniques also minimize soft tissue stripping, which is of particular importance to smaller fracture fragments whose vascularity is precarious and can be damaged through open approaches.

CLINICS CARE POINTS

- With advances in technology, equipment, surgeon knowledge, and technical skill, the indications for small joint arthroscopy continue to expand. The introduction of the 1.9-mm arthroscope and low-profile surgical instruments has been important in the progression of the field.

- Arthroscopy offers direct, magnified visualization of intra-articular pathology and structures, allowing for improved articular reduction relative to fluoroscopic techniques alone.

- Arthroscopy minimizes soft tissue disruption, preserving structures critical for perfusion and stability. As such, arthroscopy may result in decreased morbidity and improved function; however, comparative studies have not yet been conducted.

DISCLOSURE

S. Kakar Consultant: Arthrex.

REFERENCES

1. Butt WD. Fractures of the hand. I. Description. Can Med Assoc J 1962;86(16):731–5.
2. van Onselen EB, Karim RB, Hage JJ, et al. Prevalence and distribution of hand fractures. J Hand Surg Br 2003;28(5):491–5.
3. Oak N, Lawton JN. Intra-articular fractures of the hand. Hand Clin 2013;29(4):535–49.
4. McElfresh EC, Dobyns JH. Intra-articular metacarpal head fractures. J Hand Surg Am 1983;8(4):383–93.
5. Chinchalkar SJ, Gan BS. Management of proximal interphalangeal joint fractures and dislocations. J Hand Ther 2003;16(2):117–28.
6. Hey HW, Chong AK, Murphy D. Prevalence of carpal fracture in Singapore. J Hand Surg Am 2011;36(2):278–83.
7. Lindau T, Adlercreutz C, Aspenberg P. Peripheral tears of the triangular fibrocartilage complex cause

distal radioulnar joint instability after distal radial fractures. J Hand Surg Am 2000;25(3):464–8.

8. Kiefhaber TR, Stern PJ. Fracture dislocations of the proximal interphalangeal joint. J Hand Surg Am 1998;23(3):368–80.

9. Leibovic SJ. Treatment of Bennett's and Rolando's fractures. Tech Hand Up Extrem Surg 1998;2(1):36–46.

10. Mrkonjic A, Geijer M, Lindau T, et al. The natural course of traumatic triangular fibrocartilage complex tears in distal radial fractures: a 13-15 year follow-up of arthroscopically diagnosed but untreated injuries. J Hand Surg Am 2012;37(8):1555–60.

11. Wolfe SW, Pederson WC, Kozin SH, et al. Green's operative hand surgery. Philadelphia, PA: Elsevier Health Sciences; 2021.

12. Goldfarb CA, Rudzki JR, Catalano LW, et al. Fifteen-year outcome of displaced intra-articular fractures of the distal radius. J Hand Surg Am 2006;31(4):633–9.

13. Knirk JL, Jupiter JB. Intra-articular fractures of the distal end of the radius in young adults. J Bone Joint Surg Am 1986;68(5):647–59.

14. Abe Y, Fujii K. Arthroscopic-Assisted Reduction of Intra-articular Distal Radius Fracture. Hand Clin 2017;33(4):659–68.

15. Yin Y, Wang Y, Wang Z, et al. Accuracy of fluoroscopic examination in the treatment of Bennett's fracture. BMC Musculoskelet Disord 2021;22(1):3.

16. Burnier M, Herzberg G, Luchetti R, et al. Dry Wrist Arthroscopy for Ulnar-Sided Wrist Disorders. J Hand Surg Am 2021;46(2):133–41.

17. Burnier M, Kakar S. Dry Wrist Arthroscopy in the Management of Ulnar Wrist Pain Disorders. Hand Clin 2021;37(4):527–35.

18. Choi AK, Chow EC, Ho PC, et al. Metacarpophalangeal joint arthroscopy: indications revisited. Hand Clin 2011;27(3):369–82.

19. Kakar S, Burnier M, Atzei A, et al. Dry Wrist Arthroscopy for Radial-Sided Wrist Disorders. J Hand Surg Am 2020;45(4):341–53.

20. Marcovici LL, Atzei A, Cozzolino R, et al. Arthroscopic Assisted Treatment of Thumb Metacarpal Base Articular Fractures. Arthrosc Tech 2021;10(7):e1783–92.

21. Camp CL, Degen RM, Sanchez-Sotelo J, et al. Basics of Elbow Arthroscopy Part I: Surface Anatomy, Portals, and Structures at Risk. Arthrosc Tech 2016;5(6):e1339–43.

22. O'Driscoll SW, Blonna D. Osteocapsular Arthroplasty of the Elbow: Surgical Technique. JBJS Essent Surg Tech 2014;3(3):e15.

23. Gupta R, Bozentka DJ, Osterman AL. Wrist arthroscopy: principles and clinical applications. J Am Acad Orthop Surg 2001;9(3):200–9.

24. Montet X, Eberlin JL, Bianchi S, et al. Assessment of intra-articular volume of the wrist: a comparative study between CT-arthrography and dissection. Surg Radiol Anat 2005;27(5):444–9.

25. Shih JG, Mainprize JG, Binhammer PA. Comparison of Computed Tomography Articular Surface Geometry of Male Versus Female Thumb Carpometacarpal Joints. Hand (N Y) 2018;13(1):33–9.

26. Munaretto N, Hinchcliff K, Dutton L, et al. Is Wrist Arthroscopy Safer with the Nanoscope? J Wrist Surg 2022;11(5):450–5.

27. del Piñal F, García-Bernal FJ, Pisani D, et al. Dry arthroscopy of the wrist: surgical technique. J Hand Surg Am 2007;32(1):119–23.

28. Frykman G. Fracture of the distal radius including sequelae–shoulder-hand-finger syndrome, disturbance in the distal radio-ulnar joint and impairment of nerve function. A clinical and experimental study. Acta Orthop Scand 1967;Suppl 108:103+.

29. Tsukazaki T, Iwasaki K. Ulnar wrist pain after Colles' fracture. 109 fractures followed for 4 years. Acta Orthop Scand 1993;64(4):462–4.

30. Lindau T, Arner M, Hagberg L. Intraarticular lesions in distal fractures of the radius in young adults. A descriptive arthroscopic study in 50 patients. J Hand Surg Br 1997;22(5):638–43.

31. Lindau T. Wrist arthroscopy in distal radial fractures using a modified horizontal technique. Arthroscopy 2001;17(1):E5.

32. Atzei A. New trends in arthroscopic management of type 1-B TFCC injuries with DRUJ instability. J Hand Surg Eur 2009;34(5):582–91.

33. Jones CM, Grasu BL, Murphy MS. Dry wrist arthroscopy. J Hand Surg Am 2015;40(2):388–90.

34. Greene RM, Kakar S. The Suction Test: A Novel Technique to Identify and Verify Successful Repair of Peripheral Triangular Fibrocartilage Complex Tears. J Wrist Surg 2017;6(4):334–5.

35. Hermansdorfer JD, Kleinman WB. Management of chronic peripheral tears of the triangular fibrocartilage complex. J Hand Surg Am 1991;16(2):340–6.

36. Ruch DS, Yang CC, Smith BP. Results of acute arthroscopically repaired triangular fibrocartilage complex injuries associated with intra-articular distal radius fractures. Arthroscopy 2003;19(5):511–6.

37. Ecker J, Andrijich C. Dry Arthroscopy Distal Radioulnar Joint and Foveal Insertion: Surgical Technique. J Wrist Surg 2022;11(1):2–5.

38. Minhas S, Kakar S, Wall LB, et al. Foveal Triangular Fibrocartilage Complex Tears: Recognition of a Combined Tear Pattern. J Hand Surg Am 2022; S0363-5023(22):00165–74.

39. Atzei A, Luchetti R, Braidotti F. Arthroscopic foveal repair of the triangular fibrocartilage complex. J Wrist Surg 2015;4(1):22–30.

40. Atzei A, Luchetti R. Foveal TFCC tear classification and treatment. Hand Clin 2011;27(3):263–72.

41. Gillis JA, Kakar S. Volar Midcarpal Portals in Wrist Arthroscopy. J Hand Surg Am 2019;44(12):e1091–4.

42. Nakamura T, Sato K, Okazaki M, et al. Repair of foveal detachment of the triangular fibrocartilage

complex: open and arthroscopic transosseous techniques. Hand Clin 2011;27(3):281–90.

43. Trehan SK, Schimizzi G, Shen TS, et al. Arthroscopic treatment of triangular fibrocartilage complex injuries in paediatric and adolescent patients. J Hand Surg Eur 2019;44(6):582–6.

44. Capo JT, Kinchelow T, Orillaza NS, et al. Accuracy of fluoroscopy in closed reduction and percutaneous fixation of simulated Bennett's fracture. J Hand Surg Am 2009;34(4):637–41.

45. Culp RW, Johnson JW. Arthroscopically assisted percutaneous fixation of Bennett fractures. J Hand Surg Am 2010;35(1):137–40.

46. Eren A, Eceviz E, Ozkan K, et al. Torus fracture of the distal radius associated with distal radioulnar joint instability: a case report. J Pediatr Orthop B 2009; 18(1):35–6.

47. Andersson JK, Lindau T, Karlsson J, et al. Distal radio-ulnar joint instability in children and adolescents after wrist trauma. J Hand Surg Eur 2014; 39(6):653–61.

48. Pomares G, Strugarek-Lecoanet C, Dap F, et al. Bennett fracture: Arthroscopically assisted percutaneous screw fixation versus open surgery: Functional and radiological outcomes. Orthop Traumatol Surg Res 2016;102(3):357–61.

49. Solomon J, Culp RW. Arthroscopic Management of Bennett Fracture. Hand Clin 2017;33(4):787–94.

50. Berger RA. A technique for arthroscopic evaluation of the first carpometacarpal joint. J Hand Surg Am 1997;22(6):1077–80.

51. Walsh EF, Akelman E, Fleming BC, et al. Thumb carpometacarpal arthroscopy: a topographic, anatomic study of the thenar portal. J Hand Surg Am 2005; 30(2):373–9.

52. Pan YW, Hung LK. The Safety of the Thenar Portal: An Anatomical Study of the Thumb Carpometacarpal Arthroscopy. J Wrist Surg 2017;6(2):152–7.

53. Hargreaves DG, Drew SJ, Eckersley R. Kirschner wire pin tract infection rates: a randomized controlled trial between percutaneous and buried wires. J Hand Surg Br 2004;29(4):374–6.

54. Mousafeiris VK, Papaioannou I, Kalyva N, et al. Horizontal (Transverse) Intraarticular Metacarpal Head Fracture in a Young Adult. Cureus 2021;13(7): e16720.

55. Nakashian MN, Pointer L, Owens BD, et al. Incidence of metacarpal fractures in the US population. Hand (N Y) 2012;7(4):426–30.

56. Wright TC, Dell PC. Avascular necrosis and vascular anatomy of the metacarpals. J Hand Surg Am 1991; 16(3):540–4.

57. Chen YC. Arthroscopy of the wrist and finger joints. Orthop Clin North Am 1979;10(3):723–33.

58. Thomsen NO, Nielsen NS, Jørgensen U, et al. Arthroscopy of the proximal interphalangeal joints of the finger. J Hand Surg Br 2002;27(3):253–5.

59. Slade JF 3rd, Gutow AP. Arthroscopy of the metacarpophalangeal joint. Hand Clin 1999;15(3):501–27.

60. Hinke DH, Erickson SJ, Chamoy L, et al. Ulnar collateral ligament of the thumb: MR findings in cadavers, volunteers, and patients with ligamentous injury (gamekeeper's thumb). AJR Am J Roentgenol 1994;163(6):1431–4.

61. Stener B. Displacement of the ruptured ulnar collateral ligament of the metacarpo-phalangeal joint of the thumb. Journal of Bone and Joint Surgery British 1962;44(4):869–79.

62. Ryu J, Fagan R. Arthroscopic treatment of acute complete thumb metacarpophalangeal ulnar collateral ligament tears. J Hand Surg Am 1995;20(6): 1037–42.

Arthroscopic-Assisted Fracture Treatment in the Wrist

Jeffrey Yao, MD[a],*, Nathaniel Fogel, MD[b]

KEYWORDS

• Distal radius • Fracture • Wrist arthroscopy • Perilunate • Wrist

KEY POINTS

- Wrist arthroscopy affords direct visualization of the articular surface and identification and treatment of concomitant soft tissue injuries with fractures about the wrist.
- Level I evidence addressing the use of arthroscopy in treatment of wrist fractures remains limited.
- Arthroscopic techniques in distal radius fractures have yielded mixed functional outcomes. Small series in perilunate injuries may have outcomes comparable to open techniques in appropriately selected patients, with some studies demonstrating improved range of motion and early pain relief with minimally invasive techniques.

INTRODUCTION

The use of wrist arthroscopy in the treatment of fractures about the wrist was first widely described in the 1990s.[1–4] The ability to obtain an anatomic reduction or identify an associated soft tissue injury under direct visualization makes wrist arthroscopy a unique means by which to treat intra-articular distal radius and perilunate fracture dislocations.[5,6] The quality of reduction with arthroscopic techniques has been shown to be superior to fluoroscopic techniques alone.[7,8] In the treatment of distal radius fractures, it has been shown that residual step-off or gap greater than 2 mm is associated with post-traumatic arthritis.[9] The degree to which residual malreduction impacts clinical outcomes remains debated in the literature,[10,11] in part as a result of historical data comparing these techniques being limited to data mostly from retrospective, non-comparative studies.

Similar to its use in distal radius fractures, the arthroscopic techniques in the treatment of perilunate fracture dislocations can be used to optimize anatomic reduction and assess the severity of associated ligamentous injury, all while theoretically limiting further capsular injury and the compromise of an already tenuous blood supply.[12] These high-energy injuries necessitate early reduction and fixation and historically have been associated with poor clinical outcomes. While limited, arthroscopic techniques have been described in the literature for a range of variations of perilunate fracture dislocations, including trans-scaphoid, trans-scaphoid transcapitate, translunate, and transradial styloid PLIND (perilunate injuries, not dislocated translunate).[12–15]

In our prior review of arthroscopic management of distal radius fractures in 2021, we discussed in depth the current literature related to minimally invasive techniques for intra-articular distal radius pathology and the associated soft tissue injuries.[16] We will provide an abbreviated summary of those findings and techniques as well as an updated review of the related recent literature. We will similarly detail the indications, contraindications, techniques, complications, and outcomes associated with arthroscopic management of perilunate injuries. As is the case with distal radius fracture, utilization of arthroscopic-assisted techniques is

[a] Department of Orthopaedic Surgery, Stanford University Medical Center, Stanford, CA, USA; [b] Department of Orthopaedic Surgery, Duke University, 10 Duke Medicine Circle, Durham, NC 27710, USA
* Corresponding author. 540 Broadway Street MC 6342, Redwood City, CA 94063.
E-mail address: jyao@stanford.edu

Hand Clin 39 (2023) 533–543
https://doi.org/10.1016/j.hcl.2023.05.004

relatively uncommon due to its steep learning curve and increased surgical times when compared with fluoroscopically assisted procedures alone. For both intra-articular distal radius fractures and perilunate injuries, the ability to directly assess the articular surface and any associated soft tissue injuries makes arthroscopy a powerful tool in the hands of an experienced practitioner.

INDICATIONS
Distal Radius

Residual intra-articular step-off or gap of greater than 2 mm on radiographs or intraoperative fluoroscopy is often cited as a relative indication for arthroscopy in the setting of distal radius fracture (**Fig. 1**).[17,18] Arthroscopy, be it diagnostic or to assist in reduction and fixation, can be performed either before or after reduction via fluoroscopy. Arthroscopy has repeatedly been found to be superior to fluoroscopy for assessing the accuracy of articular reduction.[7,19–21] A study by Omokawa and colleagues is representative of these findings, where they reported that 22% of wrists (88 of 273 in the series) evaluated by arthroscopy

after what was judged to be sufficient fluoroscopic reduction still had persistent step-off or gap of greater than 2 mm.[8] Of note, it is often beneficial to perform soft tissue releases and provisional reduction maneuvers before direct visualization, as arthroscopy is best suited for "fine tuning" the intra-articular reduction rather than more macroscopic adjustments.

Depending on the characteristics of the fracture, a variety of fixation methods can be implemented in conjunction with arthroscopic techniques, including volar locked plates, fragment-specific implants, external fixation, percutaneous Kirschner wire (K-wire) fixation, and/or dorsal spanning plates. Fractures of the radial styloid, displaced three- and four-part fractures, as well as fractures involving the central articular or "die punch" fragment are patterns particularly amenable to arthroscopic techniques and are the authors' most common indications for using arthroscopy.[22]

Intra-articular distal radius fractures are commonly associated with intercarpal ligamentous pathology, particularly injury to the scapholunate interosseous ligament (SLIL) and the lunotriquetral interosseous ligament, and triangular fibrocartilage complex (TFCC) injuries. For

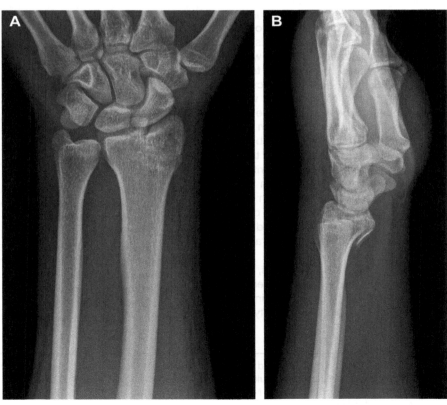

Fig. 1. PA (*A*) and lateral (*B*) radiographs of an intra-articular distal radius fracture with greater than 2 mm of intra-articular step-off.

example, a review of injuries associated with distal radius fractures across 13 studies from 1995 to 2009 reported SLIL injuries in 45% of patients, TFCC injuries in 50% of patients, and chondral injuries in 29% of patients.[23] Arthroscopy is an adjunctive technique that can be used in the evaluation of these injuries, as preoperative radiographs have been shown to have poor predictive value in the diagnosis of interosseus ligament injury, particularly of the SLIL.[2,5,24] Similarly, arthroscopy may also be indicated to evaluate the integrity of the TFCC in the setting of residual distal radial ulnar joint (DRUJ) instability after surgical fixation of the distal radius and can be used to guide decision-making with regard to ulnar styloid fixation or TFCC repair.

It is important to note that even when identified, whether or not to intervene on concomitant soft tissue injuries is not widely agreed on. Studies by Swart and colleagues and Mrkonjic and colleagues reported similar long-term outcomes between patients who were found to have soft tissue injuries by diagnostic arthroscopy at the time of initial fixation and those who did not.[23,25,26] As there is no level I or II evidence that demonstrates clinical benefit for acute intervention for most soft tissue injuries in the wrist in the setting of distal radius fractures, the decision to intervene is typically guided by the presence of signs of static carpal instability. As such, routine wrist arthroscopy without signs of static or dynamic carpal instability may not be indicated.

Perilunate Injuries

Indications for arthroscopic management of perilunate injuries are not well-defined. Patients selected in published series tend to be acute closed injuries.[27,28] Herzberg and colleagues limited patients eligible for arthroscopic-assisted techniques to patients with PLIND, dorsal perilunate dislocations, or stage 1 or 2A dorsal perilunate fracture-dislocations as defined by their modified perilunate injury classification.[13] It is important to note that this was their own criteria, and no widely agreed on set of indications is available in the literature. The authors' preference is to use arthroscopic-assisted perilunate reduction and stabilization when possible to minimize further injury to the capsular structures and the extrinsic secondary stabilizing ligaments. In practice, however, these injuries are often addressed acutely in the main trauma hospital after hours when reliably obtaining arthroscopic equipment is less predictable, and the open treatment of perilunate injuries is still reasonable and routinely performed. Particularly in the setting of perilunate injuries, it is

crucial to monitor for median nerve dysfunction and have a low threshold to release the transverse carpal ligament if there is suspicion for acute carpal tunnel symptoms that persist after initial reduction.

CONTRAINDICATIONS

Contraindications to arthroscopic techniques in the wrist are similar across pathologies. Significant capsular injury, infection, and abnormal anatomy that would preclude safe portal placement and risk neurovascular injury have all been described.[22] Dry arthroscopy techniques can be used to avoid extravasation that may occur secondary to soft tissue defects. It is important to note that some described contraindications to isolated arthroscopic reduction and percutaneous fixation such as carpal tunnel symptoms or preexisting compartment syndrome do not preclude arthroscopy from being used as an adjunct.[29]

OPERATIVE CONSIDERATIONS
Radiographic Workup

For distal radius fractures, preoperative radiographs should be obtained and scrutinized for suspicion of significant intra-articular step-off or gap as well as evidence of intercarpal injuries. Although CT has been shown to be superior to plain radiographs in elucidating involvement of the DRUJ, die punch fragments, and extent of comminution,[30] we have not found that the routine use of a computed tomogrpahy (CT) scan is of great utility and reserve its use for highly comminuted intra-articular fractures. The identification of central articular impaction is of particular importance and this is one of the authors' indications to use arthroscopic-assisted techniques. Similar to others, we have not found the routine use of a CT scan for perilunate injuries to be of significant benefit over post-reduction plain radiographs supplemented by arthroscopic direct visualization.[12]

Timing

There is relative consensus that the ideal time for arthroscopic-assisted distal radius fracture fixation is 3 to 7 days post-injury.[2,3,17] Intervening acutely within the first 72 hours of the injury may be difficult secondary to bleeding as well as increased fluid extravasation into the soft tissues if using wet arthroscopy. Mobilization of fracture fragments using arthroscopic techniques may become difficult 1 week after the injury due to callus formation. With perilunate injuries, median nerve symptoms or inability to obtain a closed reduction may necessitate urgent treatment and therefore dictate timing. Difficulties with visualization in the acute setting arthroscopically can be addressed by aggressive debridement of the radiocarpal and midcarpal joints. The timeline for the optimal treatment of associated scaphoid, capitate, or lunate fractures is similar to that of distal radius fractures. When possible, we approach treatment timing similar to Jeon and colleagues who describe arthroscopic-assisted treatment for trans-scaphoid perilunate injuries within 3 days of injury.[31] In purely ligamentous perilunate injuries, treatment 6 weeks post-injury becomes more challenging and is associated with worse outcomes regardless of technique.[32]

PROCEDURAL APPROACH
Distal Radius

- Wrist arthroscopy may be performed at the outset of the procedure, after initial open exposure in the setting of planned dorsal or volar plating, or after a provisional reduction and fixation. We prefer performing wrist arthroscopy initially unless there are soft tissue releases (ie, brachioradialis, dorsal periosteum) that must be performed beforehand to release the deforming forces on the fragments. In isolated die-punch fragments unattached to any deforming soft tissues, arthroscopic reduction may be performed before any soft tissue releases.
- We begin the arthroscopic portion by establishing the 3 to 4, 6R and midcarpal portals and we subsequently perform a standard diagnostic arthroscopy. Arthroscopy may be performed dry or with very minimal fluid ("moist arthroscopy") via gravity-fed delivery to minimize extravasation into the soft tissues. The fractures and any associated intercarpal ligament or TFCC injuries are identified and treated if appropriate.
- A 3.5 mm shaver should be used to debride and remove the associated hematoma and radiocarpal hemarthrosis to allow for clear visualization of the joint surface (**Fig. 2**). The freer elevator, probe, dental pick, trochar, osteotome, or the shaver itself may be used to manipulate each fragment. Kirschner wire (K-wire) fixation is useful both as a way to manipulate fragments as well as hold provisional fixation after arthroscopic reduction. The K-wire used for reduction may also serve as the guidewire for cannulated screw fixation (**Fig. 3**A–G).
- Abe and colleagues[33] and Del Pinal[34] have described using arthroscopy as an adjunct to standard volar locked plating. The volar

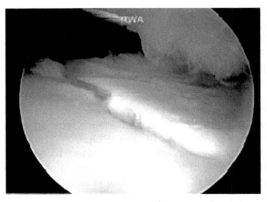

Fig. 2. Arthroscopic view demonstrating intraarticular step-off after completion of debridement.

plate can be used to obtain provisional reduction and to achieve length stability before the use of standard dorsal arthroscopic techniques to fine tune the intra-articular reduction under direct visualization.
- Arthroscopy is particularly useful in addressing articular fragments with rotated "upside-down articular fragments."[18] The orientation of the fragment is often missed on fluoroscopy alone and even if identified on preoperative imaging is challenging to reorient without manipulation under direct visualization (**Fig. 4**).

Perilunate Injuries

- Early closed reduction should be performed under conscious sedation or general anesthesia before proceeding with operative treatment. Should closed reduction fail, a probe may be used to aid in reducing the capitolunate joint.[35] Traction must be applied to help facilitate this reduction (**Fig. 5**).
- Initial 3 to 4, 6R and midcarpal portals are established to facilitate diagnostic arthroscopy and subsequent percutaneous interventions.
- Given the usual high-energy nature of these injuries, extensive debridement is often necessary to facilitate adequate visualization (**Fig. 6**). Any associated soft tissue injuries or chondral damage are cataloged and further debrided.
- For trans-scaphoid patterns, provisional guidewires are placed into either the distal or proximal segment of scaphoid (depending on pattern and surgeon preference) to aid in reduction. Reduction is then obtained under direct arthroscopic visualization. Percutaneous clamp assistance may be helpful in holding the reduction, whereas guide wire(s)

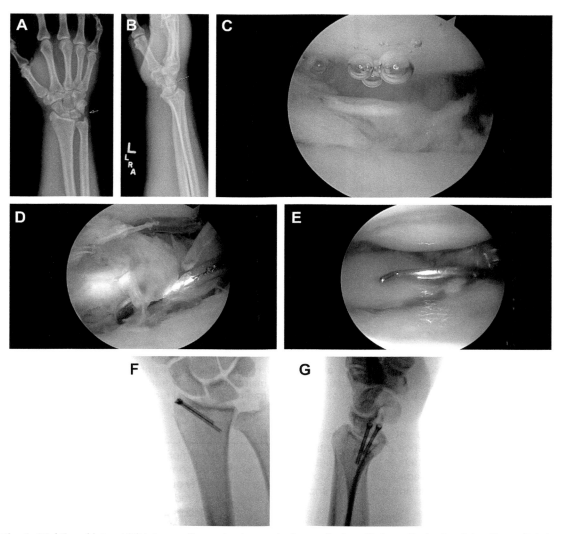

Fig. 3. PA (*A*) and lateral (*B*) injury radiographs demonstrating a displaced intra-articular involving the radial sty-loid. (*C*) Arthroscopic image demonstrating step-off at the articular surface. A probe is used to mobilize and debride (*D*), and subsequently used to obtain and temporarily hold the anatomic reduction (*E*). PA (*F*) and lateral (*G*) fluoroscopic images demonstrating cannulated screw fixation. The screws were placed over the original wires used to aid in the initial arthroscopic-assisted reduction.

are placed across the fracture site. Final fixa-tion is attained via one or two cannulated headless compression screws placed over the provisional fixation wire (**Fig. 7**).
- Using fluoroscopy, the radiolunate angle is restored. Using percutaneously placed K-wires as joysticks in the scaphoid and triquetrum, the scapholunate and lunotriquetral intervals are reduced under arthroscopic guidance and then held in place by additional K-wires (**Fig. 8**).
- If scapholunate repair is deemed necessary, a dorsal approach can be used.
- Postoperatively, patients are placed into a thumb spica splint for 2 weeks and then a

thumb spica cast for an additional 4 to 6 weeks depending on whether ligamentous repairs are performed. Following the period of immo-bilization, our patients are placed into a hand therapy protocol for 2 months and then released to full activity if their motion and strength has normalized.

OUTCOMES

Outcomes data in the arthroscopic treatment of distal radius fractures and perilunate injuries are limited to small case series and with conflicting clinical outcomes; level I studies investigating

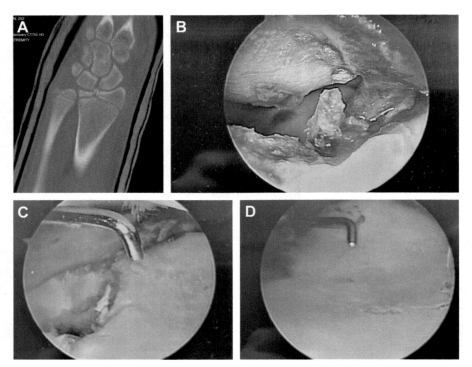

Fig. 4. (*A*) Coronal CT scan demonstrating a malrotated central articular fragment. (*B*) Arthroscopic image demonstrating articular gapping demonstrating the free malrotated central fragment. (*C*) A probe is used to obtain incremental reduction after excision of the central fragment. (*D*) Final reduction of the articular surface.

functional outcomes have yet to be published.[18] Beyond the level of evidence concerns, criticism of existing literature center on short length of follow-up that is likely inadequate when looking at post-traumatic changes and the related impact on function.[36]

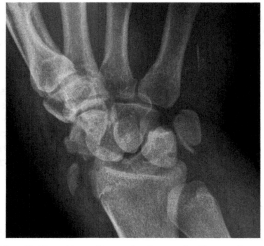

Fig. 5. Trauma radiograph demonstrating a transscaphoid perilunate fracture dislocation before reduction.

Distal Radius

The degree of improvement in articular reduction is a common outcome assessment of studies investigating the utility of arthroscopic assistance in treatment of distal radius fracture. A systematic review by Saab and colleagues[37] reported that 13 of the 16 studies evaluating the impact of arthroscopic assistance on articular reduction demonstrated arthroscopy to be advantageous in attaining a more anatomic reduction of the joint surface. In evaluating the impact of the diagnosis and treatment of interosseous ligament and TFCC injuries afforded by arthroscopy on outcomes, the authors were unable to draw conclusions, as only two studies were comparative in nature. Of note, 8 of the 12 studies reported a positive contribution of arthroscopy as it relates to the diagnosis and treatment of carpal injuries associated with distal radius fractures. The impact of arthroscopic assistance on functional outcome scores was mixed, with 6 of 12 studies reporting positive findings associated with arthroscopic techniques. The paucity of prospective comparative studies limits any strong conclusions to be drawn from the literature regarding the use of arthroscopy.

The comparative studies that have been conducted demonstrate mixed findings related to the

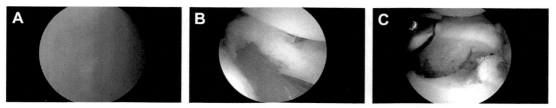

Fig. 6. (*A*) Arthroscopic image demonstrating extensive hematoma on initiation of wrist arthroscopy in setting of perilunate injury. (*B*) Radiocarpal joint after initial debridement. (*C*) Direct visualization of step-off at the scaphoid fracture site.

impact of arthroscopic assistance. Yamazaki and colleagues reported on 74 patients with unstable intra-articular distal radius fractures randomized to fluoroscopic versus arthroscopic-assisted fixation with volar locked plating and found no significant difference in radiographic step-off or gap, radial inclination, volar angulation, ulnar variance, or Disability of Arm Shoulder and Hand (DASH) scores.[30] Varitimidis and colleagues performed a prospective study of arthroscopic and fluoroscopic-assisted fixation versus fluoroscopic–assisted alone in 40 patients with C-type distal radius fractures with greater than 2 mm of articular step-off or gap after closed reduction.[38] They reported decreased pain and an earlier return to daily activities in the arthroscopic assisted group as well as statistically significant improvements in range of motion (supination, extension, and flexion) at 1-year follow-up. Abe and colleagues reported a series of 248 intra-articular distal radius fractures treated with arthroscopic-assisted techniques.[33] Of 231 fractures thought to be sufficiently reduced under fluoroscopy, 49 were found to have residual step-off or gap of greater than 2 mm when examined arthroscopically, demonstrating the improved sensitivity of arthroscopy in assessing an anatomic reduction over fluoroscopy. Although this study did not use a control group, at final follow-up, 98% of patients reported a Mayo Modified Wrist Score of excellent or good, the mean DASH score was 3.4, and mean grip strength was 91.5% of the contralateral side.

Recent outcomes data further support the improved quality of reduction possible via arthroscopic-assisted techniques. Koo and colleagues[39] performed a retrospective cohort study

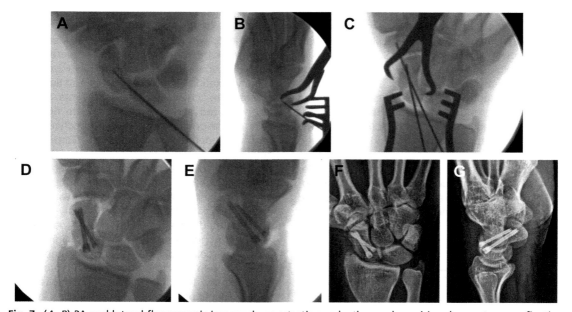

Fig. 7. (*A, B*) PA and lateral fluoroscopic images demonstrating reduction and provisional percutaneous fixation with K-wires. (*C*) PA fluoroscopic image demonstrating clamp application before headless compression screw placement. (*D, E*) PA and lateral fluoroscopic images demonstrating final fixation construct. (*F, G*) PA and lateral radiographs obtained 3-month post-op.

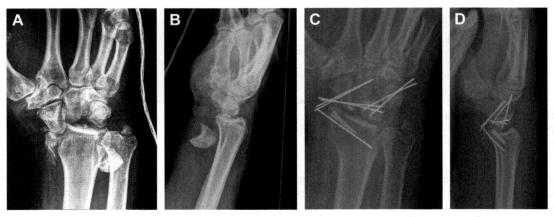

Fig. 8. (*A, B*) Trauma PA and lateral radiographs demonstrating a transradial styloid perilunate fracture dislocation. (*C, D*) Immediate postoperative PA and lateral radiographs after headless compression screw and K-wire fixation of the radial styloid, scapholunate interosseous ligament repair, and K-wire fixation of scapholunate, scaphocapitate, and lunotriquetral intervals.

evaluating 12 patients who underwent arthroscopic-assisted fixation for Arbeitsgemeinschaft für Osteosynthesefragen (AO) type C distal radius fractures alongside 12 patients who were treated with fluoroscopic-guided fixation alone. Radiographically, the arthroscopic-assisted group had statistically significant decreased articular step and gap as well as improved restoration of ulnar variance and volar tilt. At final follow-up, the range of motion and grip strength were both found to be significantly improved in the arthroscopically treated group. It is notable that these clinical outcomes have not been reproduced in many of the other similar comparative studies in the literature. Shihab and colleagues[6] performed a meta-analysis of all qualifying comparison studies published since 2015 looking at arthroscopic-assisted volar locked plating versus fluoroscopic-assisted volar locked plating that included six studies with 280 patients. Their findings reinforced prior studies that reported that arthroscopic assistance improved articular reduction and an increased rate of identification of associated soft tissue injuries. They similarly noted no difference in reported outcome measures, complications, or other radiographic outcomes with the use of arthroscopic assistance. The arthroscopic group reported longer operative time, consistent with prior literature.

Perilunate Injuries

Kim and colleagues[27] performed a retrospective review of 20 patients with perilunate injuries—15 of which were fracture dislocations involving the scaphoid-treated with arthroscopic reduction and percutaneous fixation. Thirteen of the fifteen scaphoid fractures went onto union, with no

radiographic evidence of post-traumatic arthritis at mean final follow-up of 31 months. The range of motion was found to be equivalent to previously published series using open techniques. Jeon and colleagues reported a small, four-patient series of patients with a trans-scaphoid perilunate fracture dislocation treated with arthroscopically assisted percutaneous screw fixation and bone grafting. The authors reported that all fracture went on to union. The mean flexion–extension arc was 126°, patients demonstrated no evidence of midcarpal arthritis at final follow-up (mean 17.5 months), and all patients returned to their previous occupation.[31] Liu and colleagues[35] published a series of 24 patients with dorsal perilunate injuries, 20 of which were fracture-dislocations that were treated with arthroscopically assisted mini-invasive reduction and fixation. Good or excellent functional outcomes were achieved in 19 of 24 patients. Flexion–extension arc and grip strength were 86% and 83% of the contralateral side, respectively. One scaphoid nonunion was reported. Carpal alignment was restored at the time of surgery in all patients, with no patients having subsequent loss of alignment at final follow-up. This group subsequently published a follow-on cohort with 31 patients with at least 1 year follow-up that demonstrated similar results, with no further scaphoid nonunions or loss of carpal alignment.[28]

Oh and colleagues[40] reported a comparative study of open versus arthroscopic-assisted fixation methods for trans-scaphoid perilunate fracture dislocations with 11 patients in the arthroscopic group and nine patients in the open reduction group with a minimum of 2 year follow-up. At final follow-up, the arthroscopic group had a statistically significantly greater arc of wrist flexion–extension (125° vs 105.6°) and mean DASH score. However, there was no significant difference in radiographic measures or grip strength as compared with the contralateral side, and difference in Mayo wrist scores was not significant. This small series demonstrates that arthroscopic techniques can achieve equivalent outcomes for most measures and may have benefits for range of motion and some patient-reported outcome measures as compared with open techniques.

Herzberg and colleagues[13] reported on a select series of 27 perilunate fracture dislocations treated via arthroscopic techniques over an 11-year period. All patients underwent a diagnostic arthroscopy after initial closed reduction. Seven patients underwent percutaneous pinning with arthroscopic guidance alone. The remaining 20 patients were treated with a combination of arthroscopy and a mini-open dorsal approach. Of note, all 12 scaphoid fractures reported in this series went onto union. The authors report a mean postoperative wrist flexion–extension arc of 80° and the grip strength of 69% of the contralateral side, neither of which were superior to open techniques alone.

COMPLICATIONS

Overall complication rates associated with wrist arthroscopy vary. Large review studies demonstrate the complication rates of up to 6%,[13,41] with rates of up to 13% reported among inexperienced practitioners.[42] Failure to achieve the desired outcome, iatrogenic nerve and cartilage injuries, and complex regional pain syndrome are the most commonly reported complications. Tendon injury and postoperative hematoma are rare but reported complications.[29,41] The additional operative time required by arthroscopic techniques and the associated costs and resource utilization should be considered when weighing operative strategies. Even in the most experienced of hands, arthroscopy has routinely been shown to prolong operative time compared with open reduction.

SUMMARY

Arthroscopic techniques have been demonstrated to be effective for the treatment of a variety of fracture pathology about the wrist. Arthroscopy can minimize additional capsular insult, help to minimize damage to an already tenuous blood supply, and mitigate potential soft tissue complications when compared with open techniques. In the treatment of distal radius fractures, arthroscopy can assist in minimizing residual step and gap of intra-articular fractures and can aid in the diagnosis and treatment of common associated soft tissue injuries. Percutaneous, arthroscopic-assisted techniques for reduction and fixation of perilunate fracture dislocations demonstrate acceptable results when compared with open techniques. As is the case with many arthroscopic techniques, the required level of technical proficiency to efficiently treat wrist fractures with arthroscopic methods may limit broad use. High-quality randomized control studies comparing open to arthroscopic treatment for distal radius fractures and perilunate injuries are scarce, and further investigation is warranted to better understand the functional outcome benefits associated with minimally invasive techniques.

CLINICS CARE POINTS

- Arthroscopy can allow for effective treatment of fracture treatment about the wrist while minimizing soft tissue and vascular insult.
- Arthroscopic techniques in the treatment of distal radius fractures can minimize step and gap of intra-articular fractures and identify associated soft tissue injuries.
- Multiple series have demonstrated arthroscopic assisted treatment of perilunate injuires to hae equivalent outcomes to open techniques.
- A high level of technical profeiciency with arthroscopic techniques is required for treatment of a variety of fractures about the wrist which may limit widespread adoption. Extensive debridement can be required in perilunate injuries given the usual high energy nature of these injuries.

DISCLOSURE

The authors have nothing to disclose.

REFERENCES

1. Whipple TL. The Role of Arthroscopy in the Treatment of Wrist Injuries in the Athlete. Clin Sports Med 1998;17(3):623–34.
2. Culp RW, Osterman AL. Arthroscopic reduction and internal fixation of distal radius fractures. Orthop Clin North Am 1995;26(4):739–48.
3. Geissler WB, Freeland AE, Savoie FH, et al. Intracarpal soft tissue lesions associated with an intra-articular fracture of the distal end of the radius. J Bone Joint Surg 1996;78A:357–65.
4. Savoie F, Grondel R. Arthroscopy for carpal instability. Orthop Clin North Am 1995;26(4):731–8.

5. Richards RS, Bennett JD, Roth JH, et al. Arthroscopic diagnosis of intra-articular soft tissue injuries associated with distal radial fractures. J Hand Surg Am 1997;22:772–6.

6. Shihab Z, Sivakuma B, Graham D, et al. Outcomes of Arthroscopic-Assisted Distal Radius Fracture Volar Plating: A Meta-Analysis. J Hand Surg Am 2022;47(4):330–40.

7. Abe Y, Yoshida K, Tominaga Y. Less invasive surgery with wrist arthroscopy for distal radius fracture. J Orthop Sci 2013;18(3):398–404.

8. Omokawa S, Abe Y, Imatani J, et al. Treatment of Intra-articular Distal Radius Fractures. Hand Clin 2017;33(3):529–43.

9. Knirk JL, Jupiter JB. Intra-articular fractures of the distal end of the radius in young adults. J Bone Joint Surg Am 1986;68(5):647–59.

10. Trumble TE, Schmitt SR, Vedder NB. Factors affecting functional outcome of displaced intra-articular distal radius fractures. J Hand Surg Am 1994;19:325–40.

11. Goldfarb CA, Rudzki JR, Catalano LW, et al. Fifteen-year outcome of displaced intra-articular fractures of the distal radius. J Hand Surg Am 2006;31(4):633–9.

12. Weil W, Slade W III, Trumble T. Open and Arthroscopic Treatment of Perilunate Injuries. Clin Orthop Relat Res 2006;445:120–32.

13. Herzberg G, Burnier M, Marc A, et al. The Role of Arthroscopy for Treatment of Perilunate Injuries. J Wrist Surg 2015;4:101–9.

14. Herzberg G, Cievet-Bonfils M, Burnier M. Arthroscopic Treatment of Translunate Perilunate Injuries, Not Dislocated (PLIND). J Wrist Surg 2019;8:143–6.

15. Chow E, Ho P. Three Cases of Translunate Perilunate Injury Treated with Wrist Arthroscopy. J Wrist Surg 2021;10:58–63.

16. Yao J, Fogel N. Arthroscopy in Distal Radius Fractures: Indications and When to Do It. Hand Clin 2021 May;37(2):279–91.

17. Abboudi J, Culp RW. Treating fractures of the distal radius with arthroscopic assistance. Orthop Clin North Am 2001;32(2):307–15.

18. Ardouin L, Durand A, Gay A, et al. Why do we use arthroscopy for distal radius fractures? Eur J Orthop Surg Traumatol 2018;28:1505–14.

19. Lutsky K, Boyer M, Steffen J, et al. Arthroscopic assessment of intra-articular distal radius fractures after open reduction and internal fixation from a volar approach. J Hand Surg Am 2008;33(4):476–84.

20. Auge WK, Velazquez PA. The application of indirect reduction techniques in the distal radius: the role of adjuvant arthroscopy. Arthroscopy 2000;16:830–5.

21. Edwards CC, Haraszti CJ, McGillivary GR, et al. Intraarticular distal radius fractures: arthroscopic assessment of radiographically assisted reduction. J Hand Surg Am 2001;26(6):1036–41.

22. Slutsky DJ. Portals and Methodology. In: del Pinal F, Mathoulin C, Luchetti R, editors. Arthroscopic management of distal radius fractures. Berlin: Springer; 2007. p. 13–26.

23. Swart E, Tang P. The effect of ligament injuries on outcomes of operatively treated distal radius fractures. Am J Orthop 2017;46(1):E41–6.

24. Lindau T, Arner M, Hagberg L. Intraarticular lesions in distal fractures of the radius in young adults. A descriptive arthroscopic study in 50 patients. J Hand Surg Br 1997;22(5):638–43.

25. Mrkonjic A, Lindau T, Geijer M, et al. Arthroscopically diagnosed scapholunate ligament injuries associated with distal radial fractures: a 13- to 15-year follow-up. J Hand Surg Am 2015;40(6):1077–82.

26. Mrkonjic A, Geijer M, Lindau T, et al. The natural course of traumatic triangular fibrocartilage complex tears in distal radial fractures: a 13-15 year follow-up of arthroscopically diagnosed but untreated injuries. J Hand Surg Am 2012;37(8):1555–60.

27. Kim J, Lee J, Park M. Arthroscopic Treatment of Perilunate Dislocations and Fracture Dislocations. J Wrist Surg 2015;4:81–7.

28. Liu B, Chen S, Zhu J, et al. Arthroscopic Management of Perilunate Injuries. Hand Clin 2017 Nov;33(4):709–15.

29. Wiesler ER, Chloros GD, Lucas RM, et al. Arthroscopic management of volar lunate facet fractures of the distal radius. Tech Hand Up Extrem Surg 2006;10(3):139–44.

30. Yamazaki H, Uchiyama S, Komatsu M, et al. Arthroscopic assistance does not improve the functional or radiographic outcome of unstable intra-articular distal radial fractures treated with a volar locking plate: a randomised controlled trial. Bone Joint Lett J 2015;97-B(7):957–62.

31. Jeon I, Kim H, Min W, et al. Arthroscopically Assisted Percutaneous Fixation for Trans-Scaphoid Perilunate Fracture Dislocation. J Hand Surg Eur 2010;35(8):664–8.

32. Goodman A, Harris A, Gil J, et al. Evaluation, Management and Outcomes of Lunate and Perilunate Dislocations. Orthopedics 2019;42(1):e1–6.

33. Abe Y, Fujii K. Arthroscopic-Assisted Reduction of Intra-articular Distal Radius Fracture. Hand Clin 2017;33(4):659–68.

34. Del Piñal F, Klausmeyer M, Moraleda E, et al. Arthroscopic reduction of comminuted intra-articular distal radius fractures with diaphyseal-metaphyseal comminution. J Hand Surg Am 2014;39(5):835–43.

35. Liu B, Chen S, Zhu J, et al. Arthroscopically Assisted Mini-Invasive Management of Perilunate Dislocations. J Wrist Surg 2015;4:93–100.

36. Smeraglia F, Del Buono A, Maffulli N. Wrist arthroscopy in the management of articular distal radius fractures. Br Med Bull 2016;119(1):157–65.

37. Saab M, Guerre E, Chantelot C, et al. Contribution of arthroscopy to the management of intra-articular distal radius fractures: Knowledge update based on a systematic 10-year literature review. Orthop Traumatol Surg Res 2019;105(8):1617–25.

38. Varitimidis SE, Basdekis GK, Dialiana ZH, et al. Treatment of intra-articular fractures of the distal radius: Fluoroscopic or arthroscopic reduction? J Bone Joint Surg Br 2008;90(6):778–85.

39. Koo S, Leung K, Chau W, et al. Comparing Outcomes between Arthroscopic-Assisted Reduction and Fluoroscopic Reduction in AO Type C Distal Radius Fracture Treatment. J Wrist Surg 2021;10(2):102–10.

40. Oh W, Choi Y, Kang H, et al. Comparative Outcome Analysis of Arthroscopic-Assisted Versus Open Reduction and Fixation of Trans-scaphoid Perilunate Fracture Dislocations. Arthroscopy 2017;33(1):92–100.

41. Ahsan ZS, Yao J. Complications of Wrist and Hand Arthroscopy. Hand Clin 2017;33(4):831–8.

42. Leclercq C, Mathoulin C, The members of EWAS. Complications of wrist arthroscopy: a multi-center study based on 10,107 arthroscopies. J Wrist Surg 2016;5(4):320–6.

Role for Wrist Hemiarthroplasty in Acute Irreparable Distal Radius Fracture in the Elderly

Guillaume Herzberg, MD, PhD[a],*, Marion Burnier, MD[b], Lyliane Ly, MD[c]

KEYWORDS

- Elderly • Wrist hemiarthroplasty • Fracture • Osteoporosis

KEY POINTS

- The authors provide criteria for distal radius fracture (DRF) in elderly that may not be amenable to volar plating ("irreparable DRF").
- The authors review the current results of a preliminary series of wrist hemiarthroplasty for irreparable DRF.
- Treatment of "irreparable DRF in the elderly" with wrist hemiarthroplasty may be a new viable salvage option.

INTRODUCTION

Volar locking plates are widely used to treat acute intra-articular distal radius fracture (DRF) in the elderly. However, there is evidence in the literature that complications may occur after this procedure, especially in the most comminuted osteoporotic cases. Similarly to complex proximal and distal humerus fracture management in the elderly, the use of a wrist hemiarthroplasty is emerging as an innovative treatment for these complex injuries.

Our purpose was

1. To provide criteria for a subset of complex DRF in the elderly that may not be amenable to volar plating (so-called irreparable elderly DRF) and
2. To review the current results of a single center preliminary series of wrist hemiarthroplasty for irreparable DRF in elderly.

METHODS

Between 2011 and 2019, 26 consecutive independent elderly patients (28 wrists) with irreparable intra-articular DRF were treated at the acute stage with primary wrist hemiarthroplasty. There were

96% female patients and the mean age was 79 years (minimum 65 years, maximum 92 years). A combined resection of the ulnar head was associated in 22 wrists (78%). A total of 17 wrists with a mean follow-up of 32 months were reviewed clinically and radiologically.

RESULTS

At follow-up, mean VAS pain was 1/10, mean forearm rotation arc was 148°. The mean active wrist flexion–extension arc was 60°. The mean active wrist extension was 35°. The mean grip strength was 68% of the contralateral wrist. The mean Lyon wrist score was 75% (63%–91%). Bone healing around the implants was satisfactory in all wrists with no periprosthetic osteolysis. There were 2 revisions.

CONCLUSIONS

Our current results suggest that treatment of so-called "irreparable DRF in the elderly" with wrist hemiarthroplasty may be a new viable salvage option. The authors provided a definition of this

a Clinique Parc Lyon, Val Ouest Lyon, France; b Medipole Villeurbanne France; c Hospices Civils Lyon, France
* Corresponding author.
E-mail address: profgherzberg@gmail.com

Hand Clin 39 (2023) 545–550
https://doi.org/10.1016/j.hcl.2023.05.011
0749-0712/23/© 2023 Elsevier Inc. All rights reserved.

rare injury and reported their preliminary results. Longer follow-up and comparative studies are needed to further confirm the validity of this innovative concept.

INTRODUCTION

Volar locking plates are widely used for nearly two decades to treat acute distal radius fractures (DRF) in elderly patients.[1,2]

However, several studies have shown that volar locked plating for DRF in the elderly may fail to confer a significant clinical benefit and may result in frequent complications.[3–6]

Similarly to what is done for hip, shoulder, and elbow complex fractures in the elderly, some authors[7,8] recently proposed to treat acute comminuted impacted DRF in elderly patients with a wrist hemiarthroplasty.

Since 2011, we have been using wrist hemiarthroplasty in selected elderly fractures that we considered as not amenable to volar plating due to severe impaction and comminution along with a distal epiphyseal fracture line.[9,10]

The purpose of this study was to propose a definition of acute irreparable DRF in the elderly, and to review the results of a preliminary series of wrist hemiarthroplasty for this sub-group of patients.

METHODS
Patients

Between 2011 and 2019, we treated 1861 acute DRF at a single academic institution. A total of 1179 DRFs (64%) were AO "C" fractures.

A group of 28 of the "C" fractures (2%) in 26 elderly patients (mean age 79 years, minimum 65 years, maximum 92 years, 96% female, 2 bilateral implants) were defined as acute irreparable fractures and treated with wrist hemiarthroplasty at the acute stage. The average time from injury to surgery was 4 days (minimum 1, maximum 7 days).

The inclusion criteria were as follows: According to the P.A.F. classification chart[11,12] of DRF (patient–accident–Fracture), all patients in this group were defined as older than 65 years and 2 to 2, that is, presenting with comorbidities but independent at home, able to perform activities of daily living by themselves. All fractures were produced by a low energy injury. Regarding the pathology of the fractures, all were defined as irreparable with volar plate fixation because of a combination of the following criteria: type "C" complete intra-articular fracture with high extra- and intra-articular P.A.F. displacement scores, main fracture line distal to the watershed line, impaction and circumferential comminution.

Exclusion criteria were irreparable DRF in dependent patients and failure of a previous treatment for acute DRF. All patients meeting the inclusion and exclusion criteria comprised the cohort of this study. This retrospective study was approved by our institutional review board.

Follow-up

A total of 20 wrists in 19 patients with more than 9 months of follow-up were assessed. Three patients reported satisfactory outcomes on the phone but denied a follow-up visit. A total of 17 wrists in 16 patients were assessed clinically and radiologically at an average follow-up of 32 months (maximum 57 months).

Follow-up clinical evaluation included VAS pain on a 10 points scale, evaluation of the functional status, active range of motion, and grip strength (Jamar dynamometer). The Lyon wrist score[13] including information about pain, functional limitation with forearm rotation/wrist flexion–extension, active forearm rotation/wrist flexion–extension, and grip strength was used.

The radiological follow-up evaluation used the Centricity Enterprise 3.0 software (General Electrics) and consisted of standard anteroposterior and lateral radiographs. A control computed tomographic scan was performed in 2 wrists.

Implants and Surgical Technique

At the beginning of series (10 of 28 wrists), we used the radial component of the press-fit remotion total wrist arthroplasty Small Bone Innovation Company (SBI). Then we designed a specific trauma implant Cobra 1 Groupe Lepine with a longer stem and orientation flanges to help rotational control that we used in 18 of 28 wrists (16 press-fit and 2 cemented). The Cobra 1 implant includes a volar offset to replicate the shape of the distal radial epiphysis. Two intra-flange holes may help peripheral bone fixation with sutures if necessary.

Both Remotion and Cobra implants are provided in right and left versions.

A resection of the ulnar head was associated in 22 of 28 wrists (78%).

The detailed operative technique and postoperative management were described elsewhere.[9,10] The wrist approach was dorsal. An osteotome entered the dorsal aspect of fracture into the third compartment. Osteoperiosteal flaps were elevated radially and ulnarly in a "book-opening like" manner keeping the second and fourth extensor compartments intact. While the wrist was flexed at 90° using several towels, the comminuted distal radius epiphyseal and articular fragments were excised.

Care was taken to preserve thick peripheral dorsal, lateral, and volar osteo-periosteal flaps to save the remaining bone stock of the distal radius and optimize bony surrounding of the implant at the end of the procedure. If the sigmoid notch remnants were reparable with trans-osseous non-absorbable sutures, the ulnar head was left intact for Distal Radiounlar Joint (DRUJ) salvage. If the sigmoid notch remnants were irreparable, or if there was an associated ulnar head or neck fracture, the ulnar head was removed. We used an oblique distal ulna resection.[9]

The implant stem was then introduced into the radial diaphysis with critical attention to restoring distal radius length according to preoperative planning.[9] Depending on the bone quality and implant stem press-fit, intra-diaphyseal cancellous bone from the epiphysis or cement may be used. Stabilization of the ulnar stump was then performed using the volar DRUJ capsule that was secured to the dorsal part of the ulnar stump with trans-osseous non-absorbable sutures.[9] The 2 osteo-periosteal flaps were then brought back together and sutured so as to close like a book the osteoperiosteal flaps around the implant.

During the whole procedure, all the extensor compartments but the third were left intact. The dorsal retinaculum was closed. If the closure of the dorsal retinaculum was too tight, the extensor pollicis longus tendon was left out of the dorsal retinaculum.

The wrist is immobilized in 20° extension and neutral ulno-radial deviation in a long-arm cast for 3 weeks. Then a volar wrist splint in 20° wrist extension was applied for 3 weeks and patient's self-rehabilitation was initiated. Immobilization was discarded at day 45.

RESULTS
Complications

In this series, we did not observe any loosening or superficial/deep infection of the implants.

We observed 3 reflex sympathetic dystrophies that resolved in less than 18 months. We performed revision surgery in 2 cases.

One wrist displayed a satisfactory implant alignment on the immediate postoperative radiographs but the implant was too small for the big wrist of this male patient and a progressive ulnar subluxation of the whole carpus with respect to the implant was observed during the first postoperative months. The implant was successfully revised to a larger one providing a satisfactory result (Lyon wrist score 81% = good) at 2 years of follow-up.

One wrist was reoperated 20 months after the index operation because she presented a significant stiffness (marked loss of flexion) due to tendon adhesions along with a tendency to radial deviation of the wrist. Through a dorsal approach, we performed extensor tendons tenolysis combined with tendon transfer of extensor carpi radialis longus (ECRL) to extensor carpi radialis brevis (ECRB). At final follow-up of 31 months her clinical status was markedly improved (Lyon wrist score 72% = good).

Clinical Results

At final follow-up among the 17 wrists in 16 patients who could be reviewed, the average VAS pain was 1/10 (range 0–3). The mean forearm rotation arc was 148° (range 120°–170°). The mean active wrist flexion–extension arc was 60° (range 35°–100°). The mean active wrist extension was 35° (range 15°–50°). The mean grip strength was 14 kg that was 68% of the contralateral wrist (range 36%–100%). The mean Lyon wrist score was 75% (good) with a range from 63 (fair) to 91 (excellent).

Among the 14 of 17 wrists in which we had to combine an ulnar head resection in combination with the wrist hemiarthroplasty, no patient complained about painful radio-ulnar impingement.

Radiological Results

Bone healing around the implants at follow-up was satisfactory in all wrists. Sagittal orientation of the implant was satisfactory in all cases. An example is provided in **Figs. 1–3**. Apart from the wrist of the male patient which displayed an early ulnar subluxation revised with a larger implant, we did not observe any abnormal ulnar or volar translation of the carpus relative to the implant. Each implant remained well seated within the distal cup of the implant. There was no subsidence of the implants or erosion of the carpus, nor peroprosthetic osteolysis.

DISCUSSION

Our current data suggest that treatment of so-called irreparable DRF in the independent elderly patient with a bone-preserving wrist hemiarthroplasty may be a viable innovative option.

An independent elderly patient is able to perform all activities of daily living (ADLs) at home without any help. She or he may present several comorbidities and may need the use of crutches.[11,12] This is why it would be so important, should an irreparable DRF occur, to provide a one-stage treatment with early rehabilitation and use of the wrist in a functional position including at least 20° to 30° of active extension.

Because there is no current definition available to characterize these fractures, we proposed to define

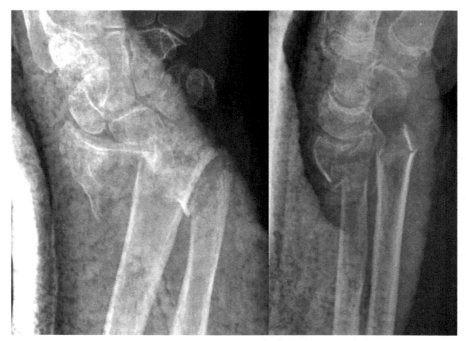

Fig. 1. Irreparable distal radius fracture in a 83 year old woman, independent at home. There is marked intra- and extra-articular displacements, distal fracture line, impaction separation with circumferential comminution.

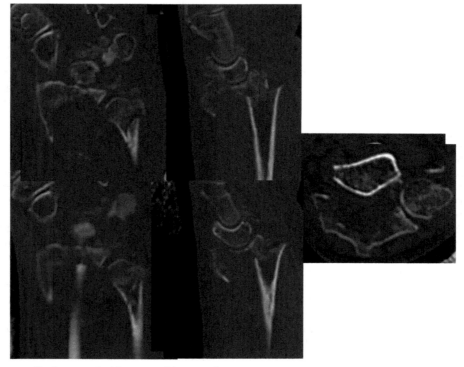

Fig. 2. Same patient, computed tomographic scan views.

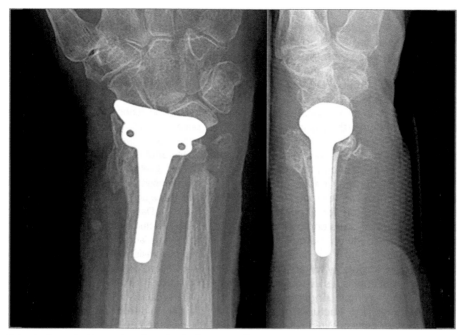

Fig. 3. Radiological result 5 months after the index procedure.

them according to simple radiological criteria available on initial standard postero - anterior (PA) and lateral views. An irreparable DRF would be a type "C" complete intra-articular fracture with high extra- and intra-articular P.A.F. displacement scores,[9] main fracture line distal to the watershed line, impaction and circumferential comminution.

There are no really good therapeutic options to treat these complex osteoporotic fractures.

Closed reduction and casting may leave significant deformity and unpredictable functional impairment.[2,14]

Percutaneous pinning often fails due to the limited purchase of pins into osteoporotic fractured fragments.[2,15]

External fixation is a cumbersome treatment of elderly patients and may cause complications as pin tract infections.[16]

Volar plating may be in some cases a satisfactory option.[2] However, in Orbay's study[2] only 33% were classified as AO type "C" fractures. In our experience, successful volar plating is difficult to achieve in so-called "irreparable" DRF in elderly and secondary displacement frequently occurs. Moreover, Arora and Gabl[4] showed in a level I study that ORIF with volar plating in this group of patients did not convey any improvement in terms of function and range of motion when compared with closed reduction and cast immobilization.

Distraction plating is a new validated treatment of complex DRF REF which was proposed for

elderly patients presenting with the equivalent of irreparable DRF.[17] However, the long (average 4 months) post-operative time before plate removal in this study[17] and a potential for skin complications over the metacarpal area in elderly patients may limit its use.

Roux[8] was the first to propose to treat acute comminuted impacted DRF in elderly patients with a massive wrist hemiarthroplasty replacing both the radiocarpal and distal radioulnar joints. His preliminary series included 6 wrist operated on at the acute stage. The hypothesis was that some complex impacted intra-articular DRF in the elderly would be amenable wrist hemiarthroplasty. This surgery would obviate hardware removal in the absence of complications and would be followed by early mobilization. Using the same implant, Vergnenègre[18] subsequently reported satisfactory results with no implants removal in 8 patients presenting with irreparable DRF. However, the implant used in these two series is no longer available.

Another radiocarpal hemiarthroplasty including a long pin-shaped radial stem was recently proposed for irreparable DRF[7] with satisfactory results. However, it is the authors opinion that the long pin-stem of the implant may jeopardize the radial head in case of further falls that are not unusual in elderly patients.

The implants used in our series preserve as much as possible the distal radius bone stock and have a reasonable stem length. At the beginning of our experience, we used the radial component of a remotion total wrist arthroplasty. However, we found that its stem was too short to provide a constantly straight orientation with respect to the radial diaphysis. This is why we designed a specific fracture implant (Cobra Groupe Lepine) with a similar ellipsoid distal surface but a longer stem and 2 lateral flanges to help rotational stability.

Whatever the type of hemiarthroplasty, it is well accepted that metal on cartilage is not the best contact for an arthroplasty. We recognize that the contact between the implant and the convexity of the proximal carpal row may cause cartilage wear in the long-term. However, the metal on cartilage contact is well accepted for shoulder and elbow salvage treatments in acute complex osteoporotic fractures in the elderly as the advantages outweight the drawbacks.

Similarly, wrist hemiarthroplasty for acute irreparable DRF in elderly patients is a salvage procedure aimed at providing a simple single operation with quick rehabilitation for fractures that are barely amenable to volar plating. Wrist hemiarthroplasty was also was recently proposed for treatment of wrist arthritis.[19,20]

Longer-term follow-ups and comparative studies are needed to confirm the usefulness of the wrist hemiarthroplasty concept for irreparable DRF in the independent elderly patients as well as the fate of the cartilage of the first carpal row against the implant.

CLINICS CARE POINTS

- Volar locking plates for DRF in the elderly may show complications in the most comminuted osteoporotic cases
- Wrist hemiarthroplasty may be a novel option to treat irreparable DRF not amenable to volar locking plates
- Our results suggest that treatment of "irreparable DRF in the elderly" with wrist hemiarthroplasty may be a new viable salvage option.

DISCLOSURE

G. Herzberg Royalties from Groupe Lepine.M. Burnier & L. Ly, nothing to disclose.

REFERENCES

1. Martinez-Mendez D. Prospective study of comminuted articular distal radius fractures stabilized by volar plating in the elderly. Int Orthop 2018;42(9):2243–8.
2. Orbay JL, Fernandez DL. Volar fixed angle plate fixation for unstable distal radius fractures in the elderly patient. JHSA 2004;29A:96–102.
3. Arora R. Complications following internal fixation of unstable distal radius fracture with a palmar locking plate. J Orthop Trauma 2007;21(5):316–22.
4. Arora R, Gabl M. A prospective randomized trial comparing nonoperative treatment with volar locking plate fixation for displaced and unstable DRF in patients 65 years and older. J Bone Joint Surg Am 2011;93A(20):2146–53.
5. Chen Y. Safety and efficacy of operative vs nonsurgical management of DRF in the elderly patients: a systematic review and meta-analysis. JHSA 2016;41(3):404.
6. Day CS, Daly MC. Management of geriatric distal radius fractures. JHSA 2012;37A(12):2619–22.
7. Martins A, Facca S, Liverneaux P. Isoelastic resurfacing prosthesis for DRF; outcomes in 24 cases with at least 2 years followup. OTSR 2020;106(8):1613.
8. Roux JL. Treatment of intra-articular fractures of the distal radius by wrist prosthesis. J Orthop Traumatol: Surgery and Research 2011;97S:S46–53.
9. Herzberg G, Burnier M, Marc A, et al. Primary wrist hemiarthroplasty for irreparable distal radisu fracture in the independent elderly. J Wrist Surg 2015;4:156–63.
10. Herzberg G, Merlini L, Burnier M. Hemi-arthroplasty for distal radius fracture in the independent elderly. Orthop Traumatol Surg Res 2017;103(6):915–8.
11. Herzberg G, Izem Y, Al Saati M, et al. PAF analysis of acute distal radius fractures in adults. Preliminary results. Chir Main 2010;29:231–5.
12. Herzberg G. Acute distal radius fracture: PAF analysis. J Wrist Surg 2012;1(1):81–2.
13. Herzberg G, Burnier M, Nakamura T. A new wrist clinical evaluation score. J Wrist Surg 2018;7(2):109.
14. Beumer A, McQueen MM. Fractures of the distal radius in low-demand elderly patients: closed reduction of no value in 53 of 60 wrists. Acta Orthop Scand 2003;74(1):98–100.
15. Glickel SZ, Catalano LW, Raia FJ. Long term outcomes of closed reduction and percutaneous pinning for the treatment of distal radius fractures. JHSA 2008;33(10):1700–5.
16. Capo JT. External fixation of distal radius fractures: effect of distraction and duration. JHSA 2009;34A: 1605.
17. Richard MJ, Ruch DS. Distraction plating for the treatment of highly comminuted DRF in elderly patients. JHSA 2012;37A(5):948–56.
18. Vergnenègre G, Mabit C, Arnaud JP, et al. Treatment of comminuted DRF by resurfacing prosthesis in elderly patients. Chir Main 2014;33(2):112.
19. Culp RW. PRC combined with wrist hemiarthroplasty. J Wrist Surg 2012;1(1):39–46.
20. Vance MC, Packer G, Tan D, et al. Midcarpal hemiarthroplasty for wrist arthritis: rationale and early results. J Wrist Surg 2012;1(1):61–7.

Intramedullary Nailing of Forearm Fractures

William Barritt Gilbert Jr, MD[a], Mihir Jitendra Desai, MD, MS[b],*

KEYWORDS

- Forearm fracture • Intramedullary nailing • Radius • Ulna • Intraosseous • Interlocking

KEY POINTS

- Intramedullary devices provide a viable treatment option for forearm fractures in select patients, particularly those with extensive soft tissue damge, comminution, would benefit from a minimally invasive procedure.
- Knowledge of the approrpaite antomic landmarks is critical fro using intramedullary devices for forearm fixation.
- Intra-articular fractures are not amenable to placing intrameduallry devices for forearm fractures.

INTRODUCTION/NATURE OF THE PROBLEM

The overall aim of treating forearm fractures is to restore length, rotational alignment, and the anatomic bow of the radius. Common treatment options include both open reduction internal fixation and closed reduction with immobilization. Closed treatment in adult forearm fractures quickly became regarded as unsuccessful with high rates of non-union and malunion even in minimally displaced forearm fractures.[1] Poor outcomes are attributed to deforming forces inherent in forearm motion, the relationship between the proximal and distal radioulnar articulations, and anatomic bow of the radius.[2] Therefore, outside of the pediatric population, non-operative treatment of forearm fractures is not routine and anatomic reduction is critical for bone healing and restoration of upper extremity function.[1]

Plate osteosynthesis has largely been recognized as the gold standard among orthopedic surgeons and is supported through a large body of clinical evidence.[3,4] In simple fractures, compression plates allow for absolute stability and primary bone healing due to direct cortical opposition and compression across the fracture site. In comminuted fractures plates provide a rigid construct to support length and alignment for secondary healing to occur. Though plate osteosynthesis is understood as the gold standard, it is not without its critiques. Plating often necessitates large incisions that involve soft tissue dissection, periosteal stripping, and damage to musculoskeletal vascularity. Resulting complications may include non-union, infection, synostosis, neurovascular injury, need for plate removal and subsequent refracture after the plate is removed.[5,6]

Intramedullary devices have long been successful in treating fractures of other diaphyseal long bones and offer several benefits including smaller incisions, preserved periosteum, lower refracture risk, and promotion of healing with reaming. The success in other long bones quickly led to its application as an alternative treatment in forearm fractures. Early implants included Kirshner wires, Rush pins, and Steinmann pins though results were unsatisfactory. High rates of non-union/malunion were attributed to inadequate rigidity and rotational stability of unlocked constructs.[7] Over the years, advances in implant design and interlocking capability have resulted in better functional outcomes. Thus, intramedullary nailing can be a viable treatment option in select patients, particularly those with extensive soft tissue

a Department of Orthopedic Surgery, Vanderbilt University, PGY-3, 1215 21st Avenue South Suite 3200 and 4200, Nashville, TN, USA; b Department of Orthopedic Surgery, Vanderbilt University, 1215 21st Avenue South Suite 3200 and 4200, Nashville, TN, USA
* Corresponding author.
E-mail address: mihir.j.desai@vumc.org

Hand Clin 39 (2023) 551–559
https://doi.org/10.1016/j.hcl.2023.05.012
0749-0712/23/© 2023 Elsevier Inc. All rights reserved.

hand.theclinics.com

damage, comminuted, or segmental fractures who might benefit from less invasive procedure.[6,8] In this article, the authors aim to describe current advances in intramedullary treatment of forearm fractures, the indications, surgical techniques, and outcomes associated with intramedullary fixation.

ANATOMY

Understanding anatomy and biomechanics is essential for the surgeon who treats disorders of the forearm axis. Historical difficulty in forearm intramedullary fixation is attributed to inherent anatomical barriers of forearm motion and the radial bow. The ulna is largely straight in nature and contributes to forearm axial stability while acting as a supportive strut for rotation of the radius. The radius is bowed anteriorly allowing for protonation and supination and the arc of motion is supported through ligamentous structures including the proximal and distal radioulnar joints and the interosseous membrane.[9] Any disruption in this axis may prohibit forearm motion, thus anatomic restoration is critical in operative treatment. The radial bow is defined by drawing a line between the radial tuberosity proximally and the most ulnar edge of the radius distally. A perpendicular line is then drawn at the point of maximal radial bow, and the length of this line is measured.[10] Loss of radial bow following operative fixation leads to angulation and rotational influences resulting in non-union and malunion.

HISTORY OF INTRAMEDULLARY NAILING

The use of intramedullary implants in other diaphyseal long bones led to inquiry into their potential in forearm fractures. The first description was reported by Shone in 1913 using thin silver wires.[1,11] Later Rush and Lambrinudi described the use of Steinmann pins, Kirschner and Rush rods as novel implants.[12] Though intramedullary devices demonstrated success in the femur and the tibia, their utilization in forearm fractures diminished, given unsatisfactory results. In 1949, Knight and Purvis demonstrated that over 54% of forearm fractures treated with intramedullary fixation lost rotational alignment or resulted in non-union.[13] Similarly in 1953, Bachynski and Smith, reported a cohort of 79 patients where 50% of patients treated with intramedullary forearm fixation went on to unacceptable alignment, malunion, or non-union.[14] The first large multicenter report was published by Sage and colleagues in 1957.[7] These authors reported on 338 patients with 555 forearm fractures that were treated with Rush pins, Kirschner wires, Steinmann pins, Kunschner V nails, and Lottes nails. The overall rate of non-union in this cohort was approximately 21% with the highest rate of non-union belonging to those fractures treated with kirschner wires (38%). Sage and colleagues attributed the lack of success of forearm intramedullary fixation to the challenges of balancing strength with malleability of the implant. Stiff nails, although biomechanically sound, might distort the radial bow or distract the fracture site. Conversely, malleable implants, capable of spanning the fracture and maintaining radial bow, might not overcome the deforming forces of forearm motion over time. These problems are compounded by the small diameters of forearm medullary canals. In hope to improve nail design, Sage performed a cadaveric study of over 100 radii looking at the anatomy of the medullary canal, and developed a pre-bent triangular nail that demonstrated improvements in primary union rate.[14]

Despite these challenges, Sage noted the utility of intramedullary fixation as a simple and relatively quick treatment option for patients with mangled extremities or significant soft tissue defects. Intramedullary implants in these situations resulted in superior reduction and motion when compared to traditional skeletal traction, external fixation, or conservative treatment.[7]

CURRENT NAIL DESIGN AND OUTCOMES

As described, traditional unlocked nails were not ideal in overcoming biomechanical barriers of forearm motion. In response, the development of interlocking nails aimed to improve rotational and axial control.

In 1990, Lefevre introduced one of the first locking nails for ulna fractures.[15] It was approximately 6 mm in diameter with proximal and distal interlocking screws. De Pedro and colleagues reported the results of the Lefevre nail in 20 patients with displaced ulna fractures.[16] Outcomes were defined as time to clinical and radiographic union, post-operative flexion–extension, pronation, and supination. Of the patients treated, 20% had an excellent result, 70% had a good result, and 10% had a fair result. The Lefevre nail was not applicable for radial shaft fractures and patients with concurrent radial shaft fractures, required treatment with Kirschner wires or plating.

A new locking nail with the ability to treat both radial and ulnar shaft fractures was introduced by Crenshaw in 1999.[17] The ForeSight nail was stainless steel with diameter options of 4.0 and 5.0 mm, slightly smaller than the prior Lefevre nail. The nail was straight but malleable, allowing the surgeon to contour the nail to the desired radial bow.

Multiple groups reported outcomes on patients treated with the ForeSight nail. Goa and colleagues evaluated 18 patients with 32 displaced diaphyseal forearm fractures.[18] All patients treated went on to fracture union. Based on the Grace and Eversmann rating system, 13 patients had an excellent or good result, 3 had an acceptable result, and 2 had an unacceptable result. Of the 32 fractures treated, 12 required open reduction and when compared with fractures treated in a closed manner there was a significant difference in time to healing (10 vs 14 weeks). Mean loss of rotation was 32° and the mean Disabilities of the Arm, Shoulder, and Hand (DASH) index scores were 19 indicating mild-to-moderate residual impairment when compared with the uninjured extremity. The incidence of complications was high at 22% and included synostosis, superficial wound infections, without progression to deep infection, and loosening of distal interlocking screws.

Weckbach and colleagues reported the results of 32 patients treated with the ForeSight nail.[19] Radiographic union was seen on average at 3.5 months with union rate of 82%. Complications included nonunion in one patient, delayed union in 2 patients, and radioulnar synostosis in 2 patients. There were no reports of infection. Functionally, 79% demonstrated restoration of motion to greater than 90% of the uninjured extremity. DASH scores in this patient group averaged 13.7. Similarly, Vinsa and colleagues demonstrated the results of the ForeSight nail in 78 patients. Of note, all fractures went on to union with an average time to union of 14.2 weeks.[20] Complications included radioulnar synostosis in 3%, superficial infection in 1 patient and compartment syndrome in 1 patient. Twenty-seven patients ultimately underwent hardware removal with no evidence of refractures. Reported disadvantages of the ForeSight nail included increased operative time required to appropriately contour the nail and the fact that nail insertion often disrupted the desired contour. In addition, authors cited technical difficulty with distal interlock insertion due to the small size of the interlocking screws that may add to operative time needed for free hand placement.

Acumed introduced a radial and ulnar nail with modifications aimed to reduce the challenges reported in the use of the ForeSight nail. Smaller than the Foresight nail, it is available in 3.0 and 3.6 mm diameters and made from titanium rather than stainless steel. The nail was not interchangeable between the radius and ulna but came prebent for either radial or ulnar insertion. It contained only proximal interlocks and in lieu of distal interlocks the nail was fluted with a paddle tip blade to allow for rotational control. This removed the need for a separate distal interlock incision and sought to element the risk of mechanical irritation from prominent distal screws. The prebent nature of the nail aimed to decrease operative time required for nail adjustment reported with the Foresight nail.[19]

Lee and colleagues reported on 38 fractures treated with the Acumed nail and all but one resulted in union with an average time to healing of 14 weeks.[21] Mean pronation and supination was of 85 and 87° in isolated ulna fractures, 84 and 87° in isolated radial fractures and 79 and 81° in both bone fractures. There were no deep infections, radioulnar synostosis, or mechanical irritation. According to the Grace and Eversmann rating system, 81% had an excellent result, 11% had a good result, and 8% had an acceptable result. DASH scores averaged 15 points. Lee noted higher DASH scores were seen in patient's containing concomitant injuries such as humeral fractures and nerve injuries.

He and colleagues looked at 86 adult patients with both bone forearm fractures treated with the Acumed nail.[22] Among them, 85 cases healed successfully with mean time to union of 13.3 weeks. Complications included one hypertrophic nonunion, one radioulnar synostosis, and one extensor pollicis longus injury. Mean DASH score was 15.6 and according to Grace-Eversman criteria, results were excellent in 65 cases, good in 15, acceptable in 5, and poor in 1.

In Germany, Blazevic and colleagues described the use of a novel intramedullary implant with compression screw capability (Treu-Instrumente GmbH, Neuhausen ob ECK, Germany).[8] The compression screw is inserted after interlock insertion and as the screw is tightened it provides tension and compression of the fracture. In the 21 patients reported, overall union rate was 95.24%. Unlike other reports requiring post-operative immobilization, theoretical compression across the fracture allowed for immediate mobilization. Complications included one nonunion, one postoperative rupture of the extensor pollicis longus tendon, and 1 postoperative transitory radial nerve palsy. They did not report on post-operative range of motion or DASH scores.

INDICATIONS

Though plate osteosynthesis remains the gold standard of treatment in adult diaphyseal forearm fractures, it requires additional soft tissue destruction and periosteal stripping disrupting blood supply at the fracture site. Therefore, intramedullary fixation is an adequate alternative in select populations such as mangled extremities, comminuted or segmental fractures, or burns (**Fig. 1** A, B).

Fractures treated with intramedullary implants demonstrate a higher value of whole bone and fracture site blood flow than those treated with plates.[5] In patients with open injuries, severe swelling, mangled limbs, or extensive burns, a traditional extensile excision may not be desirable. In such a population, intramedullary osteosynthesis provides an advantage in quick operative time, a small operative incision and minimal disruption in periosteal blood supply.[5,8,21,23–26] The surgical field is distanced from the site of injury and hardware remains protected in comparison to extraosseous plates. In a similar light, segmental or comminuted fractures require an extensive surgical incision, and the surgeon is often limited by the length of plates available to span the fracture. The working length of an intramedullary implant is superior to plate fixation and can effectively span comminuted or segmental fractures with acceptable restoration of alignment (**Fig. 2** A, B).

Post-operatively, the need for plate removal and subsequent refracture after removal has been described as a disadvantage to plate osteosynthesis.[27,28] If needed, intramedullary nails can be removed at ease with small incisions and decreases the risk of re-fracture as multiple drill holes are not required. It must be noted that intramedullary

implants are biomechanically inferior to plate fixation and may require post-operative immobilization for an extended period that prevents early post-operative range of motion.[21]

Intramedullary fixation has also been described as an alternative indication in the treatment of non-union. Davis and colleagues looked at 9 patients with infected non-union of diaphyseal forearm fractures treated with serial debridement, antibiotic spacers, and staged reconstruction using allograft and intramedullary fixation.[29] They found all patients achieved union without recurrence of infection with substantial improvement of pain and function. Yet, patients often required additional debridement and autologous bone grafting.

Blazevic and colleagues described the use of intermedullary nailing in a small subset of patients who went onto non-union following plate fixation. All included patients went onto union, though the time to union was longer averaging approximately 17 weeks.[8] Hong and colleagues reported on 26 non-unions of diaphyseal forearm fractures that were treated with interlocking intramedullary nails and iliac bone grafts.[30] Around 96% of patients went onto union, yet functional outcomes in their patient cohort were less than those compared with plate osteosynthesis. Hong and colleagues hypothesized that the functional deficits might be related to prolonged immobilization and inadequate restoration of the radial bow. In select cases

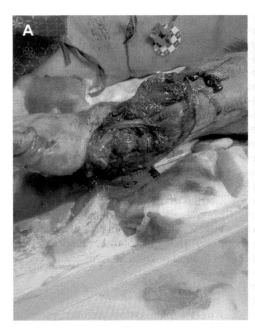
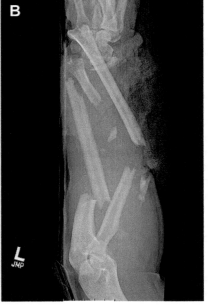

Fig. 1. (*A, B*) Clinical photo and injury film of a mangled extremity with severe degloving injury following a motor vehicle accident with underlying segmental both bone forearm fracture. This injury was treated with serial irrigation and debridement and stabilization with an ulnar intramedullary nail. Intramedullary fixation can be used in this case to prevent further soft tissue compromise with additional surgical incisions.

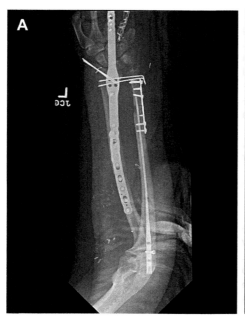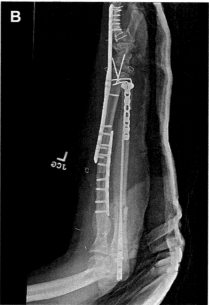

Fig. 2. (A, B) Post-operative radiographs of an intramedullary ulnar nail used to provide inherent stability for the segmental ulna fracture which was supplemented with plate fixation.

of non-union, intramedullary nailing might be an adequate option but based on the findings of Hong and colleagues, intramedullary nailing of nonunion should not be considered an adequate alternative to plate fixation.

Intramedullary implants may also be used in prophylactic fixation of pathological fractures. Prophylactic fixation is seen frequently in other long bones and allows for stability and pain relief in patients with skeletal metastases. One case report describes improved independent function after prophylactic intramedullary nailing for metastatic disease in bilateral forearms.[31]

CONTRAINDICATIONS

Several contraindications to forearm nailing have been described. Fractures extending into the proximal or distal metaphysis and articular surfaces typically are not amenable to intramedullary implants. Active infection in any long bone diaphysis is a contraindication to placing an intramedullary device. Canal size, due to the limited available implants, is often a limiting factor and intramedullary devices should not be used when the canal is less than 3 mm.

PITFALLS AND COMPLICATIONS

As mentioned, the major complication associated with intramedullary nail (IMN) of forearm fractures

is increased risk of non-union and malunion when compared with plating. Other risks described included EPL rupture, PIN palsy, transient radial nerve palsy, and radioulnar synostosis.

Non-union and malunion are often attributed to inadequate restoration of radial bow and implant stability. Historically, high complication rates were reported in unlocked nails.[7,14] Interlocked nails have improved union and malunion rate by providing greater rotational control, maintenance of length, and the ability to begin early range of motion. Mismatch between nail size and the medullary canal may increase side-to-side and rotary movements if the nail is too small. Conversely, if the implant is too large, overstuffing the canal makes insertion difficult and may lead to further comminution or fracture.[18] Malalignment may also occur and pre-bending the nail to match the patient's native anatomy must be performed carefully. Under or over bending may alter the desired radial bow affecting outcomes such as rotation and grip strength.[32] In addition, the surgeon must be conscious of changing the nail contour during insertion especially if resistance is met. Malalignment greater than 10% in any direction will lead to significant functional loss of forearm rotation as described in a biomechanical study by Matthews and colleagues.[33]

Extensor pollicis longus rupture may occur acutely during radial nail insertion and postoperatively due to the relation of the radial nail entry point and the EPL tendon, [8,32] Posterior interosseous nerve injury may occur when placing the proximal interlocking screw in the radial nail. Thus the proximal screw should be inserted with the forearm in neutral position from direct lateral entry within 3 cm from the radial head.[34] Regardless of the method of treatment, radioulnar synostosis may occur with 1% to 8% of fractures of the forearm.[35] Synostosis is more common with proximal fractures, high-energy trauma, infection, concomitant head injuries, and comminuted or open fractures.[32]

PROCEDURAL APPROACH

- *Pre-operative:* It is critical to review contralateral radiographs of the unaffected extremity prior to surgical intervention (**Fig. 3**A–O). Two view radiographs should be studied to determine length, canal diameter, and the contour of the nail. Radiographic protocols have been described to quantify the position and magnitude of radial bow.[36]
- *Positioning:* Typically the patient will be positioned supine on a radiolucent table, though lateral positioning may also be used.
- *Radial approach and insertion:*
  - A 2 to 3 cm incision is made radial to lister's tubercle between the extensor pollicis longus and extensor carpi ulnaris tendons approximately 5 mm proximal from the articular surface.
  - Dissection should be carried out carefully to avoid branches of superficial radial nerve.
- *Ulnar approach and insertion:*
  - The olecranon should be palpated and a 1 to 2 cm vertical incision is made proximal tip of the olecranon. A small vertical incision is then made splitting the triceps insertion to allow enough space for an opening awl to be used (see **Fig. 3** C, D).
- *Nail insertion:*
  - After the starting point has been identified with an awl (see **Fig. 3**B), a handheld entry reamer is used to create a portal for nail entry. A 1.9 mm Kirshner wires may also be used to create the portal.
  - A handheld reamer is then passed and may be used to aid in closed reduction of the fracture (see **Fig. 3**D, E)
- If closed reduction cannot be performed with the assistance of the handheld reamer a small incision can be made to aid in fracture reduction.
  - Manually ream should be a size of 0.5 to 1.0 mm greater than the nail diameter (see **Fig. 3**F).

- The final reamer should be left in place to maintain reduction while approaching other fractures (see **Fig. 3**G, H).
  - Of note, for fractures involving both the radius and ulna, the ulna is typically reduced first as it is largely straight and acts as a strut to aid in the reduction of the radius.
- Appropriate nail length is determined by direct measurement off the reamer and should be confirmed radiographically.
- After the appropriate nail is selected the reamer must be removed prior to nail insertion. Owing to canal size, forearm nails are not cannulated, thus reamers and guidewires must be removed. It is critical to carefully preform this step to prevent malreduction with guidewire removal or nail insertion. After removal, the nail is inserted just short of the subchondral bone distally.
- Radiographs should be taken after nail insertion and prior to interlock placement to ensure adequate nail position and fracture reduction (see **Fig. 3**K, L).
- Interlock screws are then placed with either an aiming guide or by freehand techniques depending on the implant system used, typically self-tapping 3.5 mm screws are used.
  - Radial interlocking screws are inserted dorsal to volar distally.
  - Ulnar interlocking screws are inserted lateral to medial proximally (see **Fig. 3**K, L).
- Fracture reduction, nail, and interlock position should be verified fluoroscopically through range of motion before closure (see **Fig. 3**M–O).

RECOVERY AND REHABILITATION

Multiple postoperative protocols are described and include both immediate range of motion and immobilization. Lee and colleagues immobilized all patients post-operatively and transitioned to a hinged elbow brace at the first post-operative visit with discontinuation of the brace at 6 weeks allowing patients to begin pronation and supination.[21] Hong and colleagues immobilized patients based on satisfaction of fracture fixation and fracture location. Immobilized patients underwent progressive range of motion on subsequent visits.[18] In contrast, Weckbach and colleagues allowed unlimited active and passive range of motion of elbow, wrist, and forearm post-operatively.[19] The choice to immobilize is based upon a combination of surgeon preference, injury pattern, and the perceived adequacy of fixation obtained.

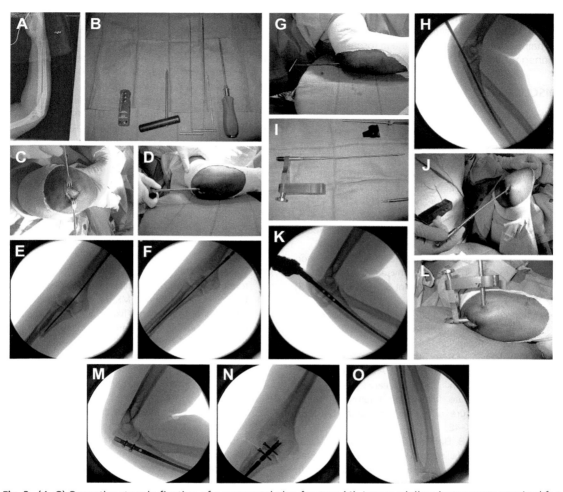

Fig. 3. (*A–O*) Operative steps in fixation of a segmental ulna fracture (*A*). Intramedullary instruments required for nail fixation are seen from left to right including a targeting device for locking screw insertion, opening awl, 3.0 and 3.7 mm hand reamers, drills bit, and screwdriver (*B*). A 2 cm incision is made over the olecranon and the triceps in split vertically to allow access to the proximal ulna, the elbow is flexed, and shoulder is abducted to 90° (*C*). The awl is inserted in line with the proximal ulna with the elbow rested on the C-arm machine (*D*). Insertion of the handheld reamed to the level of the fracture is used to aid in reduction of the fracture (*E*). Following reduction, the reamer is passed beyond the fracture to maintain reduction and left in place (*F* and *G*). A lateral XR shows the handheld reamer in proper position at the ulnar entry point and the fracture reduction is maintained (*H*). The ulnar nail with the targeting device for the proximal interlocking screws (see **Fig. 1**). Insertion of the nail after the reamer has been removed with a lateral fluoroscopic image of the nail in place and the aiming guide for proximal interlocking screws (*J, K, L*). Final fluoroscopic images of the final construct in place with maintain fracture reduction (*M, N, O*). (*From* Rehman S, Sokunbi G. Intramedullary fixation of forearm fractures. Hand Clin. 2010;26(3):391-vii; with permission.)

Prolonged immobilization may lead to inferior functional outcomes, while immediate range of motion may stress construct strength leading to an increased as non-union rate; however, this has not been formally investigated.

Summary

Intramedullary fixation of forearm fractures is an adequate option in select patients. Injuries with significant soft tissue compromise such as open fractures, mangled extremities, or significant burns may benefit from intramedullary fixation. Palliative fixation of pathologic forearm fractures may also be amenable to intramedullary implants as may segmental fractures. Outcomes continue to improve with greater control of length and rotation of newer locked implants. Surgical technique and pre-operative planning are critical to restore forearm radial bow and prevent shortening or angulation with intramedullary nails. Outside of this select patient population, plate osteosynthesis remains the treatment of choice in forearm fracture management.

DISCLOSURES

None.

REFERENCES

1. Bartonicek J, Kozanek M, Jupiter JB. History of operative treatment of forearm diaphyseal fractures. J Hand Surg Am 2014;39(2):335–42.
2. Jupiter JB, Kellam JF, Browner BD. In: Skeletal Trauma: Basic Science, Management, and Reconstruction, 1, 4th ed. Elsevier; 2009. p. 1459–98.
3. Anderson LD, Sisk D, Tooms RE, et al. Compression-plate fixation in acute diaphyseal fractures of the radius and ulna. J Bone Joint Surg Am 1975;57(3):287–97.
4. Chapman MW, Gordon JE, Zissimos AG. Compression-plate fixation of acute fractures of the diaphyses of the radius and ulna. J Bone Joint Surg Am 1989;71(2):159–69.
5. Rand JA, An KN, Chao EY, et al. A comparison of the effect of open intramedullary nailing and compression-plate fixation on fracture-site blood flow and fracture union. J Bone Joint Surg Am 1981;63(3):427–42.
6. Zhao L, Wang B, Bai X, et al. Plate Fixation Versus Intramedullary Nailing for Both-Bone Forearm Fractures: A Meta-analysis of Randomized Controlled Trials and Cohort Studies. World J Surg 2017;41(3):722–33.
7. Sage FP, Smith H. Medullary fixation of forearm fractures. J Bone Joint Surg Am 1957;39-A(1):91–8.
8. Blazevic D, Bencic I, Cuti T, et al. Intramedullary nailing of adult forearm fractures: Results and complications. Injury 2021;52(Suppl 5):S44–8. https://doi.org/10.1016/j.injury.2020.11.012.
9. Lees VC. The functional anatomy of forearm rotation. J Hand Microsurg. Dec 2009;1(2):92–9.
10. Green DP, Wolfe Scott W. Green's operative hand surgery. Philadelphia: Elsevier/Churchill Livingstone; 2011.
11. Schöne G. Zur behandlung von vorderarmfrakturen mit bolzung. Munch Med Wochenschr 1913;60:2327.
12. Lambrinudi C. Intra-Medullary Kirschner Wires in the Treatment of Fractures. Proceedings of the Royal Society of Medicine 1940;33(3):153–7.
13. Knight RA, Purvis GD. Fractures of both bones of the forearm in adults. J Bone Joint Surg Am 1949;31a(4):755–64.
14. Sage FP. Medullary fixation of fractures of the forearm. A study of the medullary canal of the radius and a report of fifty fractures of the radius treated with a prebent triangular nail. J Bone Joint Surg Am 1959;41-A:1489–516.
15. Boriani S, Lefevre C, Malingue E, et al. The Lefevre ulnar nail. Chir Organi Mov 1991;76(2):151–5.
16. De Pedro JA, Garcia-Navarrete F, Garcia De Lucas F, et al. Internal fixation of ulnar fractures by locking nail. Clin Orthop Relat Res 1992;(283):81–5.
17. Crenshaw AH, Zinar DM, Pickering RM. Intramedullary nailing of forearm fractures. Instr Course Lect 2002;51:279–89.
18. Gao H, Luo CF, Zhang CQ, et al. Internal fixation of diaphyseal fractures of the forearm by interlocking intramedullary nail: short-term results in eighteen patients. J Orthop Trauma 2005;19(6):384–91.
19. Weckbach A, Blattert TR, Weisser C. Interlocking nailing of forearm fractures. Arch Orthop Trauma Surg 2006;126(5):309–15.
20. Visna P, Beitl E, Pilny J, et al. Interlocking nailing of forearm fractures. Acta Chir Belg 2008;108(3):333–8.
21. Lee YH, Lee SK, Chung MS, et al. Interlocking contoured intramedullary nail fixation for selected diaphyseal fractures of the forearm in adults. J Bone Joint Surg Am 2008;90(9):1891–8.
22. He HY, Zhang JZ, Wang XW, et al. [Acumed intramedullary nail for the treatment of adult diaphyseal both-bone forearm fractures]. Zhong Guo Gu Shang 2018;31(9):803–7.
23. Dehghan N, Schemitsch EH. Intramedullary nail fixation of non-traditional fractures: Clavicle, forearm, fibula. Injury 2017;48(Suppl 1):S41–6.
24. Saka G, Saglam N, Kurtulmus T, et al. New interlocking intramedullary radius and ulna nails for treating forearm diaphyseal fractures in adults: a retrospective study. Injury 2014;45(Suppl 1):S16–23.
25. Al-Sadek TA, Niklev D, Al-Sadek A. Diaphyseal Fractures of the Forearm in Adults, Plating Or Intramedullary Nailing Is a Better Option for the Treatment? Open Access Maced J Med Sci 2016;4(4):670–3.
26. Schulte LM, Meals CG, Neviaser RJ. Management of adult diaphyseal both-bone forearm fractures. J Am Acad Orthop Surg 2014;22(7):437–46.
27. Rosson JW, Shearer JR. Refracture after the removal of plates from the forearm. An avoidable complication. J Bone Joint Surg Br 1991;73(3):415–7.
28. Hidaka S, Gustilo RB. Refracture of bones of the forearm after plate removal. J Bone Joint Surg Am 1984;66(8):1241–3.
29. Davis JA, Choo A, O'Connor DP, et al. Treatment of Infected Forearm Nonunions With Large Complete Segmental Defects Using Bulk Allograft and Intramedullary Fixation. J Hand Surg Am 2016;41(9):881–7.
30. Hong G, Cong-Feng L, Hui-Peng S, et al. Treatment of diaphyseal forearm nonunions with interlocking intramedullary nails. Clin Orthop Relat Res 2006;450:186–92.

31. Martin WN, Field J, Kulkarni M. Intramedullary nailing of pathological forearm fractures. Injury 2002; 33(6):530–2.

32. Yorukoglu AC, Demirkan AF, Akman A, et al. The effects of radial bowing and complications in intramedullary nail fixation of adult forearm fractures. Eklem Hastalik Cerrahisi 2017;28(1):30–4.

33. Matthews LS, Kaufer H, Garver DF, et al. The effect on supination-pronation of angular malalignment of fractures of both bones of the forearm. J Bone Joint Surg Am 1982;64(1):14–7.

34. Tabor OB Jr, Bosse MJ, Sims SH, et al. Iatrogenic posterior interosseous nerve injury: is transosseous static locked nailing of the radius feasible? J Orthop Trauma 1995;9(5):427–9.

35. Schatzker J, Tile M, Axelrod T, et al. Fractures of the Radius and Ulna. In: *The Rationale of Operative Fracture Care*. 3rd ed. Springer; 2005. p. 137–66.

36. Schemitsch EH, Richards RR. The effect of malunion on functional outcome after plate fixation of fractures of both bones of the forearm in adults. J Bone Joint Surg Am 1992;74(7):1068–78.

Proximal Interphalangeal Joint Fractures
Various Approaches to Fixation

Jeremy E. Raducha, MD, Tyler S. Pidgeon, MD*

KEYWORDS

• Proximal interphalangeal joint • Seatbelt • Fixation • Outcomes

KEY POINTS

• There are several viable options for the surgical management of proximal interphalangeal joint fractures.
• All fixation methods have similar outcomes when performed in the appropriate scenario.
• Patients with proximal interphalangeal joint injuries should be prepared for some loss of motion.

INTRODUCTION

Finger proximal interphalangeal (PIP) joint fractures and fracture dislocations can present with various patterns and chronicity. This variability necessitates multiple treatment options and fixation constructs that should be based on fracture personality and surgeon experience. It is important to understand the typical presentation of these injuries, relevant anatomy, indications for surgery, and treatment options to promptly and properly care for these difficult injuries. Even with optimal management, these injuries commonly result in decreased range of motion and grip strength.[1-3]

Relevant Anatomy

The PIP joint of the finger is a highly concentric joint, in which the bony articulation provides inherent stability. There is an intercondylar groove on the head of the proximal phalanx matching a central ridge on the base of the middle phalanx, which minimizes rotational movement.[3,4] The volar buttress of the base of the middle phalanx (**Fig. 1**), in which the articular surface extends further volarly than dorsally, is also essential to prevent dorsal dislocations of the middle phalanx. The volar buttress allows continued articulation at greater than 90° of flexion and is accommodated by the volar subcapital recess of the proximal phalanx.[5] This allows the PIP joint a 100 to 120° arc of total motion.[3] The volar buttress must be restored in the surgical management of dorsal PIP joint fracture dislocations.

The soft tissue attachments of the PIP joint are also important for its stability and function. The central slip of the extensor tendon inserts on the proximal aspect of the dorsal middle phalanx to allow for PIP joint extension. The volar plate attaches to the volar base of the middle phalanx as a thick, fibrocartilaginous structure, and proximally to the neck of the proximal phalanx via radial and ulnar checkrein ligaments with a thin membranous center.[6] This anatomy allows the volar plate to fold on itself proximally to accommodate deep flexion of the PIP joint while also having strong enough attachments to prevent hyperextension of the PIP joint. However, this anatomy also explains why the PIP joint is prone to loss of motion following injury. Scarring around the checkrein ligaments on the proximal volar plate prevents folding needed for deep flexion and can also limit extension if scarred in a flexed position. The radial and ulnar collateral ligaments prevent varus and valgus deformity of the joint. The primary collateral ligaments extend from the condyles on the proximal phalanx head to the volar third of the middle

Hand, Upper Extremity and Microvascular Surgery, Department of Orthopaedic Surgery, Duke University Medical Center, Durham, NC 27710, USA
* Corresponding author.
E-mail address: tyler.pidgeon@duke.edu

Hand Clin 39 (2023) 561–573
https://doi.org/10.1016/j.hcl.2023.05.005
0749-0712/23/

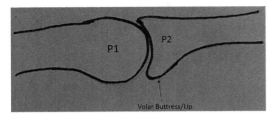

Fig. 1. Volar buttress of the middle phalanx (P2) articular surface.

phalanx base and function mostly in 30° of joint flexion. The accessory collateral ligaments extend from the proximal phalanx head to the volar plate and function in full extension.[3,6,7] Together with the volar plate, the collateral ligaments create a three-sided box around the PIP joint ensuring stability (**Fig. 2**). Understanding the importance of certain anatomic structures to PIP joint can help guide treatment to ensure the ultimate goal of a stable joint with a maximal arc of motion.

Diagnosis

Patients with PIP joint injuries commonly present with a history of a "jammed finger," which can occur frequently in ball catching and contact sports.[8,9] Patients may also describe a "crooked finger" that needed to be "put back in place." The differential diagnosis of these injuries includes collateral ligament sprain, volar plate avulsion/sprain, central slip disruptions, simple dislocations, fracture dislocations, and pilon-type fractures.[3] Unfortunately, due to this broad differential, these injuries are frequently disregarded as less severe and can present in a delayed fashion.

When a patient presents acutely with concern for a PIP joint injury, it is important to take a thorough history to determine the timing and circumstances of injury as well as any prior injuries to that joint. Long-term functional goals for work, sports, or activities of daily living should be discussed. The direction of dislocation can help narrow down which structure may be injured. Dorsal dislocations are most common and occur with an axial force applied to a slightly flexed finger. They can result in tearing of the collateral ligaments as well as soft tissue or bony avulsion of the volar plate from the base of the middle phalanx. Volar dislocations occur with axial loading of an extended or hyperextended finger and usually result in injury to the central slip. Lateral dislocations can injure the collateral ligaments, and volar rotatory dislocations occur when a rotational force is added to an axial load, resulting in buttonholing of the proximal phalanx head between the central slip and lateral band. This can block closed reduction, particularly if axial traction and joint extension are used during the closed reduction attempt.[3]

A thorough physical examination is essential to determine the stability of the joint. A range of motion examination after reduction of dislocations will allow you to determine if the joint is stable through a normal arc of motion and whether the injury can

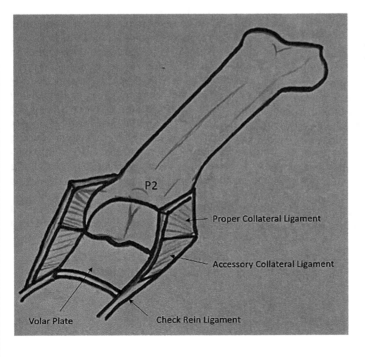

Fig. 2. The collateral ligaments and volar plate of the proximal interphalangeal joint form a three-sided "box" around joint to increase stability.

be managed nonoperatively. A digital nerve block with local anesthetic may be required to obtain an accurate examination if pain is a limiting factor.[10] The collateral ligaments should then be examined in both full extension to assess the accessory collaterals and 30° of flexion to assess the proper collaterals. In volar dislocations, the central slip should also be evaluated using the Elson test, as missed or mismanaged central slip injuries can lead to Boutonniere deformities.[11]

Imaging

PIP joint injury workup should start with plain radiographs focused on the finger of concern. Generalized hand radiographs will not likely provide adequate images particularly on the lateral. The anterior-posterior and lateral images should be assessed to evaluate primarily the congruity of the joint but also size and level of comminution of fracture fragments. The V-sign on a perfect lateral view of the finger indicates subtle dorsal subluxation of the middle phalanx[3] (**Fig. 3**). This finding is commonly missed, and incongruent joints are thought to be stable following closed reduction. If available, a live fluoroscopic view throughout a range of motion can also be useful to assess dynamic joint stability.

A computed tomography (CT) scan, while not routine, can be useful if there is a question of joint incongruity, in chronic fractures to assess bone quality, or in complex fractures to assist with surgical planning. Specifically, they can help better define fracture fragment size and orientation in pilon-type fractures and unicondylar proximal phalanx head fractures (**Fig. 4**). In general, other advanced imaging, such as MRI does not provide additional helpful information in the acute setting for these injuries.

Classification

There are several classification methods for PIP joint injuries, but the most clinically useful is to classify them by joint stability. They are then subclassified by the direction of dislocation or type of fracture as these different patterns have different stability parameters. The most commonly referenced system was described by Kiefhaber and Stern (**Table 1**). This system helps determine management. For example, dorsal fracture dislocations with less than 30% joint surface involvement are typically stable and can be managed nonoperatively, whereas fractures with greater than 50% of joint surface involvement are unstable requiring operative intervention.[12] However, it is important to note that there are always exceptions

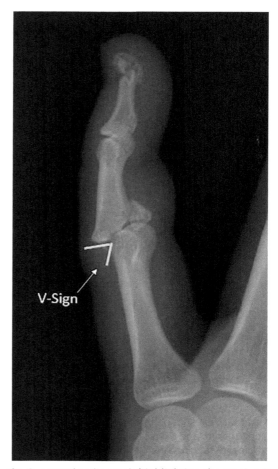

Fig. 3. Lateral radiograph highlighting the "V-sign."

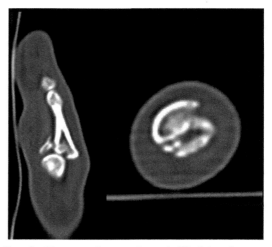

Fig. 4. CT scan of comminuted PIP joint fracture dislocation.

Table 1
Kiefhaber and Stern stability-based classification of proximal interphalangeal fracture dislocations

Pattern	% Articular Involvement	Stability	Treatment
Dorsal fracture dislocation (volar lip fragment)	<30%	Stable	Splinting
	30%–50%	Tenuous	Splinting if reduced in <30% of flexion
			Operative fixation otherwise
	>50%	Unstable	Operative fixation
Volar fracture dislocation (dorsal lip fragment)	<50%	Stable	Splinting if no volar subluxation of middle phalanx
			Operative fixation otherwise
	>50%	Unstable	Operative fixation
Pilon fracture	Any	Unstable	

Adapted from Kiefhaber TR, Stern PJ. Fracture dislocations of the proximal interphalangeal joint. J Hand Surg Am. 1998;23(3):368-380. https://doi.org/10.1016/S0363-5023(05)80454-X; with permission.

to these rules and a detailed evaluation is still necessary to determine joint stability.

TREATMENT

The first step in any treatment algorithm is to reduce any dislocations and then assess stability of the joint both clinically and radiographically. From there, a branching web of treatment options based on fracture type and direction, stability, chronicity, and surgeon preference is used (**Figs. 5** and **6**). This section briefly reviews the main surgical options and then goes into detail on a newer surgical plating technique known as the "Seatbelt" procedure.[13]

Nonoperative Management

Simple dislocations and fracture dislocations that are stable after closed reduction can be managed nonoperatively. If stable throughout an entire range of motion, they can be managed with buddy taping to prevent hyperextension and allow for immediate range of motion. Fractures that are unstable in full extension but require less than 30° of flexion to remain stable can be managed by dorsal block splinting to prevent motion beyond the stable range. These patients can also be allowed early range of motion to prevent stiffness. If the joint requires greater than 30° of flexion to remain stable then operative intervention is indicated.

Operative Management

The list of operative treatment options for PIP joint fractures, and fracture dislocations, is extensive,[3,13–20] and all of these procedures can be technically demanding. As is the case with many injuries with numerous surgical techniques, there is no consensus as to which technique is best—

most techniques produce similar outcomes. The treatment decision comes down to the characteristics of the individual patient, fracture, and surgeon to decide on the proper technique.

Kirschner wire (K-wire) only fixation can involve extension block pinning or trans-articular pinning. Extension block pinning involves a K-wire inserted percutaneously and retrograde into the proximal phalanx head between the central slip and lateral band with the PIP joint flexed to prevent joint extension beyond the stable range of motion. This is similar to dorsal block splinting but may be more reliable. This can be performed with or without pinning of the fracture fragment itself.[3] Trans-articular pinning involves passing a K-wire from the middle phalanx across the joint and into the proximal phalanx with the PIP joint reduced.[14] For both techniques, the pin is typically removed in 3 to 4 weeks. These procedures are quick and do not require an open approach to the fracture; however, trans-articular pinning does not allow for early range of motion and both techniques may not optimally restore anatomy.

Open reduction and internal fixation are a treatment option for unstable fractures that have a reconstructable joint surface. It can be performed for volar fragments, dorsal fragments, or pilon injuries. An open approach to the joint is required. For volar fractures, this typically requires "shotgunning" the joint open by releasing the volar plate and collateral ligaments allowing for visualization of the entire articular surface. Fixation constructs range from 1 to 1.5 mm inter-fragmentary screws alone, to plate and screw constructs, to cerclage wiring.[3,13,14,18,21] This allows for more anatomic fixation of the fracture with the opportunity to directly evaluate the articular surface reduction. The "Seatbelt" procedure is performed through a shotgun approach and is designed to restore and

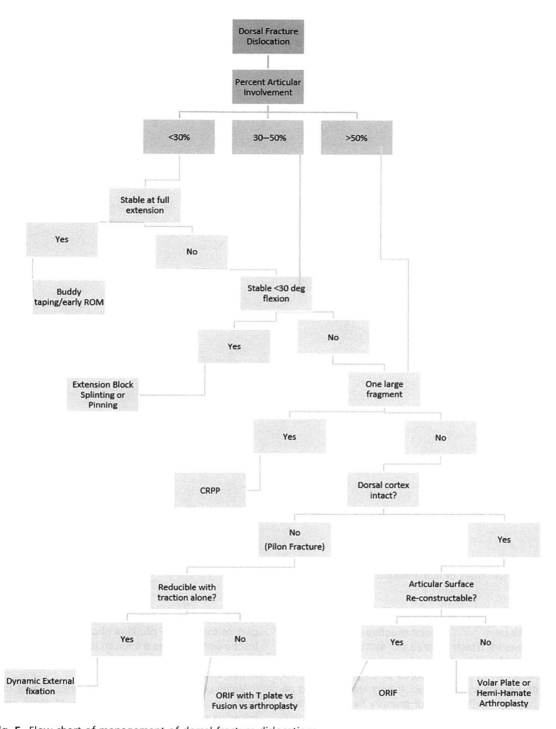

Fig. 5. Flow chart of management of dorsal fracture dislocations.

buttress the volar lip of the base of the middle phalanx as well as raft the articular surface after reduction. This provides stable fixation using a low-profile construct (**Fig. 7**). The detailed surgical technique for this procedure will be described in the next section.

Dynamic external fixation (**Fig. 8**) uses ligamentotaxis to reduce the articular surface in fractures

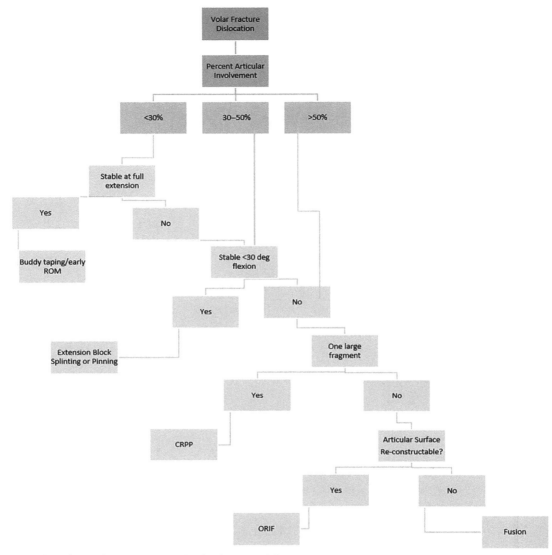

Fig. 6. Flow chart of management of volar fracture dislocations.

where the joint alignment is acceptable with traction alone.[3,15,22] The joint reactive forces are thus decreased which decreases settling of articular fragments. This method is most commonly used to treat pilon-type fractures or large lip fractures with severe comminution. It can also be used as a backup method if your primary fixation method does not achieve a congruent and stable joint. The typical construct requires three K-wires and dental elastic bands. Two K-wires are inserted perpendicular to the long axis of the finger, through the rotational center of the proximal and middle phalangeal heads, respectively. The proximal wire is left long and bent into hooks so that the ends are distal to the hooks of the more distal

wire. The third wire is then inserted in the mid-axial part of the middle phalanx shaft just distal to the fracture and acts as a fulcrum to block dorsal subluxation. The rubber bands are then applied between two sets of hooks.

Volar plate and hemi-hamate arthroplasty can both be indicated in the setting of large very comminuted volar lip fractures which are not amenable to open reduction and internal fixation and also do not reduce with traction alone, negating dynamic external fixation. They are also indicated in delayed fracture presentations with chronic subluxation/dislocation but without significant arthritic changes. Both techniques require an intact dorsal cortex to accommodate fixation.

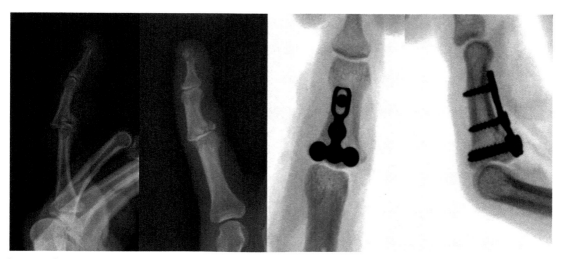

Fig. 7. Radiographs depicting a dorsal PIP fracture dislocation, which was surgically fixed using a variation of the Seatbelt technique.

Volar plate arthroplasty essentially resurfaces the comminuted portion of the volar articular surface with the volar plate. Up to 40% to 50% of the articular surface can be resurfaced using this technique.[20] This can be limited based on the size and excursion of the volar plate. Attempting to resurface too large an area will require significant joint flexion to allow the volar plate to reach the intact dorsal cortex and may result in flexion contracture. A volar approach is made to the joint and it is "shot gunned" open. The fracture fragments are excised, and a transverse groove is shaped at the edge of the intact articular surface. The volar plate is then released radially and ulnarly from the collaterals for mobilization and advanced into the transverse groove. It is tied down through two drill holes in the dorsal cortex, either outside of the skin over a dorsal button or beneath the skin on the dorsal cortex between the central slip and lateral band. Caution must be taken not to entrap the lateral bands with the sutures. The PIP joint is then typically pinned at 30° flexion for 3 weeks to protect the repair.

The hemi-hamate arthroplasty technique was first described by Hastings in 2002.[23] It can be used for fractures involving greater than 50% of the articular surface as long as there is an intact dorsal cortex for fixation and a large enough graft can be harvested. It has been shown to have fewer recurrent dislocations than volar plate arthroplasty.[24] To complete the procedure, a volar approach to the PIP joint is performed, the joint is "shot gunned" open, and the fracture fragments are removed. The autograft is then harvested from the dorsal distal hamate between the fourth and fifth metacarpals. This section of the

carpometacarpal joint has an articular surface anatomy similar to that of the volar half of the middle phalanx base. The graft is harvested with a combination of saws and osteotomes and flipped around to position in the prepared recipient site on the middle phalanx. It is important to keep the nonarticular portion of the graft thicker than the articular portion to recreate the volar buttress when the graft is positioned.[23,25] The graft is secured in place with 3 1.0 to 1.5 mm screws. The finger is then reduced and the volar plate is then reattached.

Surgical Technique (The Seatbelt Procedure)

- A volar approach to the proximal phalangeal joint is performed using a Bruner approach or a combination of a mid-lateral and Bruner incision.
  - Consider making the combination mid-lateral and Bruner flap radially based in the index and middle fingers and ulnarly based in the ring and small fingers to minimize contact hypersensitivity.
- The flexor sheath should be incised between the A2 and A4 pulleys and the flexor tendons retracted.
  - Consider raising the sheath between the A2 and A4 pulleys as a radially or ulnarly based flap (opposite direction of the skin flap), which can be used at the end of the case to help cover the plate, thereby protecting the flexor tendons.
- Both neurovascular bundles should then be liberally mobilized to prevent traction injuries with joint manipulation.

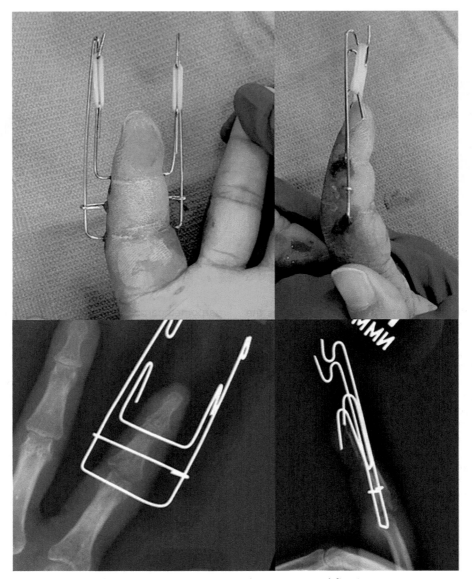

Fig. 8. Clinical and radiographic images demonstrating a dynamic external fixation construct.

- The volar plate is then released from its distal attachment on the middle phalanx, and the collaterals are released from their proximal attachments on the proximal phalanx. This will now allow the PIP joint to be hyper-extended and "shot gunned" open.
  - Extreme caution should be used to avoid fracturing the intact dorsal cortex/articular surface of the middle phalanx. If this occurs, the procedure will have to be aborted to another procedure (eg, dynamic external fixation) as the screws through the Seatbelt plate will not be able to achieve purchase.

- The entire middle phalanx articular surface should now be visible.
- The articular surface can then be elevated and the fracture fragments reduced with a dental pick.
- Cancellous bone autograft or allograft can be inserted beneath the articular surface if needed in the case of bone loss or severe impaction.
- This reduction can then be pinned in place with 0.028- or 0.035-inch K-wires if needed
  - It is sometimes helpful to apply the plate and pin through the plate with k-wires.

The k-wires can then be sequentially removed and replaced with screws.

- A three-hole 1.3- or 1.5-mm transverse plate is then made by cutting the end of a corresponding T-plate.
  - A tail can be left on the plate if more buttress effect is desired; however, the original technique calls only for a three-hole plate placed perpendicular to the long axis to the middle phalanx directly over the volar lip.
- The plate is positioned centrally on the volar surface to avoid the radial and ulnar slips of the flexor digitorum superficialis and capture the volar lip of the base of the middle phalanx.
- Three non-locking screws are then inserted through the plate to raft the articular surface and fix it to the dorsal cortex.
  - This functions similarly to a rim plate on a tibial plateau fracture.
  - The screws must be bicortical and achieve purchase through the distal cortex. Slight prominence is not a concern dorsally because this area is the insertion of the central slip; therefore, gliding of the lateral bands should not be affected.
- The joint is then reduced and alignment and range of motion assessed.
- The volar plate is then repaired to cover the plate and prevent prominence. The authors do not routinely repair the collateral ligaments.
- A lateral fluoroscopic view in flexion and extension is viewed to confirm joint congruity and stability. It must be stable enough to start early active motion.
- Place the patient in dorsal blocking splint at 30° of flexion until their first therapy visit to prevent undue stress on the volar plate repair.
- Start rehabilitation within 7 days postoperatively with the early active motion protocol of your choice.
  - An earlier start to therapy is desirable if possible.
- Tips:
  - Sharp dissection and meticulous soft tissue handling are key.
  - Have a backup plan construct in case the comminution is irreducible or the dorsal cortex/articular surface is fractured.

REHABILITATION

In general, the goal of all surgical and nonsurgical options for the treatment of PIP joint dislocation, fractures, and fracture dislocations is to restore joint congruity and alignment. Secondarily, it is optimal, if possible, to have a joint stable enough

to start early active range of motion to decrease the risk of post-traumatic joint stiffness. Patients should see a hand therapist within a few days of surgery to start their active motion protocol. Between exercises, patients are immobilized in a dorsal block splint or ulnar gutter splint.[3,13,16,18] The amount of initial extension allowed depends on the treatment method. If stable in the operating room, dynamic external fixation and open reduction and internal fixation may allow for immediate full extension and full flexion with therapy. Dorsal block pinning will prevent full extension until at least 3 to 4 weeks post-op when there is enough fracture healing to remove the pin.[3,14] Similarly, volar plate arthroplasty typically involves dorsal block pinning at 30° of flexion postoperatively to protect the volar plate repair for 3 weeks.[20] Hemi-hamate arthroplasty also limits full extension with dorsal block splinting at 10 to 20° flexion for 3 to 4 weeks to allow for early healing.[24] Even when PIP joint motion is partially restricted, full distal interphalangeal joint (DIP) and metacarpophalangeal joint (MCP) joint motion is typically allowed.

After the initial healing period of 3 to 4 weeks, patients with extension restrictions have their range of motion advanced as tolerated. K-wires are removed at this point. At 5 to 6 weeks post-op, dynamic or static progressive splinting can be started to regain full motion if there is residual stiffness.[3,20]

Athletes can expect to return to sports around 8 weeks postoperatively, but they should continue with buddy taping during sports for 4 to 6 months. The range of motion improvements can still be seen up to 1 year postoperatively.[3,20,26]

OUTCOMES

Even in cases of optimized management, PIP joint fractures and fracture dislocations still typically result in the loss of motion and potentially suboptimal outcomes.[1,2] This can be difficult for some patients to come to terms with, as many people do not consider a finger injury as a "bad problem." It is important to set realistic expectations with patients early to prepare them for potentially poor outcomes.

Demino and colleagues published a systematic review comparing the outcomes of several methods for the surgical management of PIP joint injuries.[1] They collected data from 48 studies including range of motion, grip strength, patient-reported outcome measures, and complications. They found many similarities in outcomes despite the fixation method, with no treatment being clearly superior to others. Percutaneous K-wire fixation and extension block pinning had the highest average postoperative range of motion at 86.5°

and 83.6°, respectively, whereas hemi-hamate arthroplasty had the lowest average range of motion at 79.3°. However, it can be difficult to interpret this difference as hemi-hamate arthroplasty is typically performed for more severe injuries and chronic fractures, which would be expected to have worse range of motion outcomes. Overall, dorsal fracture dislocations had better patient-reported outcomes than pilon-type fractures with an overall average range of motion of 83.2°, grip strength of 91% of the contralateral side, and Quick-Disabilities of the Arm, Shoulder, and Hand (DASH) score of 6.6.

Another systematic review by Gianakos and colleagues had similar findings (**Table 2**). They reported percutaneous pinning to have a reasonable average postoperative range of motion of 90.2°, but they found volar plate arthroplasty to have the highest average motion at 90.6°. Hemi-hamate arthroplasty and dynamic external fixation produced lower range of motion averages at 79.8° and 79.7° respectively, which is similar to other studies.[19,24] Hemi-hamate and open reduction and internal fixation had the best average DASH and Quick-DASH scores. All patients had relatively low average visual analogue score (VAS) scores and similar grip strengths.

The Seatbelt procedure was recently evaluated in 17 patients in a retrospective manner.[13] Those patients had an average delay to the operating room of 21 days after injury and had an average of 7.3 months follow-up. Average PIP and DIP joint range of motion was 77.4 and 61.5°, respectively, which is similar to other treatment options.[1,2] Sixteen out of seventeen joints remained concentric with one subtle subluxation noted on imaging, although it was not clinically symptomatic. Two patients had revision surgery for tenolysis and removal of hardware.

Complications

Postoperative complications vary based on treatment type and are fairly common overall, but most are minor.[2] All fixation methods are associated with postoperative stiffness, extension lag, and persistent pain. To a variable degree, all open surgical approaches can be associated with cold intolerance and nerve sensitivity as the "shot gun" approach can place significant stretch on neurovascular structures if not properly mobilized.

In one of the previously mentioned systematic reviews, although extension block pinning had the greatest average range of motion, it was also the fixation method with the highest rate of residual pain (38.5%) and radiographic post-traumatic osteoarthritis (46.2%). These rates were lower in patients treated with less than 21% articular

involvement, suggesting that pinning may be better suited for smaller fractures. Pinning is also associated with a 15.4% risk of recurrent subluxation and pin site infections.

Dynamic external fixation also has high rates of pin tract infection, ranging from 10% to 30%, but fewer patients complain of residual pain.[2,3,22]

Open reduction and internal fixation complications can include recurrent subluxation which has been recorded as high as 84% in one study but on average it is closer to 21.3%.[2,10] These subluxations are noted radiographically and can be subtle. They do not always correspond with clinical symptoms. However, there are few long-term studies to determine if these subtle subluxations increase the risk of post-traumatic arthritis. Open reduction and internal fixation also carry the risk of hardware prominence and intra-articular penetration of the joint with screws.[16,17] This may necessitate removal of hardware, giving this method revision surgery rates close to 20%.[2]

Volar plate arthroplasty can be associated with 4 to 6 months of postoperative swelling.[3,20,26] There is also a risk of re-displacement and joint subluxation with suture failure, which can occur with overly aggressive rehab. This is one of the reasons pinning is used to prevent early hyperextension after these repairs. The placement of this pin does also have an associated risk of pin tract infections. Suturing of the lateral bands can also occur with this technique, restricting DIP joint motion and causing a contracture.

Hemi-hamate arthroplasty has an overall complication rate as high as 35%.[2,19,24] The rates of secondary procedure for graft nonunion, screw migration, and tenolysis have been recorded at 14.3% on average. These patients can also suffer from prolonged tenderness, graft resorption, and osteoarthritis. Arthritis is likely more prevalent in these patients because this surgery is typically done for more severe injuries.

Revision Options

The main reason revision surgeries are performed is for postoperative stiffness that fails to improve with hand therapy and dynamic or progressive static splinting. Surgical options may include soft tissue release with or without distraction external fixation. These procedures can have good but short-lived results.[27,28] The surgeon and patient should always expect to retain less motion than what is gained back after release intraoperatively. Owing to the PIP joint's frustrating predilection to become stiff after surgery, even aggressive releases have been shown not to increase the risk of postoperative instability. One review of 16

Table 2
Study outcomes

Outcome Measure	Overall	Hemi-Hamate Arthroplasty	Closed Reduction and Kirschner Wire Pinning	Dynamic External Fixation	Open Reduction and Internal Fixation	Extension Block Pinning	Volar Plate Arthroplasty
Device removal(d)	26.6	NA	26 (21–28)	33 (21–49)	NA	21 (20–22)	NA
PIPJ Arc	84.7	79.8 (69–95)	90.2 (85–102)	79.7 (64–90)	82.2 (66–100)	82.7 (80–85)	90.6 (85–94)
PIPJ extension lag	10.3	12.3	8	10.2	11.0	6.9	13.4
DIPJ Arc	61.8	56.9 (39–80)	66.2 (49–78)	59.5 (47–78)	58.6 (47–65)	72.5 (68–77)	58.0 (30–85)
DASH	5.4	3.4	8	9.2	2	4.5	NR
Quick-DASH	11.4	7	NR	18.6	8.5	NR	NR
VAS	1.35	1.3	1.4	1.3	NR	1.4	NR
Grip strength (%)	90.1%	92%	NR	85.5%	91.7%	NR	9 1.3%
Complications							
Major							
Secondary procedure	6.8%	14.3%	0.0%	4.0%	19.7%	2.6%	0%
Subluxation	7.8%	0.0%	2.4%	1.8%	21.3%	15.4%	0%
Minor							
Recurring pain	15.9%	7.1%	7.3%	15.0%	21.3%	38.5%	6.3%
Infections	4.9%	0%	7.3%	16.4%	1.6%	3.8%	0%
OA	20.7%	26.2%	4.9%	18.1%	9.8%	46.2%	18.8%
Clinodactyly	6.5%	2.4%	0%	4.9%	9.8%	NR	15.6%
Rotation	1.1%	0.0%	0%	0.4%	NR	5.1%	0%

Abbreviations: DIPJ, distal interphalangeal joint; DSAH, disabilities of arm, shoulder, and hand; LOE, levelof evidence; NA, not applicable; NR, not reported; OA, osteoarthrosis; PIPI, proximal interphalanqeal joint: VAS, Visual Analoque Scale.

Adapted from Gianakos A, Yingling J, Athens CM, Barra AE, Capo JT. Treatment for Acute Proximal Interphalangeal Joint Fractures and Fracture-Dislocations: A Systematic Review of the Literature. J Hand Microsurg. 2020;12(Suppl 1):S9-S15. https://doi.org/10.1055/s-0040-1713323 with permission.

patients who underwent release of both collateral ligaments and the volar plate demonstrated a 40° improvement in total range of motion at 1 year postoperatively without any instances of postoperative instability.

Some patients may require revision for recurrent instability or progressive post-traumatic arthritis and pain. In these cases, arthroplasty or arthrodesis can be considered to improve pain control and stability. However, patients should not expect improvement of range of motion after revision surgery.

SUMMARY

There are numerous operative and nonoperative options for the management of PIP joint fractures and fracture dislocations. The treatment of choice should be guided by the fracture pattern and joint stability. The authors highlighted one of the newer described open reduction and internal fixation techniques, but all the techniques presented are viable options under the right circumstances, as is shown by the similar postsurgical outcomes. It is also important to set patient expectations early as most of these patients will have post-injury stiffness and potential functional limitations.

CLINICS CARE POINTS

- There are several viable options for the surgical management of proximal interphalangeal joint fractures.
- All fixation methods have similar outcomes when performed in the appropriate scenario.
  - For example, the Seatbelt procedure, volar plate arthroplasty, and hemi-hamate arthroplasty all require an intact dorsal cortex to adequately secure fixation.
- The ultimate goal of surgery is a congruent and stable joint that can tolerate early active range of motion to mitigate postoperative stiffness.
- Patients with proximal interphalangeal joint injuries should expect loss of motion and potentially suboptimal outcomes.

DISCLOSURE

The authors have nothing to disclose.

REFERENCES

1. Demino C, Yates M, Fowler JR. Surgical management of proximal interphalangeal joint fracture-dislocations: a review of outcomes. Hand (N Y) 2021;16(4):453–60.
2. Gianakos A, Yingling J, Athens CM, et al. Treatment for acute proximal interphalangeal joint fractures and fracture-dislocations: a systematic review of the literature. J Hand Microsurg 2020;12(Suppl 1): S9–15.
3. Yao J. Dislocations and ligament injuries of the digits. In: Wolfe SW, Pederson WC, Kozin SH, et al, editors. Green's operative hand surgery. Eighth Edi. Philadelphia, PA: Elsevier Inc.; 2022. p. 326–64.
4. Pang EQ, Yao J. Anatomy and biomechanics of the finger proximal interphalangeal joint. Hand Clin 2018;34(2):121–6.
5. Panchal-Kildare S, Malone K. Skeletal anatomy of the hand. Hand Clin 2013;29(4):459–71.
6. Pang EQ, Yao J. Anatomy and biomechanics of the finger proximal interphalangeal joint. Hand Clin 2018;34(2):121–6.
7. Leibovic SJ, Bowers WH. Anatomy of the proximal interphalangeal joint. Hand Clin 1994;10(2):169–78.
8. Rettig AC. Epidemiology of hand and wrist injuries in sports. Clin Sports Med 1998;17(3):401–6.
9. Mall NA, Carlisle JC, Matava MJ, et al. Upper extremity injuries in the National Football League: part I: hand and digital injuries. Am J Sports Med 2008;36(10):1938–44.
10. Williams CS. Proximal interphalangeal joint fracture dislocations: stable and unstable. Hand Clin 2012; 28(3):409–16.
11. Elson RA. Rupture of the central slip of the extensor hood of the finger. A test for early diagnosis. J Bone Joint Surg Br 1986;68(2):229–31.
12. Kiefhaber TR, Stern PJ. Fracture dislocations of the proximal interphalangeal joint. J Hand Surg Am 1998;23(3):368–80.
13. Federer AE, Guerrero EM, Dekker TJ, et al. Open Reduction Internal Fixation With Transverse Volar Plating for Unstable Proximal Interphalangeal Fracture-Dislocation: The Seatbelt Procedure. Hand (N Y) 2020;15(2):201–7.
14. Aladin A, Davis TRC. Dorsal fracture-dislocation of the proximal interphalangeal joint: a comparative study of percutaneous Kirschner wire fixation versus open reduction and internal fixation. J Hand Surg Br 2005;30(2):120–8.
15. Henn CM, Lee SK, Wolfe SW. Dynamic External Fixation for Proximal Interphalangeal Fracture-Dislocations. Oper Tech Orthop 2012;22(3):142–50.
16. Cheah AEJ, Tan DMK, Chong AKS, et al. Volar plating for unstable proximal interphalangeal joint dorsal fracture-dislocations. J Hand Surg Am 2012; 37(1):28–33.
17. Hamilton SC, Stern PJ, Fassler PR, et al. Mini-screw fixation for the treatment of proximal interphalangeal joint dorsal fracture-dislocations. J Hand Surg Am 2006;31(8):1349–54.

18. Weiss APC. Cerclage fixation for fracture dislocation of the proximal interphalangeal joint. Clin Orthop Relat Res 1996;327(327):21–8.

19. Frueh FS, Calcagni M, Lindenblatt N. The hemi-hamate autograft arthroplasty in proximal interphalangeal joint reconstruction: a systematic review. J Hand Surg Eur 2015;40(1):24–32.

20. Blazar PE, Robbe R, Lawton JN. Treatment of dorsal fracture/dislocations of the proximal interphalangeal joint by volar plate arthroplasty. Tech Hand Up Extrem Surg 2001;5(3):148–52.

21. Cheah AEJ, Yao J. Surgical Approaches to the Proximal Interphalangeal Joint. J Hand Surg Am 2016;41(2):294–305.

22. Ellis SJ, Cheng R, Prokopis P, et al. Treatment of proximal interphalangeal dorsal fracture-dislocation injuries with dynamic external fixation: a pins and rubber band system. J Hand Surg Am 2007;32(8):1242–50.

23. Williams RMM, Hastings H, Kiefhaber TR. PIP Fracture/Dislocation Treatment Technique: Use of a Hemi-Hamate Resurfacing Arthroplasty. Tech Hand Up Extrem Surg 2002;6(4):185–92.

24. Calfee RP, Kiefhaber TR, Sommerkamp TG, et al. Hemi-hamate arthroplasty provides functional reconstruction of acute and chronic proximal interphalangeal fracture-dislocations. J Hand Surg Am 2009;34(7):1232–41.

25. Denoble PH, Record NC. A Modification to Simplify the Harvest of a Hemi-hamate Autograft. J Hand Surg Am 2016;41(5):e99–102.

26. Eaton RG, Malerich MM. Volar plate arthroplasty of the proximal interphalangeal joint: a review of ten years' experience. J Hand Surg Am 1980;5(3):260–8.

27. Diao E, Eaton RG. Total collateral ligament excision for contractures of the proximal interphalangeal joint. J Hand Surg Am 1993;18(3):395–402.

28. Abbiati G, Delaria G, Saporiti E, et al. The treatment of chronic flexion contractures of the proximal interphalangeal joint. J Hand Surg Br 1995;20(3):385–9.

Proximal Interphalangeal Joint Arthroplasty for Fracture

Jeremy E. Raducha, MD[a], Arnold-Peter C. Weiss, MD[b],*

KEYWORDS

- Proximal interphalangeal joint • Arthroplasty • Posttraumatic osteoarthritis • Salvage

KEY POINTS

- Hemi-hamate arthroplasty is a joint salvage procedure for severely comminuted volar lip fractures.
- Implant arthroplasties are indicated in severely comminuted proximal interphalangeal joint fractures and posttraumatic arthritis.
- Each implant arthroplasty provides excellent pain relief but postoperative motion is variable.
- Complications differ with each implant slightly but they primarily include implant loosening and joint stiffness.
- Revision surgery rates are lower with silicone arthroplasties compared to the surface replacing implants.

INTRODUCTION

Fractures involving the finger proximal interphalangeal (PIP) joints can be difficult injuries to manage and often result in loss of motion, grip strength, and potentially poor patient-reported outcomes.[1,2] When these injuries present in a delayed fashion, they may not treatable with open reduction and internal fixation or pinning if the joint surfaces are not re-constructable or if they present with a healed malunion or posttraumatic arthritis. In these situations surgical treatment options become more limited to involve arthroplasty, arthrodesis, osteotomy or amputation.[3,4] Arthrodesis has historically been the gold standard for providing a stable PIP joint following a severe injury or failed fixation. However, fusing the PIP joint severely limits the finger total arc of motion which can significantly affect function, especially in the ulnar digits primarily responsible for gripping. Arthroplasty preserves motion and provides pain relief in joints requiring salvage.[5] As with all surgical implants, there have been many attempts at designing and revising PIP joint arthroplasty implants over the years with varying success. There is currently no clearly better implant option or surgical approach, with all implants having varying results and complications in the literature.[6–11] This article will discuss the pros and cons of the various arthroplasty options available in the United States as well as their indications and outcomes.

Relevant Anatomy

The finger PIP joint is a hinge joint, with highly concentric bony anatomy with an intercondylar groove on the proximal phalanx head and a corresponding ridge on the base of the middle phalanx. The volar buttress of the middle phalanx gives an asymmetric shape in the sagittal plane and helps resist dorsal dislocation. This asymmetry applies to the head of the proximal phalanx as well which is trapezoidal in shape and wider volarly in both the sagittal and axial planes. The shape of the proximal phalanx head helps increase the joint range of

[a] Department of Orthopaedic Surgery, Duke University Medical Center, 200 Trent Drive, Durham, NC 27710, USA; [b] R. Scot Sellers Scholar of Hand Surgery, Alpert Medical School of Brown University, University Orthopedics, 1 Kettle Point Avenue, East Providence, RI 02914, USA
* Corresponding author.
E-mail address: apcweiss@brown.edu

Hand Clin 39 (2023) 575–586
https://doi.org/10.1016/j.hcl.2023.06.004
0749-0712/23/© 2023 Elsevier Inc. All rights reserved.

motion and the subcapital recess accommodates the middle phalanx buttress and volar plate to allow a 100-120 deg arc of motion.[3,12] As PIP joint injures rarely allow a complete return to the normal range of motion, it is important to know that the functional arc of motion has been described as 23-87 degrees, or a 64 degree total arc of motion.[5] Even if normal motion cannot be restored, transferring the arc of motion into this functional range, e.g. decreasing extensor lag, can potentially improve patient function and outcomes.

The surrounding soft tissues of the PIP joint encompass a '3-sided box' configuration, involving the collateral ligaments and volar plate, to provide additional stability. The volar plate attaches distally as a thick fibrocartilaginous structure to the volar base of the middle phalanx, and proximally through check rein ligaments peripherally, with a thin membranous center, to the neck of the proximal phalanx.[13] The check rein ligaments allow sliding of the volar plate during joint flexion and are important in the primary function of the volar plate in resisting joint hyperextension. These structures are quick to scar after injury/surgery which is why PIP joint injuries are so prone to stiffness. The collateral ligaments are made up of the proper and accessory portions and resist radial and ulnar deviation of the joint. The proper collateral ligaments originate on the condyles of the proximal phalanx head and insert on the volar base of the middle phalanx. The accessory collateral ligaments also originate on the condyles but insert onto the volar plate.[3,13,14] The collaterals have a broad origin on the proximal phalanx which allows recession without complete release to improve articular visualization during surgical approaches. This bony congruity in addition to the surrounding soft tissues provides stability while allowing a small amount of rotation.[13]

The flexor and extensor tendon facilitate joint motion in a kinematic chain in addition to providing some additional dynamic and static stability. Dorsally the central slip inserts onto the base of the middle phalanx, and allows joint extension in addition to helping resist volar dislocation. The central slip insertion is approximately 5 mm and can be split or partially elevated during surgical approaches to allow articular visualization without complete release.[6] If the central slip is released, it must be repaired, and at the proper tension, to return anatomic motion and prevent boutonniere deformity of the finger. Radial and ulnar to the central slip, the extensor mechanism divides into the lateral bands, which continue distally to coalesce at their insertion on the dorsal distal phalanx as the terminal tendon. Their connection is stabilized by the triangular ligament distally. Radially and ulnarly the lateral bands connect to the flexor tendon sheath through the transverse retinacular ligaments.[3,6]

Volarly the flexor digitorum superficialis (FDS) and profundus (FDP) tendons run in the flexor sheath before inserting on the middle phalanx and volar base of the distal phalanx, respectively. The FDS tendon splits to insert radially and ulnarly on the middle of the middle phalanx, as the FDP runs between these two slips at Camper's chiasm. This anatomy can be utilized to approach the volar plate and joint surface by splitting the FDS tendon and retracting the FDP in a variation of the volar approach. Associated with the flexor sheath are the relevant pullies overlying the PIP joint area, A3, C1, and C2. These pullies can be divided without repair during the approach to the joint without compromising flexor tendon function.[6] Understanding the anatomy and normal function of the PIP joint is essential for successful arthroplasty. It influences implant design, surgical approaches, soft tissue balancing, and principles of rehabilitation.

PREOPERATIVE EVALUATION AND PLANNING

In the context for considering arthroplasty as a treatment option, patients will typically present in one of three scenarios: a severely comminuted fracture of the middle phalanx base or proximal phalanx head that isn't reconstructable, in a delayed fashion with deformity/malunion/nonunion or after a prior treatment with fixation failure or posttraumatic arthritis. In each of these scenarios it is important to perform a thorough history and physical examination. These patients frequently have a history of a 'jammed' finger, but either by not realizing the significance of the injury or having a delay in referral to an appropriate hand surgeon, they commonly present in a subacute or chronic fashion. Assessing the timing of the injury is important, as is hand dominance, patient occupation/recreational activities, and outcome goals. This can help guide treatment decision. An examination of the joint stability and range of motion is also important, not only to help determine arthroplasty options but also to estimate outcomes. The flexor and extensor tendon function should also be evaluated at the PIP and distal interphalangeal (DIP) joints. Due to the potentially poor outcomes in comminuted fractures, delayed presentations, and revision surgery, it is essential to set expectations early in the treatment process.

Work up should always include plain radiographs, anterior-posterior (AP) and lateral, of the affected finger. Hand radiographs are not adequate to assess PIP joint congruency, particularly on the lateral image. Close attention should be paid to fracture pattern and location, as well as joint subluxation and angulation. If the patient has had prior treatment, the original injury radiographs should also be reviewed and compared to current imaging. It is important to evaluate for implant loosening, breakage, posttraumatic arthritis, and other causes of failure.

A computed tomography (CT) scan can be useful in these complex fractures to assist with treatment decisions and surgical planning. In chronic fractures, a CT scan can also help assess bone quality, which may limit treatment options if poor. Magnetic resonance imaging (MRI) does not routinely have a role in these injuries, as the physical exam and other imaging modalities provide sufficient information for treatment.

Overall, it is important to consider the patient as a whole, as patients undergoing arthroplasty in fracture situations are usually different than a patient undergoing arthroplasty for primary degenerative or inflammatory arthritis. They are typically younger and more active than patients with degenerative arthritis.[15] Patients may also have sclerotic bone in chronic injuries, soft tissue injuries, significant scarring, etc. which can make surgery more difficult and poor outcomes more common in patients with higher functional expectations.

TREATMENT

As previously stated, arthroplasty may be indicated in acute comminuted fractures, delayed presentations, and in revision surgery for failed implants or posttraumatic arthritis. Each of these scenarios is different and should be approached with different considerations. A surgeon should be knowledgeable of the various arthroplasty options and surgical approaches available to provide the most appropriate treatment in different scenarios. The main arthroplasty options available include, hemi-hamate 'arthroplasty' or implant arthroplasty, the three main options include silicone, pyrocarbon, metal-on-polyethylene surface replacing implants. We will discuss each of these in more detail as well as the options for surgical approaches.

Surgical Approaches

There are 3 main approaches to the PIP joint that accommodate arthroplasty: volar, dorsal, and lateral. Each has pros and cons which may make it better in certain situations.

Volar approach

The volar approach allows access to the volar plate and articular surface, and is versatile as it

allows fixation or arthroplasty through the same approach without injury to the central slip. It also allows access for flexor tendon repair or FDS tenodesis if it will be part of the procedure. It can be started with a Brunner style incision, Brunner mid-lateral hybrid incision, or zig-zag incision (**Fig. 1**). The flap is typically based on the radial side of the index, long and ring finger to minimize the risk of injury to the radial digital nerve which can lead to contact hypersensitivity.[6] It is based on the ulnar side of the small finger for the same reason. The incision is carried down to the flexor sheath and the neurovascular bundles on each side are visualized and mobilized. This is particularly important if the joint will be 'shot gunned' open, to prevent excessive stretch on the bundles. The flexor sheath is then excised between the A2 and A4 pullies and the flexor tendons are retracted. Alternatively, the FDP can be retracted and the FDS splint in line with its fibers to visualize the volar plate.[6] The accessory collateral ligaments are then incised along their volar plate attachments and the proper collateral is recessed on the proximal or distal aspect. The volar plate is then released from the middle phalanx base. This now allows access to the articular surface. If more visualization is needed, the collaterals can be further recessed or released and the joint 'shot gunned' open to see the entire articular surface. During the closure, the volar plate should be repaired; however, the collaterals and flexor sheath can be left unrepaired without risking significant instability or bowstringing, respectively.[6,16]

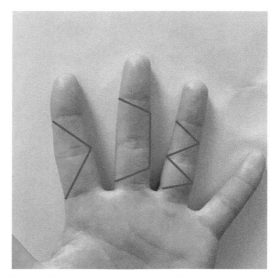

Fig. 1. Three potential skin incisions for the volar approach to the proximal interphalangeal joint.

Dorsal approach

The dorsal approach to the PIP joint allows fixation of dorsal fracture fragments and provides the best access to the proximal phalanx head, while also providing adequate exposure for arthroplasty if the collaterals are released.[6,17] The skin incision can be midline longitudinal, curvilinear, or as a lazy S (**Fig. 2**). The dorsal finger veins run just beneath the skin and should be preserved to decrease postoperative swelling and stiffness. Once flaps are raised, the extensor mechanism is visualized. There are 3 different methods for entering the joint capsule. The traditional longitudinal split incises the center of the central slip and then elevates the tendon and capsule medially and lateral off of bone to expose the articular surface.[6,18] The Chamay approach, creates a distally based triangular flap which preserves the central slip bony attachment.[19] The dorsolateral approach enters the joint between the central slip and the lateral band.[6,20] In the former 2 approaches the collaterals can then be recessed to increase joint exposure. To increase exposure in the dorsolateral approach, the ipsilateral collateral ligament is completely released and the volar plate partially released to increase exposure. During closure it is important to repair the central slip at the appropriate tension to prevent boutonniere deformity or limited function.

Lateral approach

The lateral approach to the joint has been described to further protect the extensor mechanism as well as the neurovascular bundles and flexor sheath. It is useful for unicondylar fractures but can also be extensile to perform arthroplasty.[6,21] A mid-lateral skin incision is performed from the middle of the proximal phalanx to the middle of the middle phalanx (**Fig. 3**). This is typically approached from the ulnar side of the index, long and ring fingers to preserve the radial collateral ligament for pinching.[21] Skin flaps are raised and the transverse retinacular ligament is incised at a point between the lateral band and Cleland's ligament, to protect the neurovascular bundle. The collateral ligament can then be released distally or proximally to allow exposure. If further visualization is needed for arthroplasty the joint can be 'shot gunned' open by releasing the volar plate off the middle phalanx. During closure, the volar plate and collateral ligament should be repaired.

There is debate in the literature as to which approach is best for performing arthroplasty.[17,22] Concerns about the volar approach include violation of the flexor sheath/tendon adhesions, neurovascular injury, and volar plate scarring which may limit extension. There is also concern that if the volar plate doesn't heal it could lead to a swan neck deformity. Concerns about the dorsal approach include disrupting the extensor mechanism requiring prolonged postoperative immobilization for healing which may decrease the range of motion or result in a boutonniere deformity if it doesn't heal. There is also a concern for extensor tendon adhesions which may lead to limited flexion. There is literature evaluating the outcomes of each approach and as they compare to one another,[22–24] however in general there are not significant differences in postoperative arc of motion or complications between approaches.[17] As such, the surgeon should perform whichever approach he or she finds most comfortable as long as it provides the proper visualization.

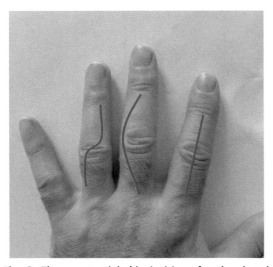

Fig. 2. Three potential skin incisions for the dorsal approach to the proximal interphalangeal joint.

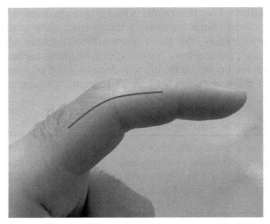

Fig. 3. The mid-lateral incision for the lateral approach to the proximal interphalangeal joint.

Arthroplasty Options

Hemi-hamate arthroplasty (**Fig. 4**) was first described by Dr Hastings in 2002 and bridges the gap between arthroplasty and fixation.[25] It is indicated for dorsal PIP joint fracture dislocations with a severely comminuted volar articular surface or a delayed presentation that prevents the joint surface from being reconstructed. In this scenario, it can reliable reconstruct the volar 50-60% of the articular surface to restore joint stability, with less risk of re-dislocation than volar plate arthroplasty.[26] Hemi-hamate arthroplasty is contra-indicated if the dorsal cortex of the middle phalanx is fractured as this is required for stable fixation. It is relatively contra-indicated if posttraumatic osteoarthritis is already present as this can lead to early failures due to increased pain and decreased function. Hemi-hamate arthroplasty is performed through a volar approach to the joint, which is 'shot gunned' open. The fracture fragments are removed and the recipient site is measured and prepared for the bone graft. The auto-graft is then harvested from the dorsal, distal hamate between the 4th and 5th metacarpal bases. The necessary size of graft is marked out on the hamate and it is harvested using a combination of saw and osteotome. A retrograde directed osteotome started at the articular surface can help guarantee the appropriate size of articular surface is harvested, as this can be more difficult to perform properly in an antegrade fashion.[25,27] In general, the graft should be oversized to allow for proper trimming, but should also be left thicker in the sagittal plan at the nonarticular surface to help recreate the volar buttress of the middle phalanx.[3,25] The graft is then secured in place with 3 screws, stability/motion is checked and the volar plate repaired.

For implant arthroplasty, there are several goals for which to aim that help ensure success.[28–30] Implants should restore functional range of motion, restore normal mechanical advantage, provide stability, facilitate easy implantation, and have good wear characteristics. There are 2 main categories for these implants: constrained or unconstrained.

Constrained implants, such as the silicone prostheses (**Fig. 5**), have an internal hinged element to allow motion in the plane of the hinge but restricts motion in other directions, which does recreate the native motion of the PIP joint.[5] The silicone implant was first described by Swanson in the 1960's.[18] It is a one piece implant of silicone elastomer, with

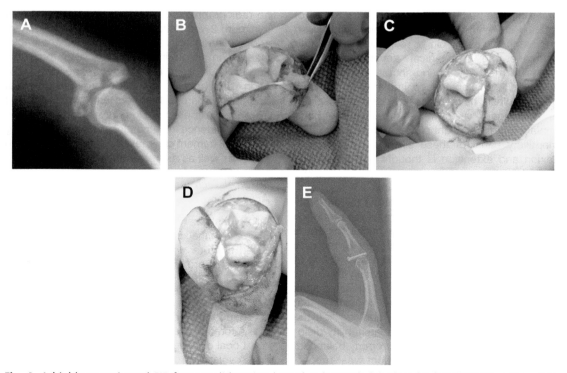

Fig. 4. A highly comminuted PIP fracture-dislocation lateral radiograph (*A*) ideal for hemihamate arthroplasty reconstruction. Via a volar exposure, the comminuted fragments are excised (*B*) and a shaped hemihamate graft is placed by two mini-screws for fixation (*C, D*). Final, lateral radiograph demonstrates a concentric PIP joint (*E*).

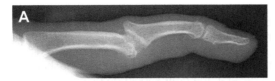
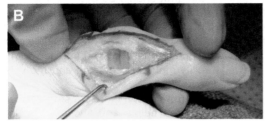

Fig. 5. A patient's lateral radiograph after 8 months following a highly comminuted PIP fracture -dislocation treated nonoperatively demonstrating complete loss of distal proximal phalanx structure (*A*). Due to significant pain, a PIP silicone implant arthroplasty was performed via a dorsal incision between the central tendon and lateral band (*B*).

intramedullary stems on each side bridged by a hinge. This material is stiff enough to maintain joint alignment but flexible enough to allow relatively easy insertion. Stability is also improved by early encapsulation of the implant.[18] The flexibility of the silicone implants also accounts for some of the hinge's motion restriction, yet the center of rotation still shifts dorsally and volar with flexion and extension of the hinge, respectively. This can decrease the mechanical advantage of the extensor mechanism and increase the risk of extensor lag.[5] Constrained implants in all types of arthroplasty have increased rates of loosening or breakage due to more stress at the bone implant interface. Slight piston motion in the intramedullary canal of these silicone implants with flexion and extension is thought to help reduce the risk of breakage by decreasing stress at the hinge; however, this can still occur.[5]

Un-constrained implants, such as the pyrocarbon (**Fig. 6**) or metal-on-polyethylene surface replacing implants (**Fig. 7**) rely on native soft tissue to provide joint stability and attempt to recreate more anatomic motion with rolling and sliding at the terminal ends of motion to maintain the center of rotation at the middle of the proximal phalanx head.[5] The risk of un-constrained implants is that they rely exclusively on the surrounding soft tissues for stability and are at risk of instability/dislocation if the soft tissue are not properly balanced. The type of material can also affect wear properties and osteointegration. Pyrolytic carbon, or pyrocarbon, is a nonmetallic material which has a low modulus of elasticity with high strength due

to its crystalline structure.[5] These properties make pyrocarbon hard yet durable, and provide excellent wear characteristics. Biomechanical evaluations have shown negligible wear after 5 million loading cycles.[5] However, pyrocarbon does not allow osteointegration and can place the implant at risk of loosening over time. In fact, it is normal to see a 0.5 mm rim of lucency around the implant on postoperative radiographs.[31–33]

Metal-on-polyethylene surface replacing implants are modeled based upon more common total hip and knee implants.[34] The metal bearing surface is typically cobalt-chrome alloy and the polyethylene is the same high molecular weight polyethylene used in other modern arthroplasties. These implants can be either cemented or cementless. The more recent implant designs have porous titanium stems or hydroxyapatite-coated stems to promote bone ingrowth with press fit implants. Studies comparing cemented to cementless arthroplasties recommend cementing all implants due to rates of radiographic loosening in the cementless implants as high as 39%.[35,36] Notably, however, the same studies showed similar functional and range of motion outcomes between the two groups and had opposite results in terms of rates of revision. These findings cast some doubt onto the superiority of cementing. Also, the newer hydroxyapatite-coated implants showed no radiographic loosening nor subsidence with a minimum 2-year follow-up in a study by Flannery and colleagues.[37] The lack of postoperative lucency in these implants was also found by Fowler, and colleagues,[21] in a retrospective evaluation of implants inserted through a lateral approach. There is therefore early optimism that advances in implant design may provide surgeons more confidence in cementless implants. Avoiding the use of cement can make revision surgery much easier as well as decrease operative time.

Surgical Technique (Silicone Arthroplasty for Acute Comminuted Fracture)

Arthroplasty can also be performed in the acute setting for the management of severely comminuted fractures involving the entire articular surface and or proximal phalanx head.

- The patient should be positioned supine with the affected extremity outstretched on a hand table
- A forearm tourniquet is placed
- Local or general anesthesia can be used.
- A volar approach is performed
  - If there is an open wound associated with the fracture, its orientation should determine your approach.

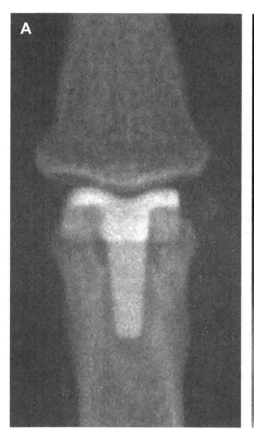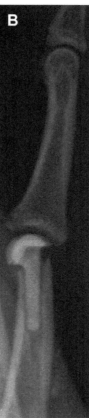

Fig. 6. An example of a hemi-arthroplasty using a pyrocarbon implant for a comminuted distal phalanx fracture in PA (*A*) and lateral (*B*) radiographs.

- ○ Other injuries requiring repair should also be taken into consideration when determining approach.
- A Brunner V-shaped incision is made
  - ○ The flap should be based radially for the index, long and ring fingers and ulnarly for the small finger to protect the contact side neurovascular bundle
- The flexor tendon sheath is encountered.
- The neurovascular bundles are then located and mobilized to minimize the risk of injury
- The flexor sheath is excised from the A2 to A4 pullies and the flexor tendons are both retracted
- The volar plate is released from the accessory collateral ligaments as well as the middle phalanx fracture fragments distally.
- The proper collateral ligaments are sharply recessed at their origin using a fresh 15 blade scalpel.
  - ○ The volar 50% of the origin should be released.
- The joint can now be hyper-extended and 'shot gunned' open.
  - ○ If this cannot be performed, the entire collateral origin can be released.

- The fracture fragments are then removed and the remaining bone stock is assessed.
  - ○ Adequate shaft bone needs to be present for the intramedullary stems to be well fixed.
- An oscillating saw is used to remove the remaining portion of the proximal phalanx head and middle phalanx base.
  - ○ The proximal phalanx head should be cut at the metaphyseal flare and the middle phalanx is typically cut just above the articular surface.
  - ○ Protect the collateral ligaments with retractors
- The middle and proximal phalanx intramedullary canals are then broached in the method according to the specification of the implant manufacturer.
- The largest implant that fits is then chosen and trialed.
  - ○ The cut end of the stem should be 1 mm shorter than then broached portion of the canal to allow piston motion.
- The joint is taken through range of motion to confirm stability and motion
- The final implant is then inserted into the prepared canals.

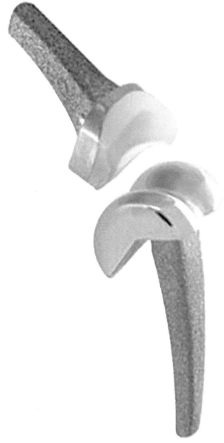

Fig. 7. An example of a proximal interphalangeal joint metal-on-polyethylene surface replacing arthroplasty implant.

- The volar plate is repaired to the accessory collateral ligaments and periosteum of the middle phalanx if able.
- The skin is then closed
  - The flexor sheath and collateral ligaments do not require repair
- The affected digit is then immobilized in an intrinsic plus position in a plaster splint.
  - If there is a wound issue, a removable orthosis can be utilized to allow for local wound care.

REHABILITATION

There is no 'gold standard' postoperative rehabilitation protocol, with varying timelines reported in the literature. There is slightly more agreement in the postoperative protocol following hemi-hamate arthroplasty, as early motion is a key goal following PIP joint fracture open reduction and internal fixation. Following hemi-hamate arthroplasty, patients are typically allowed immediate, or early active

motion a few days postoperatively, in a dorsal block splint at 10-20 degrees to protect the volar plate repair for 3-4 weeks.[26] Full DIP and metacarpophalangeal (MCP) joint motion is allowed mediately to promote tendon gliding, particularly of the lateral bands with DIP motion.

For implant arthroplasty, there is no consensus in the literature between early active motion and orthosis immobilization full time for 3-4 weeks. A couple studies describe improved postoperative range of motion with an early motion protocol. Proubasta, and colleagues,[38] immobilized patients for 7 days following silicone PIP joint arthroplasties through a volar approach, and then utilized no further splinting, allowing full motion. They reported a mean 72-degree postoperative arc of motion. Lautenbach, and colleagues[39] started active and passive joint motion on postoperative day 1, again following silicone arthroplasty through a volar approach, and reported a final arc of motion of 81 degrees on average. Unfortunately, not all early motion protocols have shown as encouraging results, with Nunley, and colleagues demonstrating e a decrease in motion, following pyrocarbon arthroplasty through a midline dorsal approach, from a mean of 32 to 30 degrees despite starting motion on postoperative day 4. The other end of the spectrum describes protocols with 3-4 weeks of full time immobilization in 0-30 degrees of flexion, resulting in the average range of motions similar to the overall literature, as will be discussed in the next section.[6,20] Postoperatively after the dorsal approach, when the central slip is released and repaired, most authors describe 3-4 weeks of postoperative immobilization with the PIP joint in full extension to allow for early healing of the central slip. This is due to the concern for boutonniere deformity with central slip deficiency. Bales and colleagues described a protocol which may be considered a middle ground with 2 weeks of full-time splinting followed by splinting in full extension between active motion exercises for 4 additional weeks.

OUTCOMES

When discussing surgical outcomes, hemi-hamate arthroplasty should be evaluated separately as it is a different procedure than implant arthroplasties. It is also typically performed in the more acute or subacute setting and in patients without preexisting arthritis. In these cases, patients have had functional and range of motion deficits for a shorter period of time prior to surgery which may explain their differential outcome scores, which are more comparable to fracture fixation than arthroplasty. Two systematic reviews evaluated the outcomes following various types of PIP fracture fixation constructs, with hemi hamate arthroplasty recording the least postoperative mean motion at 79.3 and 79.8 degrees compared to an overall average of 83.2 degrees when considering all fixation methods.[1,2] Average grip strength ranges from 91-95% of the normal side and average visual analog scale (VAS) scores are low at 1.3-1.4 out of 10.[1,2,26,40] The improved function was confirmed with improvement in patient-reported outcome measures, with average postoperative Quick DASH and DASH scores of 3.4 and 7 respectively, compared to 2 and 8.5 in open reduction and internal fixation.[1] These results are likely related to the timing of surgical intervention as Calfee, and colleagues,[26] showed worse VAS and DASH scores in patients presenting with chronic injuries, >6 weeks old.

Silicone implant arthroplasty has the longest track record. Swanson reported on his experience with 424 arthroplasties with 98% of patients reporting complete pain relief.[41] Since then numerous studies have confirmed excellent pain relief in these arthroplasties performed for degenerative arthritis, posttraumatic arthritis or inflammatory arthritis.[8–10,20,22,42] Patient satisfaction is reported at rates up to 90%.[20] Postoperative range of motion results are more variable, but the majority of studies demonstrate a mean total arc of PIP joint motion ranging from 30-61 degrees with little to no improvement compared to preoperative motion.[8,10,20,22,42] Despite these varying rates of motion, a systematic review by Yamamoto and colleagues evaluating different implants and approaches did demonstrate the highest mean postoperative motion (58 deg), improvement in motion (17 deg) and lowest extensor lag (5 deg) in silicone arthroplasties performed through a volar approach. These studies represent a mixed group of patients with varying preoperative range of motion. Notably, it is important to council patients that they should not expect an increase in motion following silicone arthroplasty. Despite limited range of motion, these implants have excellent long-term survival rates or 80-90% at 8-10 years.[7,10]

In silicone arthroplasties performed in emergent scenarios with other associated soft tissue trauma, Laurent and colleagues, and Obert, and colleagues reported their results in two small studies out of the same institution in France.[43,44] They found mean PIP joint ranges of motion from 41.8-48.8 degrees, mean VAS scores of 1/10 and a mean Quick DASH score of 24. Mean DIP joint motion and MCP joint motion were found to be 43.8 deg and 90 deg respectively. Eight of 13 patients in one of the studies were able to return to work within 6.4 months.[43] These acutely performed arthroplasties show similar outcomes to those performed for posttraumatic arthritis at a mean 2.7-4.7 years of follow up. They can be considered a viable alternative to arthrodesis or amputation in acute traumatic scenarios when the surrounding soft tissues are appropriate for salvage.

Pyrocarbon arthroplasties have also shown to have high rates of pain relief and satisfaction but variable improvements in range of motion.[15,31–33,45–48] Systematic reviews in 2012 and 2017, comparing pyrocarbon implants to silicone in PIP joint arthroplasties, showed mean postoperative range of motion for pyrocarbon implants of 44.8-51 degrees, similar to those for silicone arthroplasty. Dickson and colleagues,[32] evaluated pyrocarbon PIP implants for longevity and showed mid to long-term survival was good at 85% at 5 and 10 years. This was slightly higher than but similar to that demonstrated by Wagner, and colleagues[31] with 79% and 77% at similar time periods However, worse outcomes have been shown in patients with posttraumatic arthritis undergoing pyrocarbon PIP implant placement with 5 and 10 year survival rates of only 66% and 57% respectively.[31] Nunley and colleagues, similarly demonstrated worse outcomes in all 7 of their posttraumatic arthritis patients who underwent pyrocarbon arthroplasty reporting a decrease in postoperative range of motion with only 1 patient returning to the prior level of employment. Patients developing posttraumatic arthritis are typically younger, which some argue is the ideal patient for pyrocarbon arthroplasty due to its excellent wear characteristics, so caution is advised in this group of patients due to functional outcomes.

Metal-on-polyethylene surface replacing arthroplasty, again, shows good results with regard to pain relief and patient satisfaction.[9,21,34,35] Range of motion is variably reported in the literature with mean arcs of motion ranging from 45-65 degrees. There is limited long-term survival information reported in the literature on these implant, however one prospective randomized controlled study showed a survival greater than 70% at 42 months postoperatively.[9] Studies evaluating the newer hydroxyapatite-coated implants have shown survival rates of 82-100% with a minimum of 2 years follow up.[21,37]

Overall, all 3 implant designs have shown excellent pain relief and satisfaction with good overall mid-to long-term survival. No implant has consistently shown an ability to improve postoperative range of motion with a similar range of motion results across all implants. The implants are, however, differentiated based on their complications and revision rates.

Complications

Hemi-hamate arthroplasty is associated with an approximately 35% complication rate, including tenderness, joint contracture, posttraumatic arthritis, screw migration and graft resorption.[1,3,26,40] The rate of radiographic posttraumatic arthritis has been shown to be as high as 50% however most patients do not complain of corresponding pain or stiffness.[40] The fate of these 'arthroplasties' is tied to graft healing and preventing postoperative stiffness. Rates of reoperation have been reported at 14.3% with the majority of procedures performed for lysis of adhesions due to stiffness.

In a database review of complications of small joint arthroplasty, Billig and colleagues[11] found an overall average complication rate of 35% with a 7.3% reoperation rate. The two most commonly reported complications of silicone implants include implant breakage and peri-implant bone resorption with implant loosening or joint deformity. Rates of implant breakage range from 0-55%,[7,10,41,42] typically occurs at the hinge and is thought to be due to implant wear at the cut bone surface.[5] However, bone resorption and implant breakage do not always lead to clinical failure. Bales, and colleagues[7] reported 21 implant fractures (55%) of their study but only 3/21 patients required revision for symptomatic pain or dislocation. Similarly, other comparative studies have shown low silicone implant revision surgery rates of 4-6%.[8,22] Silicone synovitis is a theoretical risk but the actual clinical presentation is rare.[49]

Pyrocarbon arthroplasties have been associated with high rates of radiographic loosening in the literature, up to 72%.[9,15,31-33] This degree is someone difficult to interpret, as although pyrocarbon bone growth up to the sides of the implant it does not allow osteointegration. Therefore, there is always a radiolucent line around these implants, and this is not always directly addressed in the literature. The clinically important complications are progressive loosening and subsidence. These have been shown to occur in 30-48% of patients.[9,32,33] Again this does not always lead to clinical failure with previously mentioned survival rates as high as 85% at 10 years.[32] Revision rates following pyrocarbon arthroplasties range from 9-21%, with the majority occurring within 2 years of implantation.[9,31-33] Other complications include stiffness, dislocation, and implant squeaking.

Metal-on-polyethylene surface replacing arthroplasties have similar complications of instability, stiffness, implant loosening, and deformity with rates of 21-40%.[9,34] Most concerns for loosening surround the debate of cemented versus cementless implant fixation. The original implants were smooth and required cementing; however, the newer implant titanium stems are designated as press fit implants and allow bone ingrowth. Jennings, and colleagues, evaluated 43 joints with titanium stems and an average of 37 months follow up. The authors reported a 39% rate of loosening in the uncemented implants compared to 4% in the cemented group. Ten of the 11 revisions for loosening were performed in the uncemented group.[35] Fowler, and colleagues evaluated the hydroxyapatite press fit implant group and found 6 implants requiring revision out of the 33 available for review. They were revised to 4 silicone arthroplasties, 1 arthrodesis, and 1 to another hydroxyapatite-coated implant.[21]

In summary, all 3 implants have high rates of radiographic loosening that does not always lead to clinic symptoms or revision surgery. The revision surgery rate is lower with silicone implants when compared to pyrocarbon and metal-on-polyethylene surface replacement arthroplasties.

Revision Options

Since these arthroplasties are often performed in salvage or revision situations, their revision options are somewhat limited. They can either be revised to another of the same implant, another implant type (typically silicone), or undergo arthrodesis or amputation. Revision to arthrodesis can return stability to an unstable joint and allow improved pinch strength. Revision to arthrodesis is however associated with limited finger total arc of motion. This may limit overall function and the performance of some work-related activities.

SUMMARY

Proximal interphalangeal joint arthroplasties can be performed in the setting of acute comminuted fractures, chronic fracture presentations, and posttraumatic arthritis. These surgeries provide excellent pain relief and patient satisfaction but patients should be cautioned not to expect an improvement in motion. Despite high rates of minor complications and radiographic loosening, these implants have good rates of long-term survival with most revisions occurring in the early postoperative period. They provide viable alternatives to arthrodesis, osteotomy, and amputation in the appropriate patient.

CLINICS CARE POINTS

- Hemi-hamate arthroplasty is a joint salvage procedure for severely comminuted volar lip fractures

- In regards to proximal interphalangeal joint fractures, implant arthroplasties are indicated in severely comminuted fractures, delayed fracture presentations and posttraumatic arthritis.

- Each implant arthroplasty provides excellent pain relief but postoperative motion is variable

- Complications differ with each implant but they primarily include implant loosening and joint stiffness.

- Revision surgery rates are lower with silicone arthroplasties compared to the surface placing implants.

DISCLOSURE

The authors have nothing to disclose.

REFERENCES

1. Gianakos A, Yingling J, Athens CM, et al. Treatment for acute proximal interphalangeal joint fractures and fracture-dislocations: a systematic review of the literature. J Hand Microsurg 2020;12(Suppl 1): S9–15.

2. Demino C, Yates M, Fowler JR. Surgical management of proximal interphalangeal joint fracture-dislocations: a review of outcomes. Hand (N Y) 2021;16(4):453–60.

3. Yao J. Dislocations and ligament injuries of the digits. In: Wolfe SW, Pederson WC, Kozin SH, et al, editors. *Green's operative hand surgery*. Eighth Edi. Philadelphia, PA: Elsevier Inc.; 2022. p. 326–64.

4. Carroll R, Taber T. Digital arthroplasty of the proximal interphalngeal joint. J Bone Jt Surg - Am 1954;36-A(5):912–20.

5. Zhu AF, Rahgozar P, Chung KC. Advances in proximal interphalangeal joint arthroplasty: biomechanics and biomaterials. Hand Clin 2018;34(2): 185–94.

6. Cheah AEJ, Yao J. Surgical approaches to the proximal interphalangeal joint. J Hand Surg Am 2016; 41(2):294–305.

7. Bales JG, Wall LB, Stern PJ. Long-term results of Swanson silicone arthroplasty for proximal interphalangeal joint osteoarthritis. J Hand Surg Am 2014; 39(3):455–61.

8. Chan K, Ayeni O, McKnight L, et al. Pyrocarbon versus silicone proximal interphalangeal joint arthroplasty: a systematic review. Plast Reconstr Surg 2013;131(1):114–24.

9. Daecke W, Kaszap B, Martini AK, et al. A prospective, randomized comparison of 3 types of proximal interphalangeal joint arthroplasty. J Hand Surg Am 2012;37(9).

10. Takigawa S, Meletiou S, Sauerbier M, et al. Long-term assessment of Swanson implant arthroplasty in the proximal interphalangeal joint of the hand. J Hand Surg Am 2004;29(5):785–95.

11. Billig JI, Nasser JS, Chung KC. National prevalence of complications and cost of small joint arthroplasty for hand osteoarthritis and post-traumatic arthritis. J Hand Surg Am 2020;45(6):553.e1–12.

12. Williams CS. Proximal interphalangeal joint fracture dislocations: stable and unstable. Hand Clin 2012; 28(3):409–16.

13. Pang EQ, Yao J. Anatomy and biomechanics of the finger proximal interphalangeal joint. Hand Clin 2018;34(2):121–6.

14. Leibovic SJ, Bowers WH. Anatomy of the proximal interphalangeal joint. Hand Clin 1994;10(2):169–78.

15. Nunley RM, Boyer MI, Goldfarb CA. Pyrolytic carbon arthroplasty for posttraumatic arthritis of the proximal interphalangeal joint. J Hand Surg Am 2006; 31(9):1468–74.

16. Abbiati G, Delaria G, Saporiti E, et al. The treatment of chronic flexion contractures of the proximal interphalangeal joint. J Hand Surg Br 1995;20(3): 385–9.

17. Tranchida GV, Allen ST, Moen SM, et al. Comparison of volar and dorsal approach for PIP Arthroplasty. Hand (N Y) 2021;16(3):348–53.

18. Swanson AB. Finger joint replacement by silicone rubber implants and the concept of implant fixation by encapsulation. Ann Rheum Dis 1969;28(Suppl 5): 47. Available at: https://www.ncbi.nlm.nih.gov/pmc/articles/PMC2453487/. Accessed July 17, 2022.

19. Chamay A. A distally based dorsal and triangular tendinous flap for direct access to the proximal interphalangeal joint. Ann Chir Main 1988;7(2):179–83.

20. Namdari S, Weiss APC. Anatomically neutral silicone small joint arthroplasty for osteoarthritis. J Hand Surg Am 2009;34(2):292–300.

21. Fowler A, Arshad MS, Talwalkar S, et al. MatOrtho proximal interphalangeal joint arthroplasty via lateral approach: minimum 2-year follow-up. J hand Surg Asian-Pacific 2021;26(3):339–44.

22. Yamamoto M, Malay S, Fujihara Y, et al. A systematic review of different implants and approaches for proximal interphalangeal joint arthroplasty. Plast Reconstr Surg 2017;139(5):1139e–51e.

23. Bodmer E, Marks M, Hensler S, et al. Comparison of outcomes of three surgical approaches for proximal interphalangeal joint arthroplasty using a surface-

replacing implant. J Hand Surg Eur 2020;45(6): 608–14.

24. Le Glédic B, Hidalgo Diaz JJ, Vernet P, et al. Comparison of proximal interphalangeal arthroplasty outcomes with Swanson implant performed by volar versus dorsal approach. Hand Surg Rehabil 2018; 37(2):104–9.

25. Williams RMM, Hastings H, Kiefhaber TR. PIP fracture/dislocation treatment technique: use of a hemi-hamate resurfacing arthroplasty. Tech Hand Up Extrem Surg 2002;6(4):185–92.

26. Calfee RP, Kiefhaber TR, Sommerkamp TG, et al. Hemi-hamate arthroplasty provides functional reconstruction of acute and chronic proximal interphalangeal fracture-dislocations. J Hand Surg Am 2009;34(7):1232–41.

27. Denoble PH, Record NC. A modification to simplify the harvest of a hemi-hamate autograft. J Hand Surg Am 2016;41(5):e99–102.

28. Zhuang T, Wong S, Aoki R, et al. A cost-effectiveness analysis of corticosteroid injections and open surgical release for trigger finger. J Hand Surg Am 2020;45(7):597–609.e7.

29. Flatt AE, Fischer GW. Biochemical factors in the replacement of rheumatoid finger joints. Ann Rheum Dis 1969;28(Suppl 5):36. Available at: https://www.ncbi.nlm.nih.gov/pmc/articles/PMC2453495/. Accessed July 17, 2022.

30. Swanson AB. Silicone rubber implants for replacement of arthritic or destroyed joints in the hand. 1968. Clin Orthop Relat Res 1997;342(342):4–10.

31. Wagner ER, Weston JT, Houdek MT, et al. Medium-term outcomes with pyrocarbon proximal interphalangeal arthroplasty: a study of 170 consecutive arthroplasties. J Hand Surg Am 2018;43(9):797–805.

32. Dickson DR, Nuttall D, Watts AC, et al. Pyrocarbon proximal interphalangeal joint arthroplasty: minimum five-year follow-up. J Hand Surg Am 2015;40(11): 2142–8.e4.

33. McGuire DT, White CD, Carter SL, et al. Pyrocarbon proximal interphalangeal joint arthroplasty: outcomes of a cohort study. J Hand Surg Eur 2012; 37(6):490–6.

34. Linscheid RL, Murray PM, Vidal MA, et al. Development of a surface replacement arthroplasty for proximal interphalangeal joints. J Hand Surg Am 1997; 22(2):286–98.

35. Jennings CD, Livingstone DP. Surface replacement arthroplasty of the proximal interphalangeal joint using the PIP-SRA implant: results, complications, and revisions. J Hand Surg Am 2008;33(9):1565.e1–11.

36. Johnstone BR, Fitzgerald M, Smith KR, et al. Cemented versus uncemented surface replacement arthroplasty of the proximal interphalangeal joint with a mean 5-year follow-up. J Hand Surg Am 2008;33(5): 726–32.

37. Flannery O, Harley O, Badge R, et al. MatOrtho proximal interphalangeal joint arthroplasty: minimum 2-year follow-up. J Hand Surg Eur 2016;41(9):910–6.

38. Proubasta IR, Lamas CG, Natera L, et al. Silicone proximal interphalangeal joint arthroplasty for primary osteoarthritis using a volar approach. J Hand Surg Am 2014;39(6):1075–81.

39. Lautenbach M, Kim S, Berndsen M, et al. The palmar approach for PIP-arthroplasty according to Simmen: results after 8 years follow-up. J Orthop Sci 2014;19(5):722–8.

40. Frueh FS, Calcagni M, Lindenblatt N. The hemi-hamate autograft arthroplasty in proximal interphalangeal joint reconstruction: a systematic review. J Hand Surg Eur 2015;40(1):24–32.

41. Swanson AB, Maupin BK, Gajjar NV, et al. Flexible implant arthroplasty in the proximal interphalangeal joint of the hand. J Hand Surg Am 1985;10(6 Pt 1): 796–805.

42. Lin HH, Wyrick JD, Stern PJ. Proximal interphalangeal joint silicone replacement arthroplasty: clinical results using an anterior approach. J Hand Surg Am 1995;20(1):123–32.

43. Laurent R, El Rifai S, Loisel F, et al. Functional evaluation following emergency arthroplasty of the proximal interphalangeal joint for complex fractures with silicone implant. Hand Surg Rehabil 2020;39(5): 423–30.

44. Obert L, Clappaz P, Hampel C, et al. [Bone and soft tissue loss of the proximal interphalangeal joint of the long fingers: emergency treatment with a Swanson implant: prospective study of ten patients with mean 2.7 year follow-up]. Rev Chir Orthop Reparatrice Appar Mot 2006;92(3):234–41.

45. Herren DB, Schindele S, Goldhahn J, et al. Problematic bone fixation with pyrocarbon implants in proximal interphalangeal joint replacement: short-term results. J Hand Surg Br 2006;31(6):643–51.

46. Wijk U, Wollmark M, Kopylov P, et al. Outcomes of proximal interphalangeal joint pyrocarbon implants. J Hand Surg Am 2010;35(1):38–43.

47. Ono S, Shauver MJ, Chang KWC, et al. Outcomes of pyrolytic carbon arthroplasty for the proximal interphalangeal joint at 44 months' mean follow-up. Plast Reconstr Surg 2012;129(5):1139–50.

48. Storey PA, Goddard M, Clegg C, et al. Pyrocarbon proximal interphalangeal joint arthroplasty: a medium to long term follow-up of a single surgeon series. J Hand Surg Eur 2015;40(9):952–6.

49. Drake ML, Segalman KA. Complications of small joint arthroplasty. Hand Clin 2010;26(2):205–12.

Arthroscopic-Assisted Fracture Fixation About the Elbow

Abhiram R. Bhashyam, MD, PhD*, Neal Chen, MD

KEYWORDS

• Elbow fracture • Elbow arthroscopy • Coronoid fracture • Capitellar fracture • Elbow instability

KEY POINTS

• Maintain capsular distension using low pump pressures (25–30 mm Hg) to enhance visualization while minimizing risks for post-fracture compartment syndrome.
• Use inside-out techniques when establishing portals to allow for optimal placement and decrease risk of potential nerve injury.
• Targeting guides and portal "cannulas" can help maximize maneuverability inside and outside of the arthroscopic workspace while allowing for predictable placement of preliminary and final fixation.
• Elbow and fixation stability should be assessed to determine whether an open approach is required to repair ligaments or enhance fracture fixation.

INTRODUCTION

Articular fractures of the anterior elbow can be challenging to treat. Fracture visualization from classically described open approaches can be limited, and some exposures may destabilize the elbow or place neurovascular structures at risk.[1,2] Open approaches to the elbow are often complicated by stiffness due to capsular contracture or heterotopic ossification. For this reason, arthroscopic-assisted elbow fracture fixation has been increasingly advocated because of improved visualization, more limited dissection, and reduced propensity for stiffness.[3] Elbow arthroscopy provides visualization of intra-articular fractures of the anterior elbow while decreasing the likelihood of collateral ligament injury.[2–5]

Arthroscopic-assisted fracture fixation for adult elbow fractures has been described for coronoid fractures, capitellum fractures and radial head fractures. In addition, arthroscopy can be used for assessment of elbow stability before open repair or reconstruction.[3,6] Although arthroscopic radial head fracture treatment has been reported to be safe and feasible, in our experience, the arthroscopic approach is technically challenging with minimal advantage compared to open approaches.[4,7–9] In our experience, arthroscopic-assisted fracture treatment is most helpful for capitellar or coronoid fractures, and in the assessment of ligamentous stability.

CONCEPTS FOR ARTHROSCOPIC-ASSISTED REPAIR

Positioning: Elbow arthroscopy can be performed in the supine or lateral decubitus position with tourniquet control (**Fig. 1**). For supine positioning, a sterile arm holder is used to secure the elbow (McConnell arm holder, McConnell Orthopedic Manufacturing Co, Greenville, TX, USA; Spider, Smith & Nephew, Nashville, TN, USA). For lateral decubitus positioning, patients are positioned using an inflatable beanbag with an axillary roll. The arm is supported using an elbow arthroscopy arm holder attached to the side of the operating

Department of Orthopaedic Surgery, Hand & Arm Center, Massachusetts General Hospital, 55 Fruit Street, Boston, MA 02114, USA
* Corresponding author.
E-mail address: abhashyam@partners.org

Hand Clin 39 (2023) 587–595
https://doi.org/10.1016/j.hcl.2023.05.006

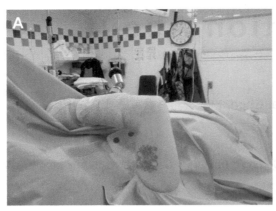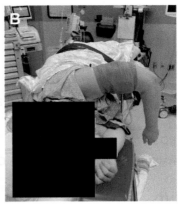

Fig. 1. Patient positioning for elbow arthroscopy. (*A*) Supine with McConnell arm positioner; (*B*) Lateral decubitus with elbow arthroscopy arm holder.

table (Western elbow holder, Smith & Nephew, Nashville, TN, USA; Elbow Arthroscopy Positioner, Alimed, Dedham, MA, USA; ElbowLOC, Hunter Medical Inc., Columbia, TN, USA). Positioning largely depends on surgeon preference as both positions permit excellent visualization of the anterior elbow joint, but supine positioning facilitates easy conversion to open approaches if needed. One disadvantage of lateral or prone positioning is that if the patient moves, the arm holder may put pressure on the anterior elbow, which may limit capsular distension.

Maintaining capsular distension: The most important difference between elbow arthroscopy and arthroscopy of other joints is that *the arthroscopic space is not supported by the surrounding bones.* In knee arthroscopy, the femur and tibia support the joint capsule; similarly, in the glenohumeral joint and the subacromial space, the arthroscopic space is supported by the humerus and glenoid, and acromion/clavicle. In the elbow, the arthroscopic space is maintained by distention of the joint capsule. Once too much of the integrity of the joint capsule is lost, the arthroscopic space becomes substantially smaller, and visualization is compromised.

The elbow capsule can maintain distension with the placement of viewing and working portals, but once the capsule loses a threshold integrity, the anterior structures, most notably the brachialis muscle, will herniate into the working space. The working space can be supported by adding accessory portals and retractors, but it is preferable if the capsular integrity is preserved. Coronoid fixation cases may last longer than an hour and maintaining capsular integrity is important to maintaining visualization. It is important to recognize the near proximity of the median nerve, radial nerve, and brachial artery anteriorly. Once the

brachialis muscle is visualized, surgeons should be aware that risk to these structures increases.

Distention of the elbow needs to be balanced with the risk of compartment swelling, especially in the setting of fracture. We prefer to keep pump pressures low (25–30 mm Hg). Excessive pump pressures can lead to forearm compartment syndrome. We do not recommend increasing pump pressures to improve visualization and if visualization is lost at these pressures, conversion to open surgery is advised. Also remember that if the patient is in lateral decubitus positioning, the visualization may be compromised if the patient and the arm moves, as the arm holder may then put pressure on the anterior elbow.

Establishing Portals: Inside Out Technique

There are 2 important considerations in portal placement: (1) What is the purpose of my portal? and (2) What are the secondary consequences of portal placement? One pitfall is to rush to put in a portal without thinking about its purpose. In general, the most advanced knee arthroscopists or shoulder arthroscopists are thinking about these 2 ideas and not focusing on named portals *per se.* In this review, we will focus on these larger questions rather than the technical exercise of portal placement, which can be found in many other excellent sources.

For arthroscopically assisted capitellar fracture fixation, the goal of portal placement is to (1) visualize the capitellar fracture and (2) adjust the reduction if necessary. For visualization, an anteromedial portal allows for the best visualization of the lateral side. When placing an anteromedial portal, the medial epicondyle can be palpated. The ulnar nerve lies posterior to the medial epicondyle, so in general, the anteromedial portal is safe for portal placement. The lateral antebrachial cutaneous nerve is at risk for injury with placement of this portal. The nerve usually lies about 1 cm distal to the tip of the medial epicondyle, but this anatomy varies widely. If the ulnar nerve has been transposed, open capitellar fixation is advised. If the ulnar nerve subluxates, usually it does not move so far anteriorly that it interferes with the medial portal placement, but in the rare event that it is very anterior, open capitellar fixation may also be preferred.

We usually prefer to use an inside-out technique to establish the working portal. This involves establishing a viewing portal, advancing a switching stick across the joint, cutting the skin, and then placing an arthroscopic cannula over the switching stick. If one uses an inside-out technique, it is important to recognize that placement of the viewing portal will dictate the position of the working portal. For instance, if the anteromedial viewing portal is established proximally relative to the joint space, the lateral working portal will be constrained by the proximal boundaries of the joint and forced to be more distal than intended. For an arthroscopic-assisted capitellar fixation, it is preferable for the viewing portal to be slightly distal to the medial epicondyle so the working portal can be placed slightly proximal. If a capitellar fracture needs to be adjusted, usually the capitellum needs to be slightly "pushed" from superior to inferior. Proximal-lateral portal placement makes this reduction maneuver easier.

For arthroscopic coronoid fixation, the viewing portal should be a lateral portal. The inside-out considerations for arthroscopic coronoid fixation are arguably more important than those for capitellar fixation. Working portal placement for arthroscopic coronoid fixation is unforgiving and needs to be placed as best as possible. The working portal in arthroscopic coronoid fixation needs to (1) allow for reduction of the coronoid fragment, (2) allow for a grasper to hold a guidewire to prevent unintended advancement, and (3) suture passage and exchange. In general, there is a bias to place anterolateral working portals slightly proximally and relatively close to the humerus to avoid injury to the radial nerve. This position forces the medial working portal to be too anterior that makes it harder to reduce the coronoid fragment. It is helpful to place the anteromedial working portal as "centered" as possible relative to proximal-distal positioning. Secondly, the working portal needs to be anterior enough to be functional. One trick is before establishing the medial working portal, see if the camera can reduce the coronoid fragment from the lateral side. If it cannot, the lateral viewing portal needs to be adjusted.

EQUIPMENT

Basic equipment: A standard 4 mm 30° arthroscope is routinely used, but a 70° arthroscope can be helpful for some coronoid and capitellar fractures.[2,5] An arthroscopic 3.5 mm or 4.0 mm shaver is used to clear the joint of clot and fracture debris. It is important to minimize suction. An elbow arthroscopy instrument tray is essential to provide flexibility in selecting an appropriate reduction and fixation technique. It should ideally include a large probe, elevators, ring curettes, suture retrievers, and graspers (eg, Elbow Arthroscopy Instrument Set, Arthrex, Inc., Naples, FL, USA).

Specialized equipment: Arthroscopic-assisted elbow fracture fixation is particularly challenging due to the need to transition inside and outside the arthroscopic environment while reducing and fixating fractures. An additional variable is the need to obtain fluoroscopic images using a C-arm or mini C-arm that enters and exits the operative field. During these transitions, it is easy to "lose" a portal or struggle to place a reduction wire in the appropriate position. To minimize these challenges, targeting guides and portal "cannulas" can help maximize maneuverability inside and outside of the arthroscopic workspace while allowing for predictable placement of preliminary and final fixation. Targeting drill guides use an adjustable C-ring to allow for several drilling angles while maximizing accuracy of wire placement to obtain stable provisional fixation (eg, GPS Targeting Drill Guide, Arthrex, Inc., Naples, FL, USA). They also facilitate the placement of guidewires in the appropriate position for eventual replacement with a cannulated screw. Button cannulas can maximize visibility and maneuverability inside and outside of the arthroscopic workspace and being able to use shorter instruments and minimize cannula loss (eg, PassPort Cannula, Arthrex, Inc., Naples, FL, USA).

Fixation options: Arthroscopic fracture fixation in the elbow relies on 2 fixation techniques: (1) cannulated screw (headed or headless), and (2) suture "lasso" fixation. When using cannulated screws, 3 divergent guidewires should be placed prior to screw fixation. Three divergent guidewires are an important concept. If only 2 wires are placed, when the first wire is over drilled, the fragment can rotate and when the screw reaches the distal fragment, the fracture may displace. Addition of the third wire helps limit this problem. Each exiting wire should be visualized within the intra-articular space to confirm appropriate and safe positioning for stable fragment fixation. Suture "lasso" fixation can be used to reinforce screw fixation or as primary fixation in settings of comminution.

After fixation, reduction and stability should be evaluated arthroscopically and fluoroscopically with stress examination. If adequate reduction, fixation and stability cannot be obtained arthroscopically, an open technique should be utilized.

ARTHROSCOPICALLY ASSISTED REDUCTION AND INTERNAL FIXATION OF CAPITELLAR FRACTURES
Mechanism of Injury

It has been theorized that these fractures occur because of a shearing injury to the capitellum. In our view this concept is not well developed, and we offer an alternative theory. We believe that capitellar fractures occur because the posterolateral column of the distal humerus experiences an axial load. The posterolateral column compresses and fractures; however, because the capitellum is spherical, it maintains its integrity and fractures from the posterolateral column. As the elbow flexes, the capitellum then displaces anterior to the radial head.

This mechanism may result in various fracture patterns. Ring and Jupiter described various components of fracture including the capitellar fragment, lateral epicondyle, posterolateral column impaction, posterior trochlea, and medial epicondyle.[10] The Bryan Morrey classification system focuses on the thickness of the capitellar fragment as well as the comminution of this fragment.[11] The Dubberley classification focuses on the involvement of the trochlea and whether this is fragment is in continuity with the capitellum or a separate fragment.[12] With regard to arthroscopic fixation, all of these descriptions yield important information. For an arthroscopic assisted fixation to be feasible: (1) the capitellum needs to be grossly intact and large enough to be captured by the threads of a cannulated screw, (2) the posterolateral cortex of the humerus needs to be able to support cannulated screw placement, and (3) if the trochlea is involved, the trochlea must be in continuity with the capitellum or the trochlear fragment should be large enough for reasonable screw capture. We recommend a CT scan to evaluate if arthroscopic-assisted fixation is reasonable.

Arthroscopically assisted approaches for capitellar fractures and coronal shear fractures of the distal humerus are most appropriate for larger, single fragment fractures (Bryan Morrey type 1 or 4) without posterior column comminution (**Fig. 2**). The fragment must be able to be reduced and visualized adequately.[13] Arthroscopic suture lasso fixation for reducible Bryan Morrey type 2 fractures has been described, but is not commonly performed.[4] For unreducible Bryan Morrey type 2

and 3 capitellar fractures, fragment excision via an open or arthroscopic approach has been described, but we prefer to repair these fractures whenever possible.[4,14] In this section, we describe our approach to arthroscopic-assisted fixation of Bryan Morrey type 1 fractures (the most common indication).

Step 1: Closed Versus Arthroscopic-Assisted Provisional Reduction

One common question is how to reduce the capitellar fragment. An important article by Ochner and colleagues[15] demonstrated that closed treatment of capitellar fractures is possible. This serves as the basis for arthroscopic-assisted treatment. The goal of arthroscopic-assisted treatment is to reduce the fragment, but also to provide fixation to allow for early motion rather than an extended period of immobilization.

Closed reduction of the capitellar fragment can be achieved by gently placing the elbow in full extension with the forearm supinated. Usually, extension leads to spontaneous reduction because the anterior capsular attachments to the humerus are intact and will push the capitellar fragment into the right position. However, sometimes the posterior columnar fracture is impacted and flexed. Application of pressure anteriorly over the capitellar fragment while in extension will restore the anatomy of the posterolateral column in those situations. The capitellar fragment can be captured and maintained in an anatomic position by flexing the elbow at this point. Fluoroscopic films are used to confirm the reduction.[15] If the fracture cannot be reduced grossly approximated through closed means, arthroscopic-assisted fixation is likely not feasible and an open approach is recommended.

Step 2: Visualization and Fracture Manipulation

If the closed reduction captures the capitellar fracture but further refinements of the reduction are needed, an arthroscopic-assisted reduction can be performed.[4,5] Using anteromedial and anterolateral portals as described earlier, the joint can be visualized and hematoma debrided. A trocar can be placed through the proximal anterolateral portal proximal to the fragment. Usually, the capitellar fragment needs to be pushed from superior to inferior a few millimeters. A broad switching stick is usually the best instrument for reduction.

Step 3: Fracture Fixation

Three guidewires for 2.5 mm headless cannulated compression screws are then placed under

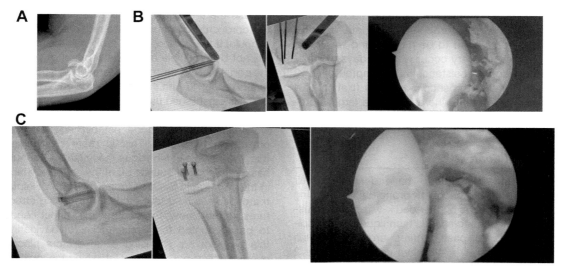

Fig. 2. Arthroscopic-assisted capitellar reduction and internal fixation. (*A*) Lateral radiograph of a capitellum fracture. (*B*) Anteroposterior and lateral fluoroscopy image and arthroscopic image showing arthroscopic-assisted and percutaneous provisional fixation of the capitellar fracture. (*C*) Anteroposterior and lateral fluoroscopy image and arthroscopic image showing final fixation of the capitellar fracture.

arthroscopic and fluoroscopic guidance ideally perpendicular to the fracture plane, from posterior to anterior. To confirm appropriate placement and maximize screw length, each wire is advanced until it is in a subchondral position on fluoroscopy. Screw lengths are measured, and the guidewires are advanced to prevent inadvertent pullout. The Kirschner wires placed for provisional fixation are then removed. Each screw is inserted sequentially in standard fashion using fluoroscopic and arthroscopic guidance. Do not drill multiple screws at one time because of risk of fragment rotation as described earlier.

Step 4: Final Evaluation

Reduction is checked with a probe and the elbow is taken through a full range of motion. Arthroscopic examination for other associated lesions is performed. A final check with fluoroscopy confirms appropriate reduction and fixation.

REHABILITATION AND RECOVERY

Postoperative care is tailored to each patient based on patient characteristics, fracture type, and fixation stability. In general, for capitellar and coronoid fractures, the elbow is splinted immediately postoperatively for 7 to 10 days followed by an active motion protocol similar to open surgery; but if there is high confidence in the fixation and the patient is compliant, motion can begin immediately. Stretching and strengthening can begin when the fracture is healed radiographically,

usually at 6 weeks. Unrestricted activity is allowed once patients recover reasonable strength compared to the contralateral side.

ARTHROSCOPICALLY ASSISTED REDUCTION AND INTERNAL FIXATION OF CORONOID FRACTURES

Most coronoid fractures are not amenable to arthroscopic-assisted fixation. Most coronoid fractures occur in the setting of a combined injury to the elbow. We generally conceptualize these patterns as (1) terrible triad injuries—a tip fracture of the coronoid, lateral collateral ligament (LCL) tear, and radial head fracture; (2) varus posteromedial rotatory instability (VPMRI)—an anteromedial facet fracture of the coronoid and LCL tear; or (3) olecranon fracture dislocation (OFD) where there is a fracture of the proximal ulna with dislocation of the intact forearm relative to the ulnohumeral joint, often accompanied by a radial head fracture. Doornberg and Ring[16] demonstrated that coronoid fracture patterns are associated with specific fracture patterns: (1) coronoid tip fractures occur with terrible triad injuries, (2) coronoid anteromedial facet fractures occur with VPMRI injuries, and (3) coronoid base fractures occur with OFD injuries.

In this context, some VPMRI injuries are amenable to arthroscopic fixation; however, the coronoid fracture fragment needs to be large enough for cannulated screw fixation. In addition, the fragment needs to be a single piece with minimal comminution. We do not feel all VPMRI injuries have coronoid fractures large enough for fixation, so the surgeon needs to be discriminating about who is an appropriate candidate. In addition, fractures need to be mobile, and we would recommend surgery occur within 5 days of injury if arthroscopic assistance is attempted. **Fig. 2** demonstrates arthroscopic-assisted fixation of a transitional fracture where there is a larger coronoid fracture accompanied by a marginal radial head fracture.

Historical Context

Adams and colleagues[17] have described their technique of arthroscopic coronoid fixation using cannulated screws or threaded k-wires; and Hausman has described a lasso technique utilizing spinal needles to pass sutures around the ulna circumferentially.[4,17] We have combined these 2 techniques to place cannulated screws, but then pass a reinforcement suture through the cannulated screw guidewire holes to provide additional fixation (**Fig. 3**).

Step 1: Portal Establishment and Fracture Evaluation

An anterolateral portal is established as described earlier. Once the anterolateral portal is established,

we use the arthroscopy camera/cannula to see if the coronoid fragment can be reduced using the cannula. If the camera is too proximal, the fracture will not be reducible and consideration of placing the portal more distal may be worthwhile. If the fracture is reducible with the cannula, the anteromedial portal is established using an inside-out technique. If the fracture is not reducible, then the medial working portal should be established using an outside in technique. This is more challenging than the inside-out technique, because the cannula has a tendency to bounce off of the capsule, which in the elbow acts like a balloon. Unlike other joints, the capsule is held taut by the surrounding structures. In the elbow, this "trampoline" effect needs to be accounted for. Some tricks for navigating this problem are (1) using serial dilators placed over a guidewire; (2) once establishing the location of the portal using a spinal needle, using a pointed, straight mosquito to dilate the portal; or (3) using an 11 blade to carefully open the capsule.

The skin incision for the medial portal should be generous. We generally aim to place a button cannula for the medial portal because standard cannulas are often too long to accommodate a targeting guide. A large, broad grasper or a switching stick is placed through the working portal. The

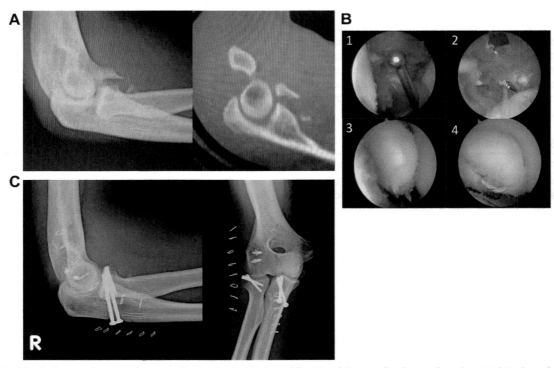

Fig. 3. Arthroscopic-assisted coronoid reduction and internal fixation. (*A*) Lateral radiograph and sagittal CT slice of a coronoid fracture. (*B*) Arthroscopic images showing fracture exposure with targeting guide (1), guidewire placement (2), reduction and fixation of the coronoid (3), and lasso augmentation of the arthroscopic-assisted coronoid fracture. (*C*) Anteroposterior and lateral radiographs showing final fixation of the coronoid fracture. (4) Final repair construct.

reduction is tested using the grasper. The coronoid tip is displaced to allow visualization of the fracture base. The fracture base is gently cleaned of any interposed tissue with a shaver or grasper.

Step 2: Posterior Incision and Placement of Guidewires

An incision is made over the posterior olecranon. The incision is usually 3 to 4 cm in length, centered with the coronoid on lateral fluoroscopic views. It is important to remember that when screws are placed, a bone bridge of about 1 cm is recommended.

A targeting guide is placed through the anteromedial working portal with the goal of placing 3 guidewires from the posterior to anterior into the fracture bed under direct visualization with the arthroscope. Usually, the primary surgeon holds the targeting guide in place, while the assistant surgeon drives the guidewire slowly until the wire tips are visualized in the fracture bed. It is important to recognize that the guidewires should not cross each other and need to be spaced in such a way that when one wire is drilled, the drill does not touch the other guidewires. The goal is to drill the most radial and most ulnar guidewires in the fracture base.

The guidewires are then measured for length. The actual screws will be the length of the guidewire added to the estimated length of the coronoid fragment. We prefer to draw a chart on the operating drapes to avoid confusion.

Step 3: Reduction of Fracture and Screw Placement

A large grasper is placed into the anteromedial portal and the coronoid fracture is reduced and held firmly opposed to the fracture base. The assistant then advances the guidewire until it is visualized in the elbow joint. There needs to be enough guidewire visible to grasp and control the guidewire during drilling to avoid inadvertent advancement of the wire through the capsule.

The first guidewire is drilled and a cannulated screw is placed. If the cannulated screw is too long, we will leave the screw prominent on the dorsal surface of the olecranon. The second cannulated screw is then drilled and placed. The third guidewire is then removed.

Step 4: Placement of Suture Lasso

A 0 polydioxanone (PDS) suture is passed into the most radial cannulated screw from the posterior incision. The PDS suture is retrieved from the medial working portal. A #2 Fiberwire suture is then tied to the 0 PDS suture and relayed through the cannulated screw. The end of the Fiberwire is then retrieved by drawing back the PDS suture. A snap is placed on the ends of the Fiberwire to prevent inadvertent suture loss. A second 0 PDS suture is placed into the other cannulated screw and the other end of the Fiberwire is then relayed into the cannulated screw. The suture ends are then tied together posteriorly. This serves as a secondary reinforcement for the coronoid fragment.

Step 5: Lateral Collateral Ligament Repair

Because most of these are VPMRI injuries, a separate lateral incision is made and the LCL is repaired. We generally use 1 or 2 GII Mitek suture anchors (DePuy Synthes, Raynham, MA, USA) and repair the LCL origin to the epicondyle.

REHABILITATION AND RECOVERY

The most important part of recovery is to avoid varus stress for the initial 6 weeks until the elbow is healed. We generally will immobilize patients for 10 to 14 days in a posterior splint and then begin active and gentle passive range of motion of the elbow while continuing to avoid varus stress. Varus stress is most commonly experienced when the arm his held away from the body, so we encourage patients to keep the elbow at the side during this period. We prefer using a posterior elbow splint during the first 6 weeks rather than a hinged elbow brace because the hinged elbow brace sometimes can slide distally and apply additional varus load to the arm if a patient is noncompliant. Stretching and strengthening can begin when the fracture is healed radiographically, usually at 6 weeks. Unrestricted activity is allowed once patients recover reasonable strength compared to the contralateral side.

CLINICAL RESULTS AND COMPLICATIONS

Arthroscopic-assisted reduction and fixation is increasingly used for intra-articular elbow fractures because of its minimally invasive nature and potential for decreased stiffness; however, most current reports are limited to retrospective case reports or series.[18,20] To better evaluate the efficacy of arthroscopic techniques compared to open approaches, further prospective and comparative trials are necessary. The available evidence does support the use of elbow arthroscopic in the management of some intra-articular elbow fractures.[19]

The evidence for arthroscopic-assisted capitellar fixation has been limited to a small series of case reports.[5,13,21,22] Open approaches to capitellar fractures are challenging and can put the posterior interosseous nerve and lateral collateral ligaments at risk.[1,21] Based on existing reports, an arthroscopic approach can minimize these risks, allow for better mobilization, facilitate earlier motion, and reduce the risk of stiffness.[4,5]

The recent evidence for arthroscopic-assisted coronoid fixation is comparatively stronger than for other arthroscopic-assisted approaches in the elbow.[2,17,23] This may be because visualization of the coronoid for fixation is especially challenging. A recent comparative study of arthroscopy-assisted versus open reduction and fixation of coronoid fractures found that the arthroscopic approach had fewer complications with similar union rates, surgical results, and patient-reported outcomes.[2]

Elbow arthroscopy is a technically challenging surgical procedure with a steep learning curve.[24,25] Although the complication rate has been reported to be as low as 2% for experienced surgeons, other studies have reported major and minor complication rates up to 12%.[26,27] Complications vary widely, but the most devastating complication is major peripheral nerve injury, particularly of the ulnar nerve.[25–29] With appropriate judgment and technique, the risk of injury to critical neurovascular structures can be minimized.[4,25,28]

CLINICS CARE POINTS

- Elbow and fixation stability should be assessed to determine whether an open approach is required to repair ligaments or enhance fracture fixation.

DISCLOSURE

No potential conflicts of interest exist with respect to the research, authorship, and/or publication of this article. This article was funded in part by the Jesse B. Jupiter/Wyss Medical Foundation Fund.

REFERENCES

1. Fram BR, Seigerman DA, Ilyas AM. Coronal Shear Fractures of the Distal Humerus: A Review of Diagnosis, Treatment, and Outcomes. Hand (N Y) 2021; 16(5):577–85.
2. Oh WT, Do WS, Oh JC, et al. Comparison of arthroscopy-assisted vs. open reduction and fixation of coronoid fractures of the ulna. J Shoulder Elbow Surg 2021;30(3):469–78.
3. Hsu JW, Gould JL, Fonseca-Sabune H, et al. The emerging role of elbow arthroscopy in chronic use injuries and fracture care. Hand Clin 2009;25(3): 305–21.
4. Fink Barnes LA, Parsons BO, Hausman M. Arthroscopic Management of Elbow Fractures. Hand Clin 2015;31(4):651–61.
5. Van Nguyen T, Kholinne E, AlSomali K, et al. Technique for Arthroscopic-Assisted Reduction and Cannulated Screw Fixation for Coronal Shear Fractures of the Distal Humerus. Arthrosc Tech 2021;10(4): e949–55.
6. Field LD, Altchek DW. Evaluation of the arthroscopic valgus instability test of the elbow. Am J Sports Med 1996;24(2):177–81.
7. Croutzet P, Guinand R, Kany J. Arthroscopic Surgery for Radial Head Fractures: A Prospective Series of 14 Cases. Arthroscopy 2015;31(6):e18.
8. Rolla PR, Surace MF, Bini A, et al. Arthroscopic treatment of fractures of the radial head. Arthroscopy 2006;22(2):233.e1–6.
9. Menth-Chiari WA, Ruch DS, Poehling GG. Arthroscopic excision of the radial head: Clinical outcome in 12 patients with post-traumatic arthritis after fracture of the radial head or rheumatoid arthritis. Arthroscopy 2001;17(9):918–23.
10. Ring D, Jupiter JB, Gulotta L. Articular fractures of the distal part of the humerus. J Bone Joint Surg Am 2003;85(2):232–8.
11. McKee MD, Jupiter JB, Bamberger HB. Coronal shear fractures of the distal end of the humerus. J Bone Joint Surg Am 1996;78(1):49–54.
12. Dubberley JH, Faber KJ, Macdermid JC, et al. Outcome after open reduction and internal fixation of capitellar and trochlear fractures. J Bone Joint Surg Am 2006;88(1):46–54.
13. Kuriyama K, Kawanishi Y, Yamamoto K. Arthroscopic-assisted reduction and percutaneous fixation for coronal shear fractures of the distal humerus: report of two cases. J Hand Surg Am 2010;35(9):1506–9.
14. Feldman MD. Arthroscopic excision of type II capitellar fractures. Arthroscopy 1997;13(6):743–8.
15. Ochner RS, Bloom H, Palumbo RC, et al. Closed reduction of coronal fractures of the capitellum. J Trauma 1996;40(2):199–203.
16. Doornberg JN, Ring D. Coronoid fracture patterns. J Hand Surg Am 2006;31(1):45–52.
17. Adams JE, Merten SM, Steinmann SP. Arthroscopic-assisted treatment of coronoid fractures. Arthroscopy 2007;23(10):1060–5.
18. Van Tongel A, Macdonald P, Van Riet R, et al. Elbow arthroscopy in acute injuries. Knee Surg Sports Traumatol Arthrosc 2012;20(12):2542–8.
19. Yeoh KM, King GJW, Faber KJ, et al. Evidence-based indications for elbow arthroscopy. Arthroscopy 2012;28(2):272–82.
20. Atesok K, Doral MN, Whipple T, et al. Arthroscopy-assisted fracture fixation. Knee Surg Sports Traumatol Arthrosc 2011;19(2):320–9.

21. Hardy P, Menguy F, Guillot S. Arthroscopic treatment of capitellum fracture of the humerus. Arthroscopy 2002;18(4):422–6.
22. Mitani M, Nabeshima Y, Ozaki A, et al. Arthroscopic reduction and percutaneous cannulated screw fixation of a capitellar fracture of the humerus: a case report. J Shoulder Elbow Surg 2009;18(2):e6–9.
23. Hausman MR, Klug RA, Qureshi S, et al. Arthroscopically Assisted Coronoid Fracture Fixation: A Preliminary Report. Clin Orthop Relat Res 2008; 466(12):3147–52.
24. Keyt LK, Jensen AR, O'Driscoll SW, et al. Establishing the learning curve for elbow arthroscopy: surgeon and trainee perspectives on number of cases needed and optimal methods for acquiring skill. J Shoulder Elbow Surg 2020;29(11):e434–42.
25. Stetson WB, Vogeli K, Chung B, et al. Avoiding Neurological Complications of Elbow Arthroscopy. Arthrosc Tech 2018;7(7):e717–24.
26. Kelly EW, Morrey BF, O'Driscoll SW. Complications of elbow arthroscopy. J Bone Joint Surg Am 2001; 83(1):25–34.
27. Reddy AS, Kvitne RS, Yocum LA, et al. Arthroscopy of the elbow: a long-term clinical review. Arthroscopy 2000;16(6):588–94.
28. Hilgersom NFJ, Oh LS, Flipsen M, et al. Tips to avoid nerve injury in elbow arthroscopy. World J Orthop 2017;8(2):99–106.
29. Desai MJ, Mithani SK, Lodha SJ, et al. Major Peripheral Nerve Injuries After Elbow Arthroscopy. Arthroscopy 2016;32(6):999–1002.e8.

Rethinking Scaphoid Fixation

Jill Putnam, MD

KEYWORDS

• Scaphoid fracture • Fixation • Double screw • Plate • Grafting • Nonunion

KEY POINTS

• Scaphoid fracture and nonunion management are controversial in part due to a variety of options for fixation and grafting, if indicated.
• Newly described double screw fixation of scaphoid fractures may allow for more robust fixation and earlier time to mobilization.
• Fixation options for nonunion include Kirschner wire, screw, and plate fixation, and the ideal choice is largely dependent on the intended graft type and nonunion characteristics.

INTRODUCTION

Scaphoid fracture fixation has long been the subject of debate, and fixation and grafting techniques continue to evolve. If indicated in an acute injury, fixation should allow for relatively early motion. In a nonunion setting, ideal fixation should achieve compression and stability without sacrificing scaphoid height and should respect the scaphoid's tenuous vascular supply.

Anatomy

The scaphoid is a cashew-shaped bone with a surface area made of 80% to 90% cartilage.[1] The dorsal ridge is non-articular and serves as the insertion for 70% to 80% of the scaphoid's primary vascular supply via a radial artery branch.[2] The distal pole includes the scaphoid tubercle and is supplied by volar branches of the radial artery and the superficial palmar branch.[2] Waist fractures make up greater than 60% of scaphoid fractures and include fractures involving the central third of the scaphoid.[3] The proximal 20% to 30% of the scaphoid is the proximal pole, which possesses relatively poor vascularity and possesses minimal surface area for fixation.[2,4] Both of these aspects put the proximal pole at a higher risk of nonunion. For this reason, surgical management is recommended for both displaced and

non-displaced proximal pole fractures to provide immediate stability while awaiting regrowth of vascular channels to the proximal pole.[5]

The scaphoid is critical in that it spans the proximal and distal rows. The scaphoid is "tethered" distally by its articulations with the trapezium and the trapezoid. Proximally, the scaphoid articulates with the scaphoid fossa of the radius. Although the primary stabilizer preventing scaphoid flexion is the scapholunate ligament, the radioscaphocapitate (RSC) ligament acts as a key secondary stabilizer. The radioscaphoid articulation, such as the scaphotrapeziotrapezoid (STT) articulation, accumulates degenerative changes as the scaphoid progressively flexes in a nonunion scenario and is the primary site for early changes in scaphoid nonunion advanced collapse (SNAC).[6] The recognition of abnormal joint kinematics in the typical SNAC scenario is critical to appreciating scaphoid fracture stability.

Diagnosis

Clinical suspicion of a scaphoid fracture should be present when a patient presents after a fall onto an outstretched wrist and has tenderness to palpation over the anatomic snuffbox.[7,8] In the absence of radiographic evidence of a scaphoid fracture, immobilization with a wrist or thumb spica orthosis is recommended initially.[9]

The Hand and Upper Extremity Center, The Ohio State University, 915 Olentangy River Road, Suite 3200, Columbus, OH 43212, USA
E-mail address: Jill.Putnam.22@gmail.com

Hand Clin 39 (2023) 597–604
https://doi.org/10.1016/j.hcl.2023.05.007

hand.theclinics.com

Advanced imaging may be pursued if an urgent diagnosis is required; Computerized tomography (CT) scan is less sensitive than MRI or bone scan for immediate diagnosis in a non-displaced scaphoid fracture.[10,11]

Management

Acute fractures can be managed nonoperatively if they are non-displaced or displaced less than 1 to 2 mm, and in patients who are low-demand, not fit for surgery, or are willing to undergo 8 to 12 weeks of immobilization.[12,13] Expedited conversion to fixation is recommended when nonoperative treatment shows signs of failure.[13] Surgical management is typically indicated for displaced fractures and allows for decreased immobilization times and faster return to work.[14]

Scaphoid nonunion is defined as failure to heal by 4 to 6 months post-injury.[15] Surgical management of symptomatic nonunion is recommended to prevent degenerative changes that typically ensue. Early-stage SNAC (type 1), in which degenerative changes are confined to the radiostyloid articulation, can be managed like other scaphoid nonunion cases with the addition of a styloidectomy.[16] Later stage SNAC cases are typically managed with a salvage procedure.[6]

Preoperative Planning

Preoperative planning for scaphoid fractures involves ruling out concurrent injuries, such as perilunate injuries, radial head fractures (up to 6%), or distal radius fractures (1%–4%).[17,18] In acute cases, a CT scan can help to evaluate for associated carpal injuries or scaphoid fracture characteristics (eg, comminution, displacement). A CT scan is often obtained in nonunion cases to evaluate humpback deformity or degenerative changes, although this modality is unlikely to change management.[19] MRI may also be used to evaluate the vascularity of the proximal pole in nonunion cases, although avascularity suggested by MRI has not been proven to correlate with intraoperative lack of punctate bleeding, histopathology consistent with avascular necrosis (AVN), nor with time to union.[20,21]

Surgical fixation of acute fractures may involve Kirschner wire (k wire), screw, or plate fixation. Screw fixation may use a dorsal or volar approach. The volar (retrograde) approach can be used for distal pole or waist fractures and can be a percutaneous procedure or an open procedure, if the direct open reduction is required. The dorsal (antegrade) approach can be performed in a percutaneous, mini-open, or open approach and is indicated for scaphoid waist or proximal pole fractures. Volar plate fixation for acute scaphoid fractures is typically reserved for small proximal pole fractures or comminuted fractures.[16,22,23]

Nonunion management is controversial, and success requires a balance of osseous stability and biology. Bone grafting is typically required for nonunions because of the osseous void created once excision of devitalized tissue is performed. This graft may be vascular or nonvascular. Nonvascular grafts include cancellous, cortical, or corticocancellous grafts typically harvested from the distal radius or iliac crest. Nonvascular grafts supplying cartilage for a proximal pole that cannot be salvaged include costochondral rib and hamate grafts. The most commonly described vascularized bone grafts include the volar carpal artery graft, the dorsal capsular-based graft, the 1,2-intercompartmental supraretinacular artery (ICSRA) or 2,3-ICSRA grafts, and the medial femoral condyle graft.[24] The medial femoral trochlear graft is a vascular graft that also provides cartilage for denuded proximal pole cases.[25]

The choice of fixation for these nonunion scenarios should be made with consideration of the graft choice. Structural grafts such as corticocancellous iliac crest graft are robust and can maintain a large segmental gap, and thus scaphoid height, despite compression and rotational forces provided by screws.[26–29] The most commonly used nonvascular cortical or corticocancellous grafts used include tricortical iliac crest or distal radius bone graft harvested in a hybrid Russe style.[28,30] The disadvantage of cortical grafts relative to cancellous grafts is the longer time to incorporation.[29,31] Nonstructural cancellous graft deserves careful management if a compression screw is used to prevent the loss of significant scaphoid height; alternatively, plate fixation can maintain length and rotation for nonstructural grafts, particularly with a large segmental defect.[32–34]

Headless central threadless shaft screws, or "Herbert" screws, have long been a gold standard for scaphoid fracture fixation.[35] Newer generation screws often have a fully threaded variable pitch to theoretically achieve further compression.[36] Although further compression may be desirable in certain scenarios with robust bone, overcompression with fully threaded screws across a segmental defect may cause loss of height or unexpected compression forces at interfragmentary gaps.[37] This difference in compression across interfragmentary gaps may be a concern in nonunion scenarios where a proximal pole/graft junction and a distal pole/graft junction are both required to heal. Further, the use of central threadless shaft screws, or "smooth shank" screws, decreases the internal volume of the scaphoid that is occupied for hardware and thus allows more area for bony healing.[38]

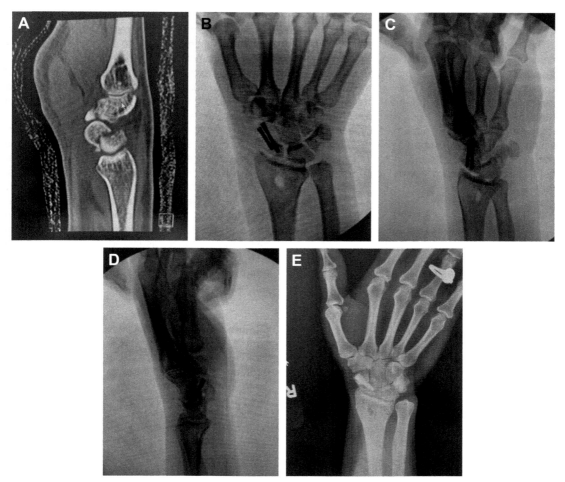

Fig. 1. (*A*) Preoperative sagittal CT image of a scaphoid waist nonunion with humpback deformity. (*B–D*) Intra-operative posteroanterior (PA), oblique, and lateral fluoroscopic images with retrograde double screw fixation with application of cancellous distal radius autograft. (*E*) Postoperative PA radiograph with union. (*Courtesy of* Christopher Chen, MD.)

Double screw fixation constructs have been increasingly described to provide superior rotational control and angular stability.[34,39,40] Hundred percent union rates have been described in three case series for acute fractures, and 90.5% to 100% union rates have been described for nonunions in two case series.[41–45] This construct may be especially well suited for proximal pole fractures, which are inherently unstable, and this technique has been successful in smaller scaphoids.[46] The use of two screws ranging from 1.5 to 3.5 mm diameters has been described; certainly, patient size and fracture location dictate what size is possible.[41,46] Fracture location and angulation will also contribute to whether a dorsal or volar approach is best indicated (**Fig. 1**). As with any screw insertion in a small target, slow insertion is critical to lower hoop stresses and decrease the

risk of fracture propagation, and sequential tightening of each screw is important to avoid gapping. Double screw fixation may allow for earlier mobilization. In their study of 21 delayed union and nonunion patients treated with two screws and cancellous bone grafting, Ek and colleagues report permitting gentle active range of motion at 10 to 14 days postoperatively, with an associated 90.5% union rate at a mean 2.8 months.[45] Further studies are needed to confirm the non-inferiority of early mobilization of for double screw fixation, but biomechanically the construct supports earlier mobilization.[34,39]

In a nonunion scenario, the volar approach is typically considered the "workhorse" for distal or waist nonunions or any nonunion with a significant humpback deformity. The volar approach allows for better visualization of the nonunion site, easier correction of the deformity, and respects the dorsal vascular supply.[2]

The necessity of vascular grafts for management of nonunion with or without AVN has not been proven.[21,47,48] Comparative studies are limited by small cohorts, heterogenous presentations of scaphoid nonunion, and different fixation methods.[48–51] Nevertheless, vascular grafts may augment healing of a nonunion. If a vascular graft is planned, the surgeon should select an approach that simplifies harvesting, and should plan for a method of fixation that will not compromise the pedicle.

Procedural Approach

All scaphoid procedures are performed with the patient positioned supine with a radiolucent hand table. Monitored anesthesia care with local anesthetic infiltration is typically sufficient for acute fracture management. Regional anesthetic blocks are frequently performed for more complex or nonunion cases.

The dorsal, or antegrade, approach for headless screw insertion is performed with the hand in a pronated position, with an incision just distal to Lister's tubercle. A percutaneous approach may be used, but the surgeon must be mindful of potential for injury to extensor tendons, in particular extensor pollicis longus (EPL) and inadequate subchondral insertion of the screw.[52] In a mini-open approach, the retinaculum is divided longitudinally approximately 1 cm distally, and the EPL tendon is brought radially. The dissection is performed between extensor carpi radialis longus (ECRL) and extensor carpi radialis brevis (ECRB), or between ECRB and the fourth dorsal compartment, depending on patient anatomy. The capsule is typically incised transversely or in a "T" fashion for improved visualization. The wrist is hyperflexed over a large roll of towels to simplify the trajectory. The proximal pole is identified, and fluoroscopy is used to select a starting point for the k-wire that allows for central trajectory.[53] If no assistant is available to aid in wrist hyperflexion, the percutaneous insertion of an antegrade .045 k-wire from the dorsal radial lip of the radius into the hyperflexed lunate will help to hold the proximal pole in a flexed position, indirectly reducing the fracture. The central positioning of the k-wire is confirmed, and a derotational wire is added to prevent scaphoid malrotation during implant insertion. The most common screw size is 20 to 22 mm for males and 18 to 20 mm for females.[54]

The volar, or retrograde approach, for headless screw insertion is typically performed as a percutaneous procedure. The wrist is hyperextended over a roll of towels, and the scaphoid tubercle is palpated. Levering the trapezium in an ulnar-dorsal direction with the use of a cannulated guide helps to protect the trapezium and gain access to the central axis of the scaphoid.[55] A k-wire is used with fluoroscopy to identify the appropriate start point, and then, a 3 to 4 mm incision is made to allow for hardware insertion.

For nonunion with little to no humpback deformity and no significant segmental defect, this investigator prefers a dorsal approach with application of cancellous bone from the distal radius. A dorsal approach to the scaphoid as previously described is performed, using a longitudinal incision to maximize visualization of the nonunion site and to allow for harvesting from the dorsal distal radius. Once visualized, the nonunion site is aggressively debrided of fibrous tissue until fresh bleeding cancellous bone is identified. The tourniquet is not deflated for this confirmation. Proximally in the incision, the retinaculum is divided longitudinally over half of the EPLs course through the retinaculum. Lister's tubercle is identified. A retinacular flap with a proximal base just proximal to Lister's tubercle is saved for closure over the bony defect after Lister's tubercle has been harvested. A quarter inch osteotome is used to create four sides of a rectangle around Lister's tubercle, which is harvested as cortical graft. Abundant cancellous graft is collected with a small curved curette. The proximally based retinacular flap is secured with absorbable suture to decrease hematoma formation. The cancellous graft is generously inserted into the nonunion site. An antegrade compression screw is then inserted as previously described.

For nonunion with a humpback deformity and/or segmental defect, this investigator typically uses a volar approach with application of cancellous bone from the dorsal distal radius and screw or volar plate fixation. A longitudinal "hockey stick" incision is made over the volar wrist, in line with the flexor carpi radialis (FCR) tendon proximally, with the apex at the volar wrist crease and coursing toward the thumb distally. The FCR sheath is incised and the tendon is swept ulnarly for exposure of the wrist capsule. The RSC ligament is incised and repaired later. The scaphoid nonunion site is identified and aggressively debrided with a curette and rongeur back to bleeding cancellous bone. The .045 k-wires are inserted in the proximal and distal poles to serve the joysticks to support nonunion site access (**Fig. 2**). This also allows for temporary correction of the humpback deformity. As previously described, cancellous distal radius fracture is harvested dorsally per this investigator's preference.

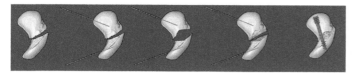

Fig. 2. Illustration of sequential identification of the segmental defect, scaphoid pole pinning, aggressive curettage of devitalized tissue, generous graft insertion, and finally fixation, with attention to maintenance of scaphoid height.

Alternatively, distal radius graft can be harvested through the proximal extension of the longitudinal volar approach, with reflection of the pronator quadratus. Abundant graft is applied to the nonunion site, with careful attention to pack in graft to the extent that the humpback deformity is "corrected." If the scaphoid is well aligned with the application of this graft, then a screw is a reasonable fixation device, with care not to "over-compress" the nonunion site to the extent that the scaphoid loses significant height. If the segmental defect is very large, or the proximal pole relatively small and at risk of fracture with screw placement, plate fixation may be considered. This investigator prefers a pre-contoured six-hole volar locking plate (Medartis, AG, Basel, Switzerland). The contour of the plate is typically a good template if the alignment of distal and proximal poles is challenging. The plate is applied proximally and distally, using the previously described k-wires as joysticks. K-wires are then driven through the plate into the proximal and distal poles for provisional plate application. A single cortical screw is inserted distally to compress the plate to bone, and a single cortical screw is inserted similarly in the proximal pole. Unicortical locking screws are used to fill the remainder of the holes, and then the cortical screws are replaced with unicortical locking screws. Fluoroscopy and wrist manipulation should confirm that there is no impingement of the plate proximally. If there is impingement, the proximal most screw and screw hole may be removed (**Fig. 3**). This also facilitates the use of plate for smaller proximal pole fractures, where the plate can be used in a buttress fashion. Finally, the RSC is closed with nonabsorbable suture to prevent flexion of the scaphoid.

The heterogenous fixation and grafting methods for scaphoid fixation clearly demonstrate that no universal method has been accepted for scaphoid nonunion management. Although it is useful for the surgeon to have many techniques in his or her armamentarium for these challenging cases, this investigator recommends using the simplest technique that allows for earliest time to union. The use of nonvascular grafting techniques and length-stable fixation methods may be less technically demanding and allow for shorter operative times than alternatives.[21,45,47,56]

Postoperative Management

The timing of wrist mobilization postoperatively depends on the scaphoid injury and fixation method. In compliant patients with minimally displaced acute fractures status post screw fixation, active wrist motion is often permitted between 1 and 3 weeks postoperatively, with weight-bearing restrictions typically maintained until 6 weeks postoperatively.[41,57,58]

In nonunion scenarios, mobilization is typically deferred until radiographs or CT confirm greater than 50% healing, and until the patient is nontender over the anatomic snuffbox.[24] CT scan is often obtained to follow scaphoid healing before liberating a patient from immobilization.[59] However, the likelihood of CT to change the management of the patient has been questioned; radiographs may be just as reliable to "confirm" scaphoid union.[60]

Outcomes

Average time to union for acute scaphoid fractures managed with screw fixation is typically reported

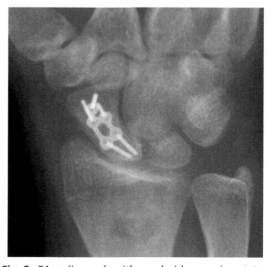

Fig. 3. PA radiograph with scaphoid nonunion status post plate fixation with removal of the proximal-most hole of the plate, to prevent impingement. (*Courtesy of* Scott Edwards, MD.)

from 4 to 8 weeks versus 8 to 12 weeks for acute fractures managed nonoperatively.[14,57,58,61,62] Time to union for nonunion scenarios varies dramatically between 4 weeks and 6 months, largely dependent on the nature of the nonunion, fixation and grafting technique used, and definition of union.[16,63]

Although patients with surgical management of acute scaphoid injuries return to work and sports faster than those managed without surgery, the complication rate is higher with surgical management.[13,64] The most common complications reported include delayed union or nonunion (1%–5%), hardware complications (2%–4%), and sensory nerve irritation (1%–2%).[13,14]

Salvage procedures are reserved for symptomatic degenerative changes associated with missed scaphoid fractures or failed management of nonunion cases.[65] Depending on the degree of degenerative changes, patients may be a candidate for excision of the distal pole of the scaphoid, styloidectomy, limited arthrodesis, proximal row carpectomy, or total wrist arthrodesis.

SUMMARY

There is a lack of consensus regarding scaphoid fracture and nonunion management. Recent literature suggests that more stable fixation, such as dual screw fixation or plate fixation, when indicated, may allow for earlier mobilization or faster time to union. Stability and biology are important to fracture healing. The need for vascularized bone grafting has not been proven, and less demanding techniques may yield similar outcomes. The quality of available literature on scaphoid fracture and nonunion outcomes is limited by heterogenous cases and reporting. Future studies could better guide surgeons by clearly reporting definitions of nonunion and dysvascularity, fracture and nonunion characteristics, and clear definition of union.

CLINICS CARE POINTS

- Successful surgical management of scaphoid nonunion requires attention to both biology and stability.
- Clinical evidence and reported outcomes for scaphoid nonunion management is limited by a predominance of Level IV and V evidence, the heterogeneity of the nonunion characteristics, and a patient population that can be challenging to follow.

DISCLOSURE

Dr J. Putnam has nothing to disclose.

REFERENCES

1. Kawamura K, Chung KC. Treatment of scaphoid fractures and nonunions. J Hand Surg 2008;33(6): 988–97.
2. Gelberman RH, Menon J. The vascularity of the scaphoid bone. J Hand Surg 1980;5(5):508–13.
3. Garala K, Taub NA, Dias JJ. The epidemiology of fractures of the scaphoid: impact of age, gender, deprivation and seasonality. Bone Jt J 2016;98-B(5):654–9.
4. Luchetti TJ, Hedroug Y, Fernandez JJ, et al. The morphology of proximal pole scaphoid fractures: implications for optimal screw placement. J Hand Surg Eur 2018;43(1):73–9.
5. Chong HH, Kulkarni K, Shah R, et al. A meta-analysis of union rate after proximal scaphoid fractures: terminology matters. J Plast Surg Hand Surg 2021; 22:1–12.
6. Vender MI, Watson HK, Wiener BD, et al. Degenerative change in symptomatic scaphoid nonunion. J Hand Surg 1987;12(4):514–9.
7. Kodumuri P, McDonough A, Lyle V, et al. Reliability of clinical tests for prediction of occult scaphoid fractures and cost benefit analysis of a dedicated scaphoid pathway. J Hand Surg Eur 2021;46(3): 292–6.
8. Dias JJ, Ring D, Grewal R, et al. Acute scaphoid fractures: making decisions for treating a troublesome bone. J Hand Surg Eur 2022;47(1):73–9.
9. Clay NR, Dias JJ, Costigan PS, et al. Need the thumb be immobilised in scaphoid fractures? A randomised prospective trial. J Bone Joint Surg Br 1991;73(5):828–32.
10. Brydie A, Raby N. Early MRI in the management of clinical scaphoid fracture. Br J Radiol 2003; 76(905):296–300.
11. Beeres FJP, Hogervorst M, den Hollander P, et al. Outcome of routine bone scintigraphy in suspected scaphoid fractures. Injury 2005;36(10):1233–6.
12. Arsalan-Werner A, Sauerbier M, Mehling IM. Current concepts for the treatment of acute scaphoid fractures. Eur J Trauma Emerg Surg 2016;42(1):3–10.
13. Dias JJ, Brealey SD, Fairhurst C, et al. Surgery versus cast immobilisation for adults with a bicortical fracture of the scaphoid waist (SWIFFT): a pragmatic, multi-centre, open-label, randomised superiority trial. Lancet Lond Engl 2020;396(10248):390–401.
14. Alnaeem H, Aldekhayel S, Kanevsky J, et al. A Systematic Review and Meta-Analysis Examining the Differences Between Nonsurgical Management and Percutaneous Fixation of Minimally and

Nondisplaced Scaphoid Fractures. J Hand Surg 2016;41(12):1135–44.e1.

15. Capo JT, Shamian B, Rivero S. Chronic scaphoid nonunion of 28-year duration treated with nonvascularized iliac crest bone graft. J Wrist Surg 2013;2(1):79–82.

16. Putnam JG, Mitchell SM, DiGiovanni RM, et al. Outcomes of Unstable Scaphoid Nonunion With Segmental Defect Treated With Plate Fixation and Autogenous Cancellous Graft. J Hand Surg 2019;44(2):160.e1–7.

17. Wildin CJ, Bhowal B, Dias JJ. The incidence of simultaneous fractures of the scaphoid and radial head. J Hand Surg Edinb Scotl 2001;26(1):25–7.

18. Gürbüz Y, Sügün TS, Kayalar M. Combined Fractures of the Scaphoid and Distal Radius: Evaluation of Early Surgical Fixation (21 Patients with 22 Wrists). J Wrist Surg 2018;7(1):11–7.

19. Gvozdenovic R, Presman B, Larsen MB, et al. Can CT-Scan Measurements of Humpback Deformity, Dislocation, and the Size of Bony Cysts Predict Union after Surgery for Scaphoid Nonunion? J Wrist Surg 2021;10(5):418–29.

20. Günal I, Ozçelik A, Göktürk E, et al. Correlation of magnetic resonance imaging and intraoperative punctate bleeding to assess the vascularity of scaphoid nonunion. Arch Orthop Trauma Surg 1999;119(5–6):285–7.

21. Rancy SK, Swanstrom MM, DiCarlo EF, et al. Success of scaphoid nonunion surgery is independent of proximal pole vascularity. J Hand Surg Eur 2018;43(1):32–40.

22. Quadlbauer S, Pezzei C, Jurkowitsch J, et al. [Palmar angular stable plate fixation of nonunions and comminuted fractures of the scaphoid]. Oper Orthopadie Traumatol 2019;31(5):433–46.

23. Leti Acciaro A, Lana D, Fagetti A, et al. Plate fixation in challenging traumatic carpal scaphoid lesions. Musculoskelet Surg 2022;106(2):179–85.

24. Moon ES, Dy CJ, Derman P, et al. Management of nonunion following surgical management of scaphoid fractures: current concepts. J Am Acad Orthop Surg 2013;21(9):548–57.

25. Bürger HK, Windhofer C, Gaggl AJ, et al. Vascularized medial femoral trochlea osteocartilaginous flap reconstruction of proximal pole scaphoid nonunions. J Hand Surg 2013;38(4):690–700.

26. Jarrett P, Kinzel V, Stoffel K. A biomechanical comparison of scaphoid fixation with bone grafting using iliac bone or distal radius bone. J Hand Surg 2007;32(9):1367–73.

27. Gire JD, Thio T, Behn AW, et al. Rotational Stability of Scaphoid Waist Nonunion Bone Graft and Fixation Techniques. J Hand Surg 2020;45(9):841–9.e1.

28. Shapiro LM, Roe AK, Kamal RN. Clinical and Patient-Reported Outcomes After Hybrid Russe

Procedure for Scaphoid Nonunion. Hand N Y N 2022;17(1):13–22.

29. Hegazy G, Massoud AH, Seddik M, et al. Structural Versus Nonstructural Bone Grafting for the Treatment of Unstable Scaphoid Waist Nonunion Without Avascular Necrosis: A Randomized Clinical Trial. J Hand Surg 2021;46(6):462–70.

30. Robbins RR, Ridge O, Carter PR. Iliac crest bone grafting and Herbert screw fixation of nonunions of the scaphoid with avascular proximal poles. J Hand Surg 1995;20(5):818–31.

31. Sanjeev K, Thomas E, Bruce B, et al. Biology and enhancement of skeletal repair. In: Skeletal trauma. 4th edition. Philadelphia: Saunders; 2009. p. 33–50.

32. Goodwin J, Castañeda P, Drace P, et al. A Biomechanical Comparison of Screw and Plate Fixations for Scaphoid Fractures. J Wrist Surg 2018;7(1):77–80.

33. Goodwin JA, Castañeda P, Shelhamer RP, et al. A Comparison of Plate Versus Screw Fixation for Segmental Scaphoid Fractures: A Biomechanical Study. Hand N Y N 2019;14(2):203–8.

34. Mandaleson A, Tham SK, Lewis C, et al. Scaphoid Fracture Fixation in a Nonunion Model: A Biomechanical Study Comparing 3 Types of Fixation. J Hand Surg 2018;43(3):221–8.

35. Herbert TJ, Fisher WE. Management of the fractured scaphoid using a new bone screw. J Bone Joint Surg Br 1984;66(1):114–23.

36. Patel S, Tiedeken N, Qvick L, et al. Interfragmentary Compression Forces Vary Based on Scaphoid Bone Screw Type and Fracture Location. Hand N Y N 2019;14(3):371–6.

37. Koh IH, Kang HJ, Kim JS, et al. A central threadless shaft screw is better than a fully threaded variable pitch screw for unstable scaphoid nonunion: a biomechanical study. Injury 2015;46(4):638–42.

38. Gholson JJ, Bae DS, Zurakowski D, et al. Scaphoid fractures in children and adolescents: contemporary injury patterns and factors influencing time to union. J Bone Joint Surg Am 2011;93(13):1210–9.

39. Nicholson LT, Sochol KM, Azad A, et al. Single Versus Dual Headless Compression Screw Fixation of Scaphoid Nonunions: A Biomechanical Comparison. Hand N Y N 2021. https://doi.org/10.1177/1558944720974111. 1558944720974111.

40. Jurkowitsch J, Dall'Ara E, Quadlbauer S, et al. Rotational stability in screw-fixed scaphoid fractures compared to plate-fixed scaphoid fractures. Arch Orthop Trauma Surg 2016;136(11):1623–8.

41. Yildirim B, Deal DN, Chhabra AB. Two-Screw Fixation of Scaphoid Waist Fractures. J Hand Surg 2020;45(8):783.e1–4.

42. Quadlbauer S, Beer T, Pezzei C, et al. Stabilization of scaphoid type B2 fractures with one or two headless compression screws. Arch Orthop Trauma Surg 2017;137(11):1587–95.

43. Acar B, Köse Ö, Turan A, et al. Single versus double screw fixation for the treatment of scaphoid waist fractures: Finite element analysis and preliminary clinical results in scaphoid nonunion. Jt Dis Relat Surg 2020;31(1):73–80.

44. Garcia RM, Leversedge FJ, Aldridge JM, et al. Scaphoid nonunions treated with 2 headless compression screws and bone grafting. J Hand Surg 2014;39(7):1301–7.

45. Ek ET, Johnson PR, Bohan CM, et al. Clinical Outcomes of Double-Screw Fixation with Autologous Bone Grafting for Unstable Scaphoid Delayed or Nonunions with Cavitary Bone Loss. J Wrist Surg 2021;10(1):9–16.

46. DiPrinzio EV, Dieterich JD, Walsh AL, et al. Two Parallel Headless Compression Screws for Scaphoid Fractures: Radiographic Analysis and Preliminary Outcome. Hand N Y N 2022. https://doi.org/10. 1177/15589447221081879. 15589447221081880.

47. Rancy SK, Schmidle G, Wolfe SW. Does Anyone Need a Vascularized Graft? Hand Clin 2019;35(3): 323–44.

48. Braga-Silva J, Peruchi FM, Moschen GM, et al. A comparison of the use of distal radius vascularised bone graft and non-vascularised iliac crest bone graft in the treatment of non-union of scaphoid fractures. J Hand Surg Eur 2008;33(5):636–40.

49. Ribak S, Medina CEG, Mattar R, et al. Treatment of scaphoid nonunion with vascularised and nonvascularised dorsal bone grafting from the distal radius. Int Orthop 2010;34(5):683–8.

50. Pinder RM, Brkljac M, Rix L, et al. Treatment of Scaphoid Nonunion: A Systematic Review of the Existing Evidence. J Hand Surg 2015;40(9):1797–805. e3.

51. Aibinder WR, Wagner ER, Bishop AT, et al. Bone Grafting for Scaphoid Nonunions: Is Free Vascularized Bone Grafting Superior for Scaphoid Nonunion? Hand N Y N 2019;14(2):217–22.

52. Adamany DC, Mikola EA, Fraser BJ. Percutaneous fixation of the scaphoid through a dorsal approach: an anatomic study. J Hand Surg 2008;33(3):327–31.

53. McCallister WV, Ambrose HC, Katolik LI, et al. Comparison of pullout button versus suture anchor for zone I flexor tendon repair. J Hand Surg 2006; 31(2):246–51.

54. Meermans G, Verstreken F. Influence of screw design, sex, and approach in scaphoid fracture fixation. Clin Orthop 2012;470(6):1673–81.

55. Vaynrub M, Carey JN, Stevanovic MV, et al. Volar percutaneous screw fixation of the scaphoid: a cadaveric study. J Hand Surg 2014;39(5):867–71.

56. Cohen MS, Jupiter JB, Fallahi K, et al. Scaphoid waist nonunion with humpback deformity treated without structural bone graft. J Hand Surg 2013; 38(4):701–5.

57. Schädel-Höpfner M, Marent-Huber M, Gazyakan E, et al. Acute non-displaced fractures of the scaphoid: earlier return to activities after operative treatment. A controlled multicenter cohort study. Arch Orthop Trauma Surg 2010;130(9):1117–27.

58. Papaloizos MY, Fusetti C, Christen T, et al. Minimally invasive fixation versus conservative treatment of undisplaced scaphoid fractures: a cost-effectiveness study. J Hand Surg Edinb Scotl 2004;29(2):116–9.

59. Hackney LA, Dodds SD. Assessment of scaphoid fracture healing. Curr Rev Musculoskelet Med 2011;4(1):16–22.

60. Matzon JL, Lutsky KF, Tulipan JE, et al. Reliability of Radiographs and Computed Tomography in Diagnosing Scaphoid Union After Internal Fixation. J Hand Surg 2021;46(7):539–43.

61. Inoue G, Tanaka Y, Nakamura R. Treatment of transscaphoid perilunate dislocations by internal fixation with the Herbert screw. J Hand Surg Edinb Scotl 1990;15(4):449–54.

62. Bond CD, Shin AY, McBride MT, et al. Percutaneous screw fixation or cast immobilization for nondisplaced scaphoid fractures. J Bone Joint Surg Am 2001;83(4):483–8.

63. Ghoneim A. The unstable nonunited scaphoid waist fracture: results of treatment by open reduction, anterior wedge grafting, and internal fixation by volar buttress plate. J Hand Surg 2011;36(1):17–24.

64. Ibrahim T, Qureshi A, Sutton AJ, et al. Surgical versus nonsurgical treatment of acute minimally displaced and undisplaced scaphoid waist fractures: pairwise and network meta-analyses of randomized controlled trials. J Hand Surg 2011;36(11):1759–68. e1.

65. Moritomo H, Tada K, Yoshida T, et al. The relationship between the site of nonunion of the scaphoid and scaphoid nonunion advanced collapse (SNAC). J Bone Joint Surg Br 1999;81(5):871–6.

Advances in Soft Tissue Injuries Associated with Open Fractures

Andrew W. Hollins, MD[a], Suhail K. Mithani, MD[b],*

KEYWORDS

- Soft tissue • Flap reconstruction • Traumatic wounds • Grafts

KEY POINTS

- Soft tissue reconstruction is a critical step in management of open fractures.
- Negative pressure wound therapy can be used as an adjunct for stabilization and healing by secondary intention.
- Dermal regenerative templates provide a tool for treatment of soft tissue injury without additional donor site morbidity.
- Understanding the anatomy of the upper extremity and goals of functional reconstruction allows for planning of local and free tissue flap reconstruction.

INTRODUCTION

Management of soft tissue injury of the upper extremity is a common challenge for practicing hand surgeons. This is a complex topic because there are multiple approaches and solutions to each defect. These soft tissue deficits can result from trauma, burns, oncologic resection, or infection. The upper extremity is unique because of the intricate underlying anatomy and need for coverage of vital structures including nerves, arteries, and tendons. The soft tissue coverage is managed in tandem with treatment of the deep structures. It is important to select the reconstructive option that provides the patient the most durable coverage with the least donor site morbidity. Soft tissue coverage should be thin and pliable and accommodate the importance of sensation, gliding of tendons, and range of motion of multiple joints. The best reconstructive choice not only provides soft tissue coverage but also optimizes the patient's hand function.

The timing of soft tissue coverage in upper extremity trauma is critical. Adequate surgical debridement of open fractures and wounds is a principle in management. Highly contaminated or infected wounds may require serial surgical debridement before definitive reconstruction. The earlier soft tissue coverage is attained, the more favorable the outcome of osseus healing of underlying fractures and earlier range of motion.[1–3] Without adequate source control, patients are at risk of nonunion and secondary complications. The final soft tissue coverage should take place after the deeper structure injuries are treated.

The options for soft tissue reconstruction of the upper extremity have evolved with advances in the field. Negative pressure wound therapy provides a sterile dressing that results in macro-deformation of the wound, improved granulation tissue, and delay in the need for soft tissue coverage.[4,5] The advent of dermal regenerative templates (DRTs) has provided a new option for the coverage of wounds not amenable to immediate skin grafting without additional donor site morbidity.[6] Improved microsurgical techniques have created refined free tissue options that allow for soft tissue options that better match the upper extremity anatomy.[7]

[a] Division of Plastic Surgery, Department of Surgery, Duke University Medical Center, Box 3974 Duke Medical Center, Durham, NC 27710, USA; [b] Division of Plastic Surgery, Department of Surgery, Duke University Medical Center, 2301 Erwin Road, Durham, NC 27705, USA
* Corresponding author. North Carolina Orthopaedic Clinic, 3609 Southwest Durham Drive, Durham, NC 27707.
E-mail address: suhail.mithani@duke.edu

Hand Clin 39 (2023) 605–616
https://doi.org/10.1016/j.hcl.2023.05.008

hand.theclinics.com

Patient Evaluation

A comprehensive assessment and evaluation of the patient and their injuries is a vital initial step. This includes obtaining a full history of the patient and their medical comorbidities. Hand dominance and occupation will help formulate the goals of treatment in discussions with the patient. Patients with associated uncontrolled diabetes are at a higher risk of postoperative infection.[8,9] Active smokers have a significantly higher rate of skin graft failure and delayed wound healing.[10] Some limb salvage and reconstruction options require multiple surgeries and longer hospital stays. Discussing the long-term treatment trajectory and expected recovery time will help formulate patient expectations and decisions. A full physical examination should be performed to rule out any concomitant injuries in the trauma population. Patients presenting with life-threatening injuries or critical illnesses should be triaged appropriately. Management of upper extremity fractures and associated soft tissue injuries should be delayed or temporized if the patient is not a candidate for surgical intervention.

The mechanism of the injury will often reflect the suspected extent of involvement and steps in management. Crush injuries to the hand and upper extremity can cause a wide zone of injury with significant inflammation. These can be associated with difficult to manage fractures along with significant neurologic and vascular compromise.[11] Patients with oncologic pathologies may present with unique large defects from en-bloc resection. Preparing for the expected margins of resection and involved structures helps dictate the reconstruction. The patient's prognosis or need for additional adjuvant treatments, such as radiation therapy, will affect the need for more durable coverage.[12] The operative plan for fixation of bony fractures will also play a role in soft tissue reconstruction.

Reconstructive Ladder

The reconstructive ladder can be used as a guide for soft tissue coverage of upper extremity injuries. The base of the reconstructive ladder is healing by secondary intention. Secondary intention is indicated for injuries without any exposed bone or implants, soft tissue injuries that do not cross a joint space, or in critically ill patients that are not candidates for surgery. Secondary intention healing of fingertip injuries has demonstrated superior return of sensation.[13] A study evaluating defects of the dorsum of the hand found that healing by secondary intention resulted in satisfactory esthetic outcomes in a time period similar to surgical recovery.[14] It is important to recognize when a wound can be treated with wound care alone. This option should be presented to patients as an alternative to surgical intervention if possible. Secondary intention requires maintenance dressing care and may require longer healing time depending on the size of the defect. It can provide an esthetic and functionally acceptable result without additional donor site morbidity or added expense of surgery.

Split-thickness skin graft (STSG) or full-thickness skin graft (FTSG) is also options for wounds without exposed critical structures. Skin grafts can be adjuncts to expedite the process of epithelialization and healing in large wounds. FTSGs require greater metabolic demand for survival compared with STSGs, but they lead to less secondary contracture. When considering wounds near joints, it is important to avoid contractures that may limit function. Skin grafts can be harvested from the ipsilateral upper arm using an area of excess skin from the ulnar aspect of the upper arm at the bicep ulnar aspect. This donor site can often be closed primarily with minimal morbidity. Larger grafts can be harvested from the outer thigh region.

The application of DRTs has greatly expanded in upper extremity reconstruction. Integra and Matriderm are commonly used bilayer dermal templates sometimes referred to as DRTs. DRTs refer to a variety of products that can help stimulate growth of granulation tissue in a wound bed that would not be amenable to skin grafting. These adjuncts can be used to facilitate closure of wounds through secondary intention or to bridge a wound to secondary successful skin graft a few weeks after application. Understanding the role for DRT is helpful to avoid complications from skin grafts and morbidity of flap reconstruction. **Fig. 1** shows a simplified algorithm for deciding between STSG, FTSG, or DRT depending on the wound characteristics.

DRT can be used in a wound bed with exposed tendon or bone without paratenon or limited periosteum (**Fig. 2**).[14,15] DRT should not be applied to any wound with active infection or contamination, absent vascularity, exposed hardware, or an open joint. The use of DRT can also prevent secondary contracture of wounds often seen with split-thickness skin grafting.[16,17] This secondary contracture may result in the significant loss of function of the hand.

Negative Pressure Wound Therapy

NPWT was popularized as innovative method for secondary intent healing by Argenta and

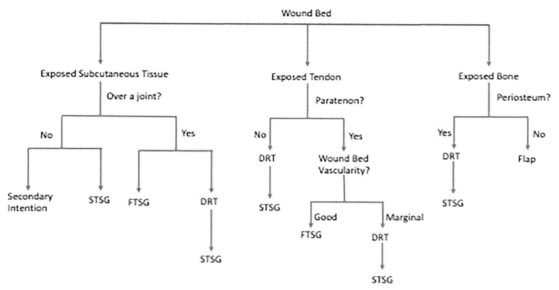

Fig. 1. Proposed algorithm for decision-making process for treatment with secondary intention, split-thickness skin graft (STSG), full-thickness skin graft (FTSG), dermal regenerative template (DRT), or flap reconstruction.

colleagues.[18] NPWT contributes to wound healing via multiple mechanisms including wound macro-deformation, fluid drainage, and stabilization of wound environment.[19] NPWT is an important tool in the hand surgeon's armamentarium. A foam or gauze wound dressing is covered and sealed with an impermeable polyurethane outer layer. This helps prevent bacterial colonization of the wound compared with standard dressings. Open fractures of the upper extremity can be treated with NPWT after initial surgical treatment if soft tissue coverage is not available. Open fractures treated with NPWT have demonstrated a

significantly lower infection rates compared with standard dressings.[20,21]

NPWT is contraindicated in wounds with active infection or contamination, ischemic tissue, malignancy, or vital structures including organs, blood vessels, or grafts.[22] It can be applied to open fractures with or without exposed hardware. The use of NPWT can continue until granulation tissue builds up for adequate coverage of deeper structures. This continued wound vac therapy prevents the need for larger flap coverage. For example, an open forearm fracture with skin loss can be treated with serial applications of NPWT. This treatment

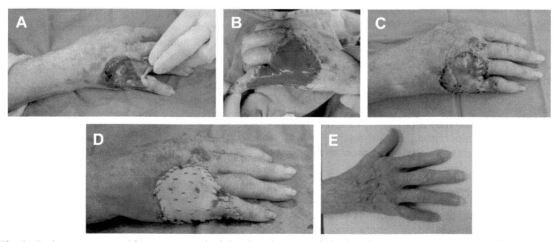

Fig. 2. Patient presents with open wound of the dorsal aspect of the hand with exposed paratenon (A). The patient was treated with bilayer dermal regenerative template (Integra) (B). Integra had appropriate take at 3 weeks (C) and subsequent staged skin grafting (D). Long-term results demonstrate a well-healed skin graft (E).

will decrease the size of needed coverage and can be treated with a staged local muscle flap or skin grafting alone.

FIXATION METHODS

Exposed hardware is a high risk for contamination and bony infection. The selection of fixation method for upper extremity fractures may dictate the need for flap reconstruction. Fractures that can be treated with intramedullary fixation eliminate exposed hardware that needs soft tissue coverage. If fractures require a plate and screw construct, thoughtful location of plate placement may reduce the need for flap coverage.

External fixation is a useful tool in treatment of upper extremity injuries. Externalization of hardware is a safe technique to avoid contamination in an open wound. External fixators are often used in the treatment of significantly comminuted fractures. An external fixator can be readily applied in a short time and can effectively maintain length, alignment, and stability.[23] Treatment with an external fixator may reduce the need for large soft tissue coverage of internally placed hardware. However, this treatment method has significant associated complications including loosening, pin site infections, malreduction, stiffness, and the possible need for revision surgeries.[24,25] This is not an ideal method of fixation but has a role in mangled upper extremity trauma and can temporize or obviate flap reconstruction.

Thoughtful implant selection and/or adjusting treatment fixation method can alter the need for flap reconstruction. Although volar locking plates are the most common implant choice for the surgical treatment of distal radius fractures, their use may be limited in some situations.[26] For example, although the use of dorsal bridge plating requires a second surgery for hardware removal, it remains a viable option for the treatment of certain distal radius fractures.[27] Having and using multiple treatment and fixation options based on soft tissue coverage may affect the reconstructive needs. For example, for patients with distal radius fractures and associated volar soft tissue defects, a dorsal bridge plate may be a better fixation option to prevent wound healing issues related to an already compromised volar soft tissue envelope (**Fig. 3**).

Flap Reconstruction

Flap coverage is indicated for wounds that are not amenable for skin grafting, DRT, or healing by secondary intent. Thorough surgical debridement remains the first step before any reconstructive coverage. Flap coverage over a contaminated or infected field will result in postoperative infections and unstable wounds. Selecting the ideal flap reconstruction depends on each specific clinical assessment. The anatomic location of each defect will limit the available local pedicled flap options. In addition, wound size, location, comorbidities, or recipient vessel availability will guide decision for possible free flap reconstruction.

Pedicled Flaps of the Upper Extremity

Posterior interosseous artery flap

The posterior interosseous artery (PIA) flap was first described by Zancolli and Angrigiani.[28] This is a fasciocutaneous flap based on the vascular pedicle of the PIA that is located between the septum of the extensor carpi ulnaris and extensor digiti minimi. The flap can be raised either based on the antegrade or retrograde flow of the PIA. Antegrade-based PIA flap can be used for coverage of defects of the proximal forearm or elbow.[29] The flap is more commonly described as a reverse flow flap for coverage of defects of the wrist or first web space. However, modifications in technique have demonstrated additional reach for distal defects of the thumb and digits.[30]

The flap template is designed based on a line drawn from the ulnar head to the lateral epicondyle. The flap width and location are determined by the defect and application of antegrade or reverse flow flap. Flap widths of greater than 6 cm (cm) often require skin graft closure of the donor site. For a reverse flow PIA flap, the flap island can be located at the middle third of the forearm with an arc of rotation usually centered 3 cm proximal to distal radial-ulnar joint. The antegrade PIA flap is located more distally at the forearm with the distal most aspect about 4 cm proximal from the dorsal wrist crease.

An osteocutaneous PIA flap has previously been described for successful treatment of nonunions of the humerus or ulna.[31,32] The thin and pliable nature of this flap makes it ideal for contouring defects of the wrist and web space. It can be used both as a local and free tissue transfer. The pedicle can be smaller in caliber and more superficial at the distal aspect making it susceptible to injury during harvest. The location of the perforator can also limit pedicle length of the reverse PIA flap. Dissection of the pedicle can sometimes be tedious as it courses between the Extensor Carpi Ulnaris (ECU) and Extensor Digiti Minimi (EDM). Despite these challenges, this flap is an excellent choice for many soft tissue defects of the upper extremity, including first web space reconstruction to maintain the depth needed for functional thumb opposition.

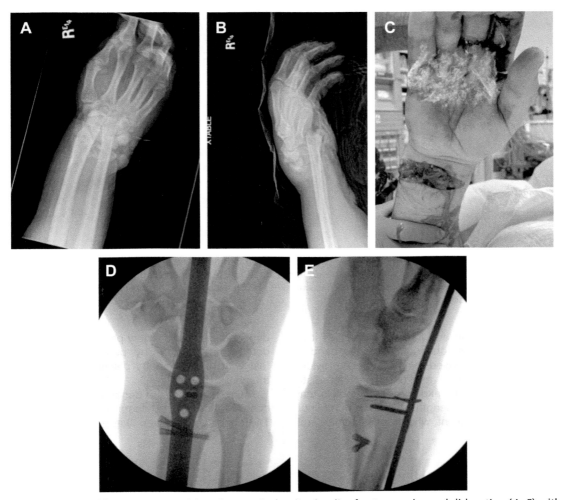

Fig. 3. A 42-year-old man presents with an intra-articular distal radius fracture and carpal dislocation (*A*, *B*) with volar soft tissue defect (*C*). He was treated with open reduction and internal fixation with dorsal bridge plate (*D*, *E*). The volar soft tissue wound healed by secondary intent.

Radial forearm flap

The radial forearm flap (RFF) was first described as a free flap by Yang and colleagues.[33] Modifications of this flap have been described as local options for elbow coverage or reverse flow for hand and wrist defects (**Fig. 4**). The RFF is based on the blood supply from perforators of the radial artery located in the septum between the brachioradialis (BR) and flexor carpi radialis (FCR). This can also be raised as an innervated flap based on the lateral antebrachial cutaneous nerve. The flap can be harvested as a fasciocutaneous or adipofascial flap depending on the need for coverage.

The design of the RFF depends on the location of the defect. The flap is centered over the radial artery which can be identified using a hand-held Doppler. The more distal the skin island on the forearm, the greater pedicle length and reach can be obtained for proximal defects. The perforators supplying the skin island are found in the septum between the BR and FCR. The radial artery can be dissected to its proximal takeoff from the brachial artery to provide maximal pedicle length. Inclusion of the cephalic vein within the flap can help assist with superficial venous drainage.

The reverse flow flap variant (**Fig. 5**) can be designed at the middle aspect of the forearm. The placement of the flap island too proximal at the forearm runs the risk of inadequate skin island perfusion due to fewer perforators at this proximal portion as the radial artery dives deep at its origin. The RFF has also been described as an osteocutaneous flap for hand reconstruction.[34] Rates of radius fracture with composite flap have been reported as high as 17%, but this fracture rate may be reduced with prophylactic fixation.[35,36] The

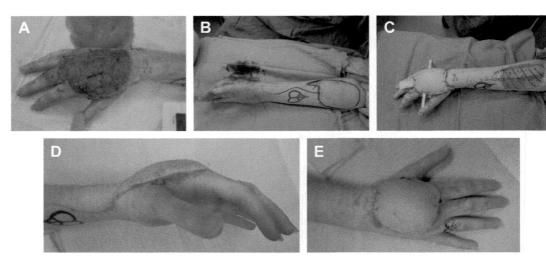

Fig. 4. The patient presented with significant hypergranulation wound of the dorsum of the hand (*A*). A reverse flow RFF was designed at the proximal forearm (*B*) and rotated for coverage of the dorsal defect with donor site closure with split-thickness skin graft (*C*). The flap and skin graft healed well with long-term follow-up and good overall contour of dorsal hand (*D, E*).

pliability of the flap and its thinness makes it an ideal soft tissue reconstruction for the hand or elbow. Its axial based blood supply provides robust perfusion with minimal issues for distal flap ischemia or breakdown. The pedicle can reach up to 20 cm in length. This flap is contraindicated for any patient who has a palmar arch dependent on radial artery perfusion. This can be determined clinically by performing an Allen's test with pulse oximetry placed on the patients thumb.

The morbidity of the donor site is the greatest consideration when determining the use of RFF. The donor site requires skin grafting for closure

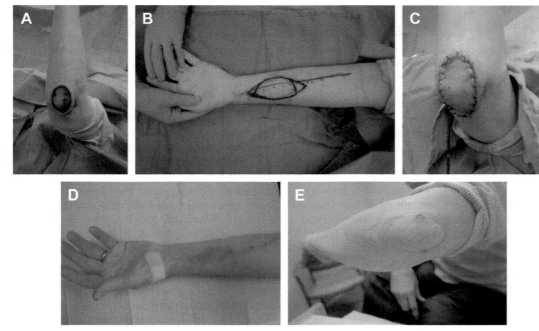

Fig. 5. Patient presented with open defect of the elbow (*A*). A pedicled radial forearm free flap was designed and inset for coverage with split thickness skin graft of the donor site (*B, C*). The posterior elbow wound healed well with appropriate take of the donor skin graft (*D, E*).

which may lead to partial graft take and exposed tendons. Patients may experience the loss of sensation and cold intolerance.[36] Studies have demonstrated that postoperatively, patients have increased Disability of the Shoulder and Hand scores that resolve after 2 years. They also have a loss of grip strength persist after long-term follow-up.[37,38]

Flexor carpi ulnaris flap

The flexor carpi ulnaris (FCU) flap is a muscle flap based on the posterior ulnar recurrent artery. This flap is described based on a proximal arc of rotation for coverage of antecubital and elbow wounds.[39,40] Before muscle harvest, a line is drawn from the medial epicondyle to the pisiform. An incision is made along this line overlying the muscle belly of the FCU. The tendinous portion of the FCU is released at its distal insertion. The pedicle is located immediately deep to this muscle belly and preservation of the proximal perforator will dictate the arc of rotation. This perforator is usually located within 5 to 6 cm of the medial epicondyle, providing adequate length for elbow coverage.[39] Although this flap can be smaller in width with a 2 to 4 cm muscle belly, the muscle fascia can be released longitudinally to allow the muscle to fan out for a larger area of coverage. The FCU was noted to have the most versatile and robust coverage in an anatomic study when compared with the BR and FCR.[41]

Care must be taken to preserve injury to the adjacent ulnar nerve during flap harvest. The FCU is a powerful flexor and aids with ulnar deviation of the wrist.[42] Reports have shown that there is some evidence of weakness associated with wrist flexion following surgery.[43] Splitting the muscle or keeping the distal tendon intact may be helpful in reducing the loss of wrist flexion.[44] Despite these potential limitations, this muscle flap is an excellent choice for antecubital and proximal forearm reconstruction.

Anconeus flap

Another local muscle flap option for elbow coverage is the anconeus flap. The anconeus flap was first described by Cardany.[45] This elbow stabilizer muscle originates at the dorsum of the lateral epicondyle and inserts at the lateral aspect of the olecranon. This flap is perfused by the recurrent PIA (RPIA) and is approximately 8 × 4 cm in size.[46] A previous study evaluating this flap demonstrated reliable coverage with posterior elbow defects averaging 4 × 3 cm in size.[47] To use this flap, a 5-cm incision is made over the lateral epicondyle and is carried distal for exposure of the muscle belly as it inserts on the

olecranon. The anconeus muscle is then sharply released from its entire insertion on the ulna under tourniquet.[48] The RPIA is a branch of the PIA and travels along the intraosseous membrane entering the muscle at its posterior surface. Studies have shown that patients note minimal deficits in elbow extension and range of motion following anconeus harvest.[46,47] Coverage with this option is limited to the posterior elbow and does not have adequate reach for antecubital defects.

Groin flap

The groin flap was first described in 1972 for soft tissue coverage of the hand.[49] The groin flap is a fasciocutaneous flap based on the superficial circumflex iliac artery and can be used to cover soft tissue defects of the hand. The flap is approximately 6 to 10 cm in width and centered over a parallel line 3 cm inferior to the inguinal ligament. The flap is raised in a lateral to medial fashion. The flap is elevated superficial to the investing fascia until the sartorius muscle is encountered, and then the dissection is converted deep to the investing fascia. The medial skin bridge is left intact and the flap is inset at the defect of the hand.[50,51] The patient must keep their hand adducted at the groin until the pedicle is ready for division. Some surgeons may use a body wrap postoperatively for immobilization of the operative arm. A Penrose drain can be applied to the pedicle in clinic before flap elevation to ensure adequate collateral blood flow has developed. The flap pedicle can be divided at approximately 3 weeks postoperatively.[52] The groin flap is a good bail out option for defects of the upper extremity. It requires multiple stages for reconstruction and fixates the operative hand position until flap division. The flap requires collateral ingrowth from the recipient site; therefore, contaminated or dysvascular wounds are not amenable for coverage.

Lateral arm flap

The lateral arm flap was first described by Song and colleagues.[53] This is a fasciocutaneous flap perfused by the radial collateral artery. This can be raised as a sensate flap based on the posterior brachial cutaneous nerve. A line is drawn from the deltoid insertion to the lateral epicondyle. The flap can be designed up to 20 × 14 cm in size and is located at the distal aspect of the upper arm (**Fig. 6**).[54] The flap is elevated distal to proximal with the pedicle running adjacent to the radial nerve at the lateral intermuscular septum. This flap can also be raised as a composite flap with inclusion of the distal humerus.[55] This lateral arm flap can be used as a free tissue transfer or used

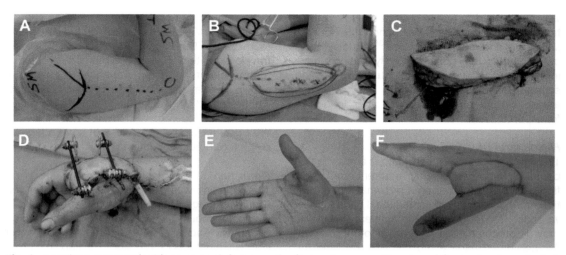

Fig. 6. A patient presented with an open defect over the first web space with external fixator in place. An ipsilateral lateral arm free flap was designed from the ipsilateral extremity (*A, B*). The flap was isolated on the recurrent posterior intraosseous artery (*C*) anastomosed to the radial artery for first web space coverage (*D*). The patient went on to heal with good overall contour and appearance (*E, F*).

as a pedicled flap for shoulder and axilla coverage.[56,57] The pedicle of the lateral arm flap is about 4 to 8 cm in length, limiting its mobility. A modified extended lateral arm flap moves the skin paddle distal to the proximal third of the lateral forearm. This modification of the flap is helpful in providing additional pedicle length of up to 12 cm.[58] A reverse lateral arm flap can be used for soft tissue coverage of the elbow and antecubital fossa.[59] This flap is supplied by the collateral blood flow through the radial recurrent artery.

The lateral arm flap tends to provide bulky coverage that may require secondary thinning depending on the patient's donor site. The donor site can often be closed primarily and is in an acceptable cosmetic location. Most of the patients do experience some loss of sensation over the dorsal forearm. This flap is an excellent option for ipsilateral upper extremity reconstruction for moderately sized defects.

Common Free Flaps of the Upper Extremity

Latissimus dorsi flap
The latissimus dorsi flap was the first described by Tansini for breast reconstruction.[60] The latissimus muscle is the largest surface muscle in the body measuring 25 × 35 cm, originating from the thoracolumbar fascia and inserting on the humeral groove. This muscle contributes to arm adduction, extension, and external rotation. The muscle can be used as a pedicled muscle flap or myocutaneous flap for coverage of the upper arm (**Fig. 7**).[61] The latissimus flap can also be harvested as a

free flap for larger soft tissue deficits. The pedicle for both of these options is the thoracodorsal artery. An elliptical skin paddle with width up to 10 cm can be closed primarily.[62,63] The donor site morbidity with harvest of this shoulder stabilizer should be considered when counseling patients. Overall, patients can expect to have decreased range of motion of the shoulder and weakness that typically does not interfere with activities of daily living.[63] Several modifications of this flap have been proposed to reduce the associated morbidity. Harvest of a muscle sparing split latissimus flap for small defects is associated with less donor site morbidity.[64] A thoracodorsal artery perforator flap can be harvested for a similar elliptical skin paddle without any muscle harvest.[65]

When harvested as a muscle flap alone, the thin nature of the latissimus flap creates a smooth contour for the distal arm. This muscle flap atrophies over time with denervation and may resolve bulkiness without the need for secondary thinning procedures. This flap is a reliable option for free tissue transfer of significantly larger soft tissue defects. The latissimus dorsi flap can provide coverage of degloving injuries of the forearm or upper arm with exposed hardware or critical vascular structures.

Anterolateral thigh flap
The anterolateral thigh (ALT) flap was described by Song and colleagues.[66] This fasciocutaneous flap can be harvested as an ellipse designed along a line from the anterior superior iliac spine to the lateral border of the patella. This flap can be an

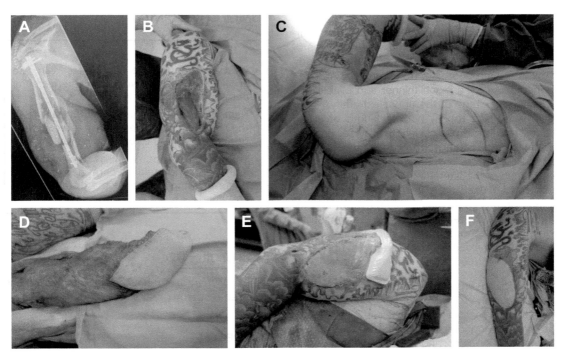

Fig. 7. This patient presented with open fracture of the humerus with large soft tissue defect of the upper arm (*A, B*). A myocutaneous pedicled latissimus flap was designed for coverage (*C, D*). It is not uncommon for the immediate postoperative period to have some transient venous congestion on clinical examination (*E*), but this improved postoperatively with well-healed contour at long-term follow-up (*F*).

alternative option for large soft tissue defects of the upper extremity in free flap reconstruction. The flap is supplied by the descending branch of the lateral femoral circumflex artery as it courses between the septum of the rectus femoris and vastus lateralis. It can be harvested with a skin paddle of up to 25 × 35 cm in size with skin grafting of the donor site. The donor site can often be

Table 1
Anatomic considerations of regional flap reconstruction

Local Flap	Coverage	Pedicle	Innervation	Pros	Cons
Latissimus	shoulder, axilla, bicep	Thoracodorsal	Thoracodorsal	Large muscle for coverage	Loss of shoulder ROM
Lateral Arm	shoulder, axilla	Radial Collateral	Posterior brachial	Large fasciocutaneous	Bulky, transient radial nerve palsy
Anconeus	elbow	Recurrent posterior interosseus artery	Radial nerve	Minimal morbidity	Smaller zone of coverage
RFF	antecubital, elbow	Radial artery	Lateral antebrachial	Thin, reliable	Donor site scar and morbidity
PIA	proximal forearm, elbow	Posterior interosseus artery	Dorsal antebrachial	Thin, pliable	dependent on perforator location
FCU	proximal forearm, elbow	Ulnar artery	Ulnar nerve	Versatile arc of rotation	Loss of wrist flexion, smaller muscle
Reverse PIA	wrist and hand	Posterior interosseus	Dorsal antebrachial	Thin, minimal morbidity	Tedious pedicle dissection
Reverse RFF	wrist and hand	Radial artery	Lateral antebrachial	Thin, reliable	Donor site scar and morbidity
Groin Flap	wrist and hand	Superficial circumflex iliac	none	Versatile, reliable	Morbidity, need for second stage

closed primarily with width up to 10 cm in size.[67,68] The vastus lateralis can also be included for additional bulk and chimeric design. The bulkiness of this flap is directly related to the patient's body habitus at the donor site. A suprafascial ALT can be harvested for a much thinner and pliable flap to match coverage of the upper extremity.[69] The ALT provides a robust pedicle length of up to 12 cm. This longer pedicle length provides an ideal option for large zones of injury and reaching recipient vessels in free tissue transfers. The descending branch of the lateral femoral circumflex artery can also be used as a flow through flap in the setting of large soft tissue defects with need for grafts in vascular reconstruction.[70] The versatility, minimal donor morbidity, and reliable anatomy of the ALT flap make it a workhorse flap in upper extremity reconstruction.

Anatomic considerations in regional flap reconstruction

The size and location of soft tissue injury dictate the available options of local flap reconstruction (**Table 1**). Shoulder and axilla defects can be covered with the pedicled latissimus or lateral arm flaps. The extended lateral arm flap provides additional pedicle length for more proximal wounds. The latissimus flap can also be used for coverage of the anterior or posterior upper arm. Anconeus, FCU, RFF, or PIA all are available options for local reconstruction of the elbow. The PIA and FCU flap provide a reliable arc of rotation to reach defects of the proximal forearm and antecubital region. The reverse PIA flap is the classic description for first web space local reconstruction. Reverse RFF has been described for soft tissue reconstruction of the wrist and distal aspects of the hand. The versatility of the groin flap can be used for varying coverage of the wrist and distal hand.

SUMMARY

There are many options for solving complex upper extremity soft tissue defects in the setting of underlying fractures. Understanding the patient's injuries and exposed structures is critical for selecting the appropriate reconstruction. DRT has allowed for a bridging of many wounds that are not amenable to skin graft coverage. If a flap is required for coverage, the defect size and location are the greatest factors for the appropriate operative treatment. Often times, multiple options are available for reconstruction and the decision must be made in conjunction with the patient for each specific clinical encounter.

CLINICS CARE POINTS

- Dermal regenerative templates can be applied to wounds with intact periosteum, paratenon, and clean wound beds.
- Negative pressure wound therapy can delay the need for definitive soft tissue reconstruction in the setting of open fractures.
- Thin pliable flaps, such as the extended lateral arm and radial forearm flap, are ideal for resurfacing defects of the distal forearm and hand.

DISCLOSURE

Dr S.K. Mithani is a consultant for Integra and has received research grant support from KCI.

REFERENCES

1. Freeland AE, Jabaley ME. Stabilization of fractures in the hand and wrist with traumatic soft tissue and bone loss. Hand Clin 1988;4(3):425–36.
2. Ruta D, Ozer K. Open fractures of the hand with soft tissue loss. Hand Clin 2013;29(4):551–67.
3. Sundine M, Scheker LR. A comparison of immediate and staged reconstruction of the dorsum of the hand. J Hand Surg Br 1996;21(2):216–21.
4. Lesiak AC, Shafritz AB. Negative-pressure wound therapy. J Hand Surg Am 2013;38(9):1828–32.
5. Cherubino M, Valdatta L, Tos P, et al. Role of Negative Pressure Therapy as Damage Control in Soft Tissue Reconstruction for Open Tibial Fractures, J Reconstr Microsurg, 33 (S 01), 2017, S08-S13.
6. Burke JF, Yannas IV, Quinby WC, et al. Successful use of a physiologically acceptable artificial skin in the treatment of extensive burn injury. Ann Surg 1981;194(4):413–28.
7. King EA, Ozer K. Free skin flap coverage of the upper extremity. Hand Clin 2014;30(2):201–9, vi.
8. Sharma K, Pan D, Friedman J, et al. Quantifying the Effect of Diabetes on Surgical Hand and Forearm Infections. J Hand Surg Am 2018;43(2):105–14.
9. Federer AE, Baumgartner RE, Cunningham DJ, et al. Increased Rate of Complications following Trigger Finger Release in Diabetic Patients. Plast Reconstr Surg 2020;146(4):420e–7e.
10. Rinker B. The evils of nicotine: an evidence-based guide to smoking and plastic surgery. Ann Plast Surg 2013;70(5):599–605.
11. Goodman AD, Got CJ, Weiss AC. Crush Injuries of the Hand. J Hand Surg Am 2017;42(6):456–63.

12. Vetter M, Germann G, Bickert B, et al. Current strategies for sarcoma reconstruction at the forearm and hand. J Reconstr Microsurg 2010;26(7):455–60.

13. Martin-Playa P, Foo A. Approach to Fingertip Injuries. Clin Plast Surg 2019;46(3):275–83.

14. Lateo SA, Langtry JA. A prospective case series of secondary intention healing for surgical wounds on the dorsum of the hand. Clin Exp Dermatol 2013; 38(6):606–11.

15. Shores JT, Hiersche M, Gabriel A, et al. Tendon coverage using an artificial skin substitute. J Plast Reconstr Aesthet Surg 2012;65(11):1544–50.

16. Frame JD, Still J, Lakhel-LeCoadou A, et al. Use of dermal regeneration template in contracture release procedures: a multicenter evaluation. Plast Reconstr Surg 2004;113(5):1330–8.

17. Di Giuli R, Dicorato P, Kaciulyte J, et al. Donor Site Wound Healing in Radial Forearm Flap: A Comparative Study Between Dermal Substitute and Split-Thickness Skin Graft Versus Full-Thickness Skin Graft Primary Coverage. Ann Plast Surg 2021; 86(6):655–60.

18. Argenta LC, Morykwas MJ. Vacuum-assisted closure: a new method for wound control and treatment: clinical experience. Ann Plast Surg 1997; 38(6):563–76. discussion 577.

19. Normandin S, Safran T, Winocour S, et al. Negative Pressure Wound Therapy: Mechanism of Action and Clinical Applications. Semin Plast Surg 2021; 35(3):164–70.

20. Stannard JP, Volgas DA, Stewart R, et al. Negative pressure wound therapy after severe open fractures: a prospective randomized study. J Orthop Trauma 2009;23(8):552–7.

21. Bhattacharyya T, Mehta P, Smith M, et al. Routine use of wound vacuum-assisted closure does not allow coverage delay for open tibia fractures. Plast Reconstr Surg 2008;121(4):1263–6.

22. White RA, Miki RA, Kazmier P, et al. Vacuum-assisted closure complicated by erosion and hemorrhage of the anterior tibial artery. J Orthop Trauma 2005; 19(1):56–9.

23. Capo JT, Rossy W, Henry P, et al. External fixation of distal radius fractures: effect of distraction and duration. J Hand Surg Am 2009;34(9):1605–11.

24. Williksen JH, Frihagen F, Hellund JC, et al. Volar locking plates versus external fixation and adjuvant pin fixation in unstable distal radius fractures: a randomized, controlled study. J Hand Surg Am 2013; 38(8):1469–76.

25. Weber SC, Szabo RM. Severely comminuted distal radial fracture as an unsolved problem: complications associated with external fixation and pins and plaster techniques. J Hand Surg Am 1986;11(2):157–65.

26. Orbay J. Volar plate fixation of distal radius fractures. Hand Clin 2005;21(3):347–54.

27. Brogan DM, Richard MJ, Ruch D, et al. Management of Severely Comminuted Distal Radius Fractures. J Hand Surg Am 2015;40(9):1905–14.

28. Zancolli EA, Angrigiani C. Posterior interosseous island forearm flap. J Hand Surg Br 1988;13(2):130–5.

29. Robinson LP, Usmani RH, Hazel A, et al. Use of the Antegrade Posterior Interosseous Artery Flap for Coverage of Complex Elbow Wounds. Plast Reconstr Surg 2021;148(6):1316–9.

30. Kocman EA, Kavak M, Kaderi S, et al. An extended distally based reverse posterior interosseous artery flap reconstruction for the thumb and distal defects of the fingers. Microsurgery 2021;41(5):430–7.

31. Pagnotta A, Taglieri E, Molayem I, et al. Posterior interosseous artery distal radius graft for ulnar nonunion treatment. J Hand Surg Am 2012;37(12): 2605–10.

32. Kamrani RS, Farhadi L, Farhoud AR. Forearm as a valuable source of vascularized bone graft for the distal humerus. J Shoulder Elbow Surg 2018;27(3):435–43.

33. Yang GF, Chen PJ, Gao YZ, et al. Forearm free skin flap transplantation: a report of 56 cases. 1981. Br J Plast Surg 1997;50(3):162–5.

34. Yajima H, Tamai S, Yamauchi T, et al. Osteocutaneous radial forearm flap for hand reconstruction. J Hand Surg Am 1999;24(3):594–603.

35. Satteson ES, Satteson AC, Waltonen JD, et al. Donor-Site Outcomes for the Osteocutaneous Radial Forearm Free Flap. J Reconstr Microsurg 2017; 33(8):544–8.

36. Richardson D, Fisher SE, Vaughan ED, et al. Radial forearm flap donor-site complications and morbidity: a prospective study. Plast Reconstr Surg 1997; 99(1):109–15.

37. Liu J, Liu F, Fang Q, et al. Long-term donor site morbidity after radial forearm flap elevation for tongue reconstruction: Prospective observational study. Head Neck 2021;43(2):467–72.

38. Calotta NA, Chandawarkar A, Desai SC, et al. An Algorithm for the Prevention and Treatment of Pain Complications of the Radial Forearm Free Flap Donor Site. J Reconstr Microsurg 2020;36(9):680–5.

39. Payne DE, Kaufman AM, Wysocki RW, et al. Vascular perfusion of a flexor carpi ulnaris muscle turnover pedicle flap for posterior elbow soft tissue reconstruction: a cadaveric study. J Hand Surg Am 2011;36(2):246–51.

40. Sharpe F, Barry P, Lin SD, et al. Anatomic study of the flexor carpi ulnaris muscle and its application to soft tissue coverage of the elbow with clinical correlation. J Shoulder Elbow Surg 2014;23(1):82–90.

41. Avashia YJ, Shammas RL, Poveromo LP, et al. Forearm-Based Turnover Muscle Flaps for Elbow Soft-Tissue Reconstruction: A Comparison of Regional Coverage Based on Distal Flap Perfusion. Plast Reconstr Surg 2018;142(1):152–7.

42. Kreulen M, Smeulders MJ. Assessment of Flexor carpi ulnaris function for tendon transfer surgery. J Biomech 2008;41(10):2130–5.

43. Okamoto S, Tada K, Ai H, et al. Flexor carpi ulnaris muscle flap for soft tissue reconstruction after total elbow arthroplasty. Case Rep Surg 2014;2014: 798506.

44. Lingaraj K, Lim AY, Puhaindran ME, et al. Case report: the split flexor carpi ulnaris as a local muscle flap. Clin Orthop Relat Res 2007;455:262–6.

45. Cardany C MP, Gilbert A. Pedicle flaps of the upper limb. The antecubital forearm flap. New York: Martin Dunitz; 1992.

46. Schmidt CC, Kohut GN, Greenberg JA, et al. The anconeus muscle flap: its anatomy and clinical application. J Hand Surg Am 1999;24(2):359–69.

47. Elhassan B, Karabekmez F, Hsu CC, et al. Outcome of local anconeus flap transfer to cover soft tissue defects over the posterior aspect of the elbow. J Shoulder Elbow Surg 2011;20(5):807–12.

48. Ruch DS, Orr SB, Richard MJ, et al. A comparison of debridement with and without anconeus muscle flap for treatment of refractory lateral epicondylitis. J Shoulder Elbow Surg 2015;24(2):236–41.

49. McGregor IA, Jackson IT. The groin flap. Br J Plast Surg 1972;25(1):3–16.

50. Abdelrahman M, Zelken J, Huang RW, et al. Suprafascial dissection of the pedicled groin flap: A safe and practical approach to flap harvest. Microsurgery 2018;38(5):458–65.

51. Chow JA, Bilos ZJ, Hui P, et al. The groin flap in reparative surgery of the hand. Plast Reconstr Surg 1986;77(3):421–6.

52. Wray RC, Wise DM, Young VL, et al. The groin flap in severe hand injuries. Ann Plast Surg 1982;9(6): 459–62.

53. Song R, Song Y, Yu Y, et al. The upper arm free flap. Clin Plast Surg 1982;9(1):27–35.

54. Kokkalis ZT, Papanikos E, Mazis GA, et al. Lateral arm flap: indications and techniques. Eur J Orthop Surg Traumatol 2019;29(2):279–84.

55. Hennerbichler A, Etzer C, Gruber S, et al. Lateral arm flap: analysis of its anatomy and modification using a vascularized fragment of the distal humerus. Clin Anat 2003;16(3):204–14.

56. Jordan SW, Wayne JD, Dumanian GA. The pedicled lateral arm flap for oncologic reconstruction near the shoulder. Ann Plast Surg 2015;74(1):30–3.

57. Kang Y, Pan X, Wu Y, et al. Subacute reconstruction using flap transfer for complex defects of the upper extremity. J Orthop Surg Res 2020;15(1):134.

58. Kuek LB, Chuan TL. The extended lateral arm flap: a new modification. J Reconstr Microsurg 1991;7(3): 167–73.

59. Morrison CS, Sullivan SR, Bhatt RA, et al. The pedicled reverse-flow lateral arm flap for coverage of complex traumatic elbow injuries. Ann Plast Surg 2013;71(1):37–9.

60. F P. Tansini Method for the Cure of Cancer of the Breast. Lancet 1908;171(4409):634–7.

61. Rogachefsky RA, Aly A, Brearley W. Latissimus dorsi pedicled flap for upper extremity soft-tissue reconstruction. Orthopedics 2002;25(4):403–8.

62. Qu ZG, Liu YJ, He X, et al. Use of pedicled latissimus dorsi myocutaneous flap to reconstruct the upper limb with large soft tissue defects. Chin J Traumatol 2012;15(6):352–4.

63. Lee KT, Mun GH. A systematic review of functional donor-site morbidity after latissimus dorsi muscle transfer. Plast Reconstr Surg 2014;134(2):303–14.

64. Muller-Seubert W, Scheibl K, Buhrer G, et al. Less is more - retrospective comparison of shoulder strength and range of motion between conventional and muscle-sparing harvesting technique of a latissimus dorsi flap. J Plast Reconstr Aesthet Surg 2021;74(10):2527–36.

65. Chen SL, Chen TM, Wang HJ. Free thoracodorsal artery perforator flap in extremity reconstruction: 12 cases. Br J Plast Surg 2004;57(6):525–30.

66. Song YG, Chen GZ, Song YL. The free thigh flap: a new free flap concept based on the septocutaneous artery. Br J Plast Surg 1984;37(2):149–59.

67. Wang HT, Erdmann D, Fletcher JW, et al. Anterolateral thigh flap technique in hand and upper extremity reconstruction. Tech Hand Up Extrem. Surg 2004; 8(4):257–61.

68. Wong CH, Wei FC. Anterolateral thigh flap. Head Neck 2010;32(4):529–40.

69. Seth AK, Iorio ML. Super-Thin and Suprafascial Anterolateral Thigh Perforator Flaps for Extremity Reconstruction. J Reconstr Microsurg 2017;33(7): 466–73.

70. Yang Z, Xu C, Zhu Y, et al. Flow-Through Free Anterolateral Thigh Flap in Reconstruction of Severe Limb Injury. Ann Plast Surg 2020;84(5S Suppl 3): S165–70.

Strategies for Perioperative Optimization in Upper Extremity Fracture Care

Thompson Zhuang, MD, MBA, Robin N. Kamal, MD, MBA, MS*

KEYWORDS

• Assessment • Optimization • Perioperative • Prehabilitation • Risk

KEY POINTS

• Short time intervals between upper extremity fracture and surgery present a challenge for perioperative optimization.
• Glycemic control in patients with diabetes, chronic anticoagulation management, smoking, nutritional status, and frailty are modifiable risk factors in the perioperative period.
• Multidisciplinary care pathways for risk stratification and modification should be designed and implemented.

INTRODUCTION

Perioperative risk evaluation and optimization is a multidisciplinary endeavor. As health care shifts toward value-based care, surgeons are assuming an increasing role in the objective evaluation and optimization of surgical risk.[1] For example, hip fracture care pathways have been developed to identify risk factors for surgical complications, readmission, and mortality,[2–5] leading to the development of patient-specific risk calculators.[6–9] These then led to standardized, multidisciplinary perioperative optimization protocols for hip fractures.[10–13] These pathways are designed to reduce surgical risk while balancing the acute demand for fracture fixation.

A role for perioperative optimization also exists for upper extremity fracture care, as these (eg, distal radius, proximal humerus) are often treated in the ambulatory setting within 1 to 2 weeks of injury,[14] creating a window for optimization. Optimization of modifiable perioperative risk factors prior to upper extremity surgery represents an opportunity to improve outcomes while reducing the overall costs of care. Here, we present a detailed review of the current state of perioperative risk assessment and optimization in upper extremity fracture care.

CURRENT EVIDENCE ON RISK ASSESSMENT AND OPTIMIZATION

The goal of perioperative risk assessment is to identify high-risk patients who may benefit from preoperative optimization (**Table 1**). Perioperative optimization in upper extremity fracture care must balance risk reduction with intervention duration and efficacy as to not cause unnecessary surgical delays. Nevertheless, surgery represents a "teachable moment" that may lead to sustained lifestyle changes that improve overall health.[15]

Glucose Control

The detrimental effects of high glucose load on bone healing have been well studied.[16] In an animal study, rats with poor glycemic control had decreased cell proliferation, mechanical stiffness, and callus bony content at fracture sites compared

Department of Orthopaedic Surgery, VOICES Health Policy Research Center, Stanford University, 450 Broadway Street MC: 6342, Redwood City, CA 94603, USA
* Corresponding author.
E-mail address: rnkamal@stanford.edu

Hand Clin 39 (2023) 617–625
https://doi.org/10.1016/j.hcl.2023.05.009

Table 1
Perioperative risk assessment and optimization strategies

Risk factor	Optimization strategies
Diabetes	• Maintain perioperative blood glucose <180–200 mg/dL • Type 1 diabetics should receive half their usual daily insulin dose even with low/no oral intake • Consider scheduling surgeries earlier in day to prevent prolonged fasting
Coagulopathy	• Decision to interrupt anticoagulation should be shared with the patient, accounting for the bleeding risk, indication for anticoagulation, and underlying coagulopathies • Patients on warfarin with INR <3 may not require interruption of warfarin
Smoking	• Preoperative tobacco use screening • Smoking cessation counseling by clinician and/or nurse • Consider referral for formal smoking cessation program and/or pharmacotherapy
Nutrition	• Preoperative nutrition assessment with laboratory markers (eg, albumin, prealbumin) and screening tools • Consider nutrition consultation for malnourished patients
Frailty	• Preoperative frailty risk assessment using clinical instruments (eg, mFI) • Consider geriatric, nutrition, and/or rehabilitation medicine consultations for frail patients to optimize comorbidities prior to surgery

to rats with tightly-controlled diabetes or without diabetes.[17] These cellular changes may be attributable to differential osteogenic growth factor expression profiles (eg, platelet-derived growth factor [PDGF], transforming growth factor-β [TGF-β], insulin-like growth factor 1 [IGF-1]) within the fracture environment as a result of diabetes.[18] For example, local delivery of platelet-enriched plasma containing enriched levels of these growth factors normalized fracture healing parameters in diabetic rats.[18]

Poor glycemic control, as measured by hemoglobin A1c or random blood glucose levels, is associated with surgical site infection and poor wound healing.[19–21] In a review of ankle fractures, patients with diabetes, especially those with neuropathy or vasculopathy, were at a higher risk for delayed union and nonunion.[22] In 2 studies of nondiabetic orthopedic trauma patients that included upper extremity fractures, perioperative hyperglycemia (blood glucose ≥200 mg/dL) was an independent risk factor for surgical site infections.[23,24] In hand surgery, diabetes is a risk factor for delayed bone healing and surgical site infections.[25–28] Although modification of long-term glycemic control may not be feasible in the acute setting, perioperative management should consist of fluid and electrolyte repletion, prevention of ketoacidosis, and avoiding the extremes of hyperglycemia or hypoglycemia.[29] Because type 1 diabetics are insulin-deficient, they are susceptible to developing ketoacidosis when long-acting insulin is held perioperatively. Thus, type 1 diabetics should receive half their usual daily insulin dose even with low or no oral intake.[29] In contrast, type 2 diabetics are less prone to ketosis but may develop a nonketotic hyperosmolar state resulting in severe hypovolemia and encephalopathy. Target perioperative blood glucose should be less than 180 to 200 mg/d to avoid hyperglycemia or hypoglycemic complications.[29] To avoid drastic blood glucose fluctuations, patients with diabetes could also be scheduled earlier in the day for surgery.

Coagulopathy

Chronic anticoagulation medications are commonly used for atrial fibrillation, mechanical heart valves, venous thromboembolism (VTE), and hypercoagulability. Perioperative anticoagulation management must balance the bleeding risk with continuation of the anticoagulant against the thrombotic risk with interruptions in anticoagulation. A meta-analysis of patients with atrial fibrillation undergoing general surgery, joint arthroplasty, vascular, urology, dental, dermatologic, or ophthalmologic procedures showed that interruption of anticoagulation did not increase the incidence of VTE, but resulted in decreased bleeding compared to continuing anticoagulation or heparin bridging.[30] Periprocedural interruption of direct oral anticoagulants is associated with an incidence of 0.4% thromboembolic and 1.8% major bleeding events within 30 days after surgery in patients with atrial fibrillation.[31] However, these studies did not include patients undergoing upper extremity fracture surgery, which typically is associated with a lower bleeding risk.

A meta-analysis of interrupting anticoagulant and antiplatelet medications in hand and wrist surgery, driven largely by carpal tunnel releases, showed that continuing anticoagulation and antiplatelet medications did not affect the incidence of reoperation for bleeding or postoperative hematoma.[32] Of the 2 studies that included open reduction internal fixation of distal radius fractures, continuing warfarin resulted in postoperative hematoma in 1 of 50 procedures and continuing antiplatelet medications resulted in 1 of 107 procedures requiring reoperation due to surgical site bleeding, compared to no complications in controls.[33,34] In another study of 55 upper extremity procedures including operative treatment of fractures, patients on warfarin with an international normalized ratio (INR) less than 3 were continued on warfarin. There were only 2 minor bleeding-related complications without long-term sequelae and no challenges with intraoperative hemostasis, leading to the conclusion that interruption in warfarin is not necessary for hand surgery patients with INR less than 3.[35] In a series of 101 patients undergoing outpatient distal radius fracture surgery who were continued on warfarin, clopidogrel, or aspirin, no bleeding complications intra- or postoperatively were reported.[36]

Given the lack of high-quality evidence on anticoagulation management in upper extremity fracture surgery, the decision to continue or interrupt anticoagulation/anti-platelet therapy should be shared between patient and physician. Factors to consider include the bleeding risk, indication for anticoagulation, history of prior VTE, and underlying coagulopathies. Warfarin may not need to be interrupted in patients with an INR less than 3. If warfarin must be discontinued, this should occur 5 days prior to the procedure where feasible; otherwise, warfarin reversal agents include prothrombin complex concentrate, phytomenadione, and vitamin K. Bridging therapy with heparin can be considered depending on VTE risk.[37] The timing of direct oral anticoagulant (DOAC) discontinuation depends on anticipated bleeding risk.[37,38] Specific reversal agents for DOACs are also available.[37] For patients on aspirin monotherapy for secondary cardiovascular prevention, aspirin can typically be continued.

Smoking

Cigarette smoking is a risk factor for delayed union and nonunion.[39] The effects of cigarette smoking on bone healing are thought to be mediated by multifactorial mechanisms involving toxic agents in cigarette smoke (eg, carbon monoxide). In cellular and animal studies, nicotine has been shown to inhibit osteoblast proliferation and expression of osteogenic growth factors including PDGF, TGF-β, bone morphogenetic protein (BMP)-2, and vascular endothelial growth factor (VEGF).[40,41] Further, an in vitro study using osteoblast-like cells found that smoke condensate exerted inhibitory effects on bone metabolic activity independently from nicotine.[42] Cigarette smoking also decreases blood oxygen delivery. Smoking a single cigarette has been shown to decrease digital blood flow velocity by over 40%.[43]

In a study of 417 patients with distal radius fractures, smokers had higher rates of hardware removal, nonunion, revision surgery, wrist stiffness, and distal radius tenderness compared to nonsmokers.[44] Another study found that smokers experienced more major surgical complications (eg, hardware removal, nonunion), worse patient-reported outcomes, and delayed radiographic healing at 3 months compared to former or never smokers after volar plate fixation of distal radius fractures.[45] A large database study found that smokers undergoing surgical fixation of distal radius fractures had higher rates of 30-day adverse events, infection, reoperation, and readmission compared to nonsmokers after propensity score matching.[46]

Smoking cessation has been shown to reduce postoperative complication rates in orthopedic surgery.[47] In a multicenter randomized, controlled trial, investigators found that a 6-week smoking cessation program after fracture surgery, consisting of weekly behavioral encouragement by nursing and nicotine substitution where necessary, reduced the incidence of postoperative complications with a number needed to treat of 5.5.[48] Within weeks of smoking cessation, immune function, wound healing, and pulmonary function improve. Former smokers have a lower risk of fracture than current smokers, but this effect may take years to become apparent, highlighting the long-term deleterious impact of smoking on musculoskeletal health.[47,49]

In light of the benefits of smoking cessation, surgery represents a "teachable" moment for lifestyle modification.[50] Smoking cessation interventions have been shown to be cost-effective in total joint arthroplasty and spine procedures.[51,52] Perioperative care pathways for smoking cessation should include preoperative tobacco use screening, cessation counseling, pharmacotherapy (if indicated), and maintenance in the postoperative period.[48,53] Behavioral counseling to stop smoking can be delivered by a clinician in the perioperative period, leveraging the "teachable" moment of surgery. Pharmacotherapy can be considered, but is most effective when combined with behavioral interventions.[54,55] Effective pharmacotherapies include nicotine replacement therapy, varenicline, and bupropion.[55] The smoking cessation intervention should be maintained in the weeks following surgery to prevent relapse.[48]

Nutrition

Adequate nutrition is critical for the metabolic demands of fracture healing.[16] In a rat model, vitamin B6 deficiency was shown to delay callus maturation and union.[56] Similarly, vitamin C deficiency in a mouse model impaired osteoblast activity and decreased bone formation.[57] In rats with tibia or femur fractures, vitamin C supplementation accelerated callus formation and increased its mechanical resistance.[58,59] Protein malnutrition in rats was shown to cause decreased callus strength and stiffness, which was rescued in rats that were renourished after their fracture.[60] The effect of protein malnutrition on fracture healing is modulated through the arginine-citrulline-nitric oxide pathway. Arginine is the only physiological precursor to nitric oxide, which plays a critical role in the inflammatory response. Additionally, arginine can be converted to ornithine, a precursor to collagen that forms the fracture callus.[61]

Nutritional status can be assessed with laboratory markers like serum albumin level, with <3.5 g/dL (hypoalbuminemia) defining poor nutrition.[62,63] A meta-analysis of studies encompassing elective joint arthroplasty, spine, and orthopedic trauma patients showed that hypoalbuminemia was associated with a 2.5-fold increase in the risk of surgical site infection.[64] In patients undergoing elective hand surgery, patients with hypoalbuminemia experienced a 3.3-fold increase in odds of surgical site infection (3.5% vs 0.9%) compared to nourished patients.[65] In patients undergoing open reduction internal fixation of distal radius fractures, hypoalbuminemia is associated with an increased risk of infectious complications, cardiac arrest, blood transfusions, reintubation, readmission, and mortality.[66] Malnutrition has also been found to be associated with less improvement in activities in daily living and increased subsequent falls after surgery for geriatric distal radius fractures.[67]

There is wide variability in the definition of malnutrition, the laboratory markers used to define malnutrition, and nutrition supplementation protocols, making clinical implementation challenging.[68] Nevertheless, given the association between malnutrition and worse surgical outcomes, we believe it is reasonable to evaluate nutrition status in patients with upper extremity fractures and consider nutritional supplementation in the perioperative period for malnourished patients. In addition to serum albumin, other laboratory (eg, prealbumin, transferrin) markers, anthropometric measurements (eg, calf circumference), and standardized screening tools (eg, Mini Nutritional Assessment) exist to elicit nutritional status.[69] Malnourished patients could then be referred for a nutrition consultation to optimize fracture healing.

Frailty

Frailty refers to a multisystem decline in physiological capacity that results in decreased physical function and, in combination with comorbidity and disability, is a key determinant of biological age.[70] Frailty is a risk factor for postoperative complications, readmissions, and mortality across a wide range of elective and emergent surgeries.[71–74] Frailty has been associated with complications and mortality after fracture surgery, total joint arthroplasty, and spine procedures.[75] Even in younger orthopedic trauma patients, frailty is associated with postoperative complications and mortality.[76] Studies using the modified frailty index (mFI) found that higher mFI scores were associated with increased complication, readmission, and reoperation rates in patients undergoing surgical treatment of distal radius or forearm fractures.[77,78]

Frailty assessment can be aided by biological age frameworks that elicit components of comorbidity, frailty, and disability to determine surgical risk.[70] Commonly used instruments for measuring frailty are the mFI,[79] frailty index,[80] and the risk analysis index.[81] The identification of frail patients in the perioperative setting provides several benefits. First, the increased surgical risk in frail patients can inform risk–benefit discussions, especially in cases of clinical equipoise (eg, geriatric distal radius fractures).[82] Second, frail patients may benefit from multidisciplinary interventions to optimize risk, including geriatric, rehabilitation medicine, and nutrition consultations.[70] Interventions targeted at correcting nutritional deficiencies, reducing the psychological impact of illness and surgery (eg, via counseling or meditation), and optimizing physical function may be beneficial in frail patients.[83]

CHALLENGES

Although the evidence suggests that the various risk factors discussed are associated with adverse outcomes after upper extremity fracture surgery, there is a lack of high-quality data on interventions for reducing surgical risk in upper extremity patients with these risk factors. Further prospective studies are needed on the efficacy of smoking cessation, renourishment, and frailty interventions for improving surgical outcomes in upper extremity fracture surgery.[84] Future studies should use standardized interventions that can be easily replicable at other sites, thereby increasing external generalizability. A key challenge to implementing perioperative interventions is the short time interval between fracture and surgery, in contrast to elective procedures such as carpal tunnel release where surgery may feasibly be delayed for optimization. This reduces the window for intervention, which brings into question to what extent these factors can be modified. For example, smoking cessation should occur at least 4 weeks prior to surgery for optimal bone healing,[85] whereas the time between fracture and surgery is typically less than that. Nevertheless, a study of surgically treated distal radius fractures showed that surgical delay did not affect patient-reported outcomes,[86] suggesting that the window for optimization may be wider than previously thought.

Although preoperative risk assessment and stratification clinics are becoming increasingly common, clinical care pathways must be redesigned to link objective risk assessments with optimization within a unified workflow.[1] Current optimization clinics are fragmented, which tend to focus on specific conditions (eg, nutrition, diabetes) as opposed to multidisciplinary, patient-centered care. Although risk assessment can inform shared decision-making, optimization advances patient-centered care by acting on risk factors to reduce surgical risk. Such clinics would provide risk assessment as well as on-site exercise, nutrition, psychological, and smoking cessation specialists to optimize the patient for surgery.[1] By streamlining the optimization process, patients can be medically optimized in the least time possible, suitable for the demands of upper extremity fracture surgery. Clinic design can be based on existing preoperative clinics that optimize nutrition and diabetes risk.[87–89] Surgeons would need to identify at-risk patients early and accept potential surgical delays in order to maximize the benefits of optimization in the fracture-to-surgery window.

SUMMARY

Strategies for perioperative optimization of the upper extremity fracture patient must balance the need for surgical fixation of the fracture with the benefits of optimization prior to surgery. Glycemic control in patients with diabetes, anticoagulation management, smoking, nutritional status, and frailty are potentially modifiable factors that can affect morbidity and mortality after upper extremity fracture surgery. Optimization of these risk factors can reduce surgical risk and complication rates in the short term and can improve musculoskeletal as well as overall health in the long term. Surgery represents a "teachable" moment in which surgeons can influence patients' health outcomes.

CLINICS CARE POINTS

- In patients with diabetes, perioperative blood glucose target should be less than 180 to 200 mg/dL.
- The decision to interrupt chronic anticoagulation therapy should be shared between patient and physician.
- Preoperative smoking cessation screening should be performed with smoking cessation interventions for smokers.
- Preoperative nutritional screening should be performed and nutritional consultations obtained in malnourished patients.
- Preoperative frailty assessment should be performed and geriatric, nutritional, and rehabilitation medicine consultations obtained for frail patients.

DISCLOSURE

The authors have nothing to disclose.

REFERENCES

1. Carli F, Baldini G, Feldman LS. Redesigning the Preoperative Clinic: From Risk Stratification to Risk Modification. JAMA Surg 2021;156(2):191–2.
2. Donegan DJ, Gay AN, Baldwin K, et al. Use of Medical Comorbidities to Predict Complications After Hip Fracture Surgery in the Elderly. J Bone Joint Surg Am 2010; 92(4). Available at: https://journals.lww.com/jbjsjournal/Fulltext/2010/04000/Use_of_Medical_Comorbidities_to_Predict.4.aspx.
3. Hu F, Jiang C, Shen J, et al. Preoperative predictors for mortality following hip fracture surgery: A systematic review and meta-analysis. Injury 2012;43(6): 676–85.
4. Sathiyakumar V, Greenberg SE, Molina CS, et al. Hip fractures are risky business: An analysis of the NSQIP data. Injury 2015;46(4):703–8.

5. Yli-Kyyny TT, Sund R, Heinänen M, et al. Risk factors for early readmission due to surgical complications after treatment of proximal femoral fractures – A Finnish National Database study of 68,800 patients. Injury 2019;50(2):403–8.

6. Schilling PL, Bozic KJ. Development and Validation of Perioperative Risk-Adjustment Models for Hip Fracture Repair, Total Hip Arthroplasty, and Total Knee Arthroplasty. J Bone Joint Surg Am 2016;98(1). Available at: https://journals.lww.com/jbjsjournal/Fulltext/2016/01000/Development_and_Validation_of_Perioperative.13.aspx.

7. Karres J, Kieviet N, Eerenberg JP, et al. Predicting Early Mortality After Hip Fracture Surgery: The Hip Fracture Estimator of Mortality Amsterdam. J Orthop Trauma 2018;32(1). Available at: https://journals.lww.com/jorthotrauma/Fulltext/2018/01000/Predicting_Early_Mortality_After_Hip_Fracture.6.aspx.

8. Pugely AJ, Martin CT, Gao Y, et al. A Risk Calculator for Short-Term Morbidity and Mortality After Hip Fracture Surgery. J Orthop Trauma 2014;28(2). Available at: https://journals.lww.com/jorthotrauma/Fulltext/2014/02000/A_Risk_Calculator_for_Short_Term_Morbidity_and.1.aspx.

9. Hornor MA, Ma M, Zhou L, et al. Enhancing the American College of Surgeons NSQIP Surgical Risk Calculator to Predict Geriatric Outcomes. J Am Coll Surg 2020;230(1):88–100.e1.

10. Swart E, Kates S, McGee S, et al. The Case for Comanagement and Care Pathways for Osteoporotic Patients with a Hip Fracture. J Bone Joint Surg Am 2018;100(15). Available at: https://journals.lww.com/jbjsjournal/Fulltext/2018/08010/The_Case_for_Comanagement_and_Care_Pathways_for.12.aspx.

11. Macfie D, Zadeh RA, Andrews M, et al. Perioperative multimodal optimisation in patients undergoing surgery for fractured neck of femur. Surgeon 2012;10(2):90–4.

12. Burton A, Davis CM, Boateng H, et al. A Multidisciplinary Approach to Expedite Surgical Hip Fracture Care. Geriatr Orthop Surg Rehabil 2020;11. https://doi.org/10.1177/2151459319898646. 2151459319898646.

13. Merloz P. Optimization of perioperative management of proximal femoral fracture in the elderly. Orthop Traumatol Surg Res 2018;104(1 Supplement):S25–30.

14. Gogna R, Armstrong D, Espag M. Time to Fixation for Distal Radius Fractures. Orthop Proc 2013;95-B:5. SUPP_12.

15. Guzman JZ, Iatridis JC, Skovrlj B, et al. Outcomes and complications of diabetes mellitus on patients undergoing degenerative lumbar spine surgery. Spine 2014;39(19):1596–604.

16. Gaston MS, Simpson AHRW. Inhibition of fracture healing. Bone Joint Lett J 2007;89-B(12):1553–60.

17. Beam HA, Russell Parsons J, Lin SS. The effects of blood glucose control upon fracture healing in the BB Wistar rat with diabetes mellitus. J Orthop Res 2002;20(6):1210–6.

18. Gandhi A, Doumas C, O'Connor JP, et al. The effects of local platelet rich plasma delivery on diabetic fracture healing. Bone 2006;38(4):540–6.

19. MHJr Marchant, Viens NA, Cook C, et al. The Impact of Glycemic Control and Diabetes Mellitus on Perioperative Outcomes After Total Joint Arthroplasty. J Bone Joint Surg Am 2009;91(7). Available at: https://journals.lww.com/jbjsjournal/Fulltext/2009/07000/The_Impact_of_Glycemic_Control_and_Diabetes.9.aspx.

20. Hogan C, Bucknell AL, King KB. The Effect of Diabetes Mellitus on Total Joint Arthroplasty Outcomes. JBJS Rev 2016;4(2). Available at: https://journals.lww.com/jbjsreviews/Fulltext/2016/02000/The_Effect_of_Diabetes_Mellitus_on_Total_Joint.3.aspx.

21. Olsen MA, Nepple JJ, Riew KD, et al. Risk Factors for Surgical Site Infection Following Orthopaedic Spinal Operations. J Bone Joint Surg Am 2008;90(1). Available at: https://journals.lww.com/jbjsjournal/Fulltext/2008/01000/Risk_Factors_for_Surgical_Site_Infection_Following.9.aspx.

22. Wukich DK, Kline AJ. The Management of Ankle Fractures in Patients with Diabetes. J Bone Joint Surg Am 2008;90(7). Available at: https://journals.lww.com/jbjsjournal/Fulltext/2008/07000/The_Management_of_Ankle_Fractures_in_Patients_with.21.aspx.

23. Richards JE, Kauffmann RM, Zuckerman SL, et al. Relationship of hyperglycemia and surgical-site infection in orthopaedic surgery. J Bone Joint Surg Am 2012;94(13):1181–6.

24. Anderson BM, Wise BT, Joshi M, et al. Admission Hyperglycemia Is a Risk Factor for Deep Surgical-Site Infection in Orthopaedic Trauma Patients. J Orthop Trauma 2021;35(12). Available at: https://journals.lww.com/jorthotrauma/Fulltext/2021/12000/Admission_Hyperglycemia_Is_a_Risk_Factor_for_Deep.13.aspx.

25. Pscherer S, Sandmann G, Ehnert S, et al. Delayed fracture healing in diabetics with distal radius fractures. Acta Chir Orthop Traumatol Cech 2017;84(1):24–9.

26. Wei C, Kapani N, Quan T, et al. Diabetes mellitus effect on rates of perioperative complications after operative treatment of distal radius fractures. Eur J Orthop Surg Traumatol 2021;31(7):1329–34.

27. Malige A, Konopitski A, Nwachuku CO, et al. Distal Radius Fractures in Diabetic Patients: An Analysis of Surgical Timing and Other Factors That Affect Complication Rate. Hand (New York, N,Y) 2020. https://doi.org/10.1177/1558944720944262. 1558944720944262.

28. Stepan JG, Boddapati V, Sacks HA, et al. Insulin Dependence Is Associated With Increased Risk of Complications After Upper Extremity Surgery in Diabetic Patients. J Hand Surg Am 2018;43(8):745–54.e4.

29. Marsland D, Colvin PL, Mears SC, et al. How to optimize patients for geriatric fracture surgery. Osteoporos Int 2010;21(4):535–46.

30. Hovaguimian F, Köppel S, Spahn DR. Safety of Anticoagulation Interruption in Patients Undergoing Surgery or Invasive Procedures: A Systematic Review and Meta-analyses of Randomized Controlled Trials and Non-randomized Studies. World J Surg 2017; 41(10):2444–56.

31. Shaw JR, Woodfine JD, Douketis J, et al. Perioperative interruption of direct oral anticoagulants in patients with atrial fibrillation: A systematic review and meta-analysis. Res Pract Thromb Haemost 2018;2(2):282–90.

32. Stone MJ, Wilks DJ, Wade RG. Hand and wrist surgery on anticoagulants and antiplatelets: A systematic review and meta-analysis. J Plast Reconstr Aesthet Surg 2020;73(8):1413–23.

33. Bogunovic L, Gelberman RH, Goldfarb CA, et al. The Impact of Uninterrupted Warfarin on Hand and Wrist Surgery. J Hand Surg Am 2015;40(11): 2133–40.

34. Bogunovic L, Gelberman RH, Goldfarb CA, et al. The Impact of Antiplatelet Medication on Hand and Wrist Surgery. J Hand Surg Am 2013;38(6):1063–70.

35. Wallace DL, Latimer MD, Belcher HJCR. Stopping Warfarin Therapy is Unnecessary for Hand Surgery. J Hand Surg Eur 2004;29(3):201–3.

36. Morris JA, Little M, Ashdown T, et al. Day case locked anterior plating for distal radial fractures is safe with uninterrupted antithrombotic therapy. J Hand Surg Eur 2021;46(2):172–5.

37. Keeling D, Tait RC, Watson H. the British Committee of Standards for Haematology. Peri-operative management of anticoagulation and antiplatelet therapy. Br J Haematol 2016;175(4):602–13.

38. Chan N, Sobieraj-Teague M, Eikelboom JW. Direct oral anticoagulants: evidence and unresolved issues. Lancet 2020;396(10264):1767–76.

39. Patel RA, Wilson RF, Patel PA, et al. The effect of smoking on bone healing. Bone Jt Res 2013;2(6): 102–11.

40. Ma L, Zwahlen RA, Zheng LW, et al. Influence of nicotine on the biological activity of rabbit osteoblasts. Clin Oral Implants Res 2011;22(3):338–42.

41. Fang MA, Frost PJ, Iida-Klein A, et al. Effects of nicotine on cellular function in UMR 106-01 osteoblast-like cells. Bone 1991;12(4):283–6.

42. Gullihorn L, Karpman R, Lippiello L. Differential Effects of Nicotine and Smoke Condensate on Bone Cell Metabolic Activity. J Orthop Trauma 2005;19(1). Available at: https://journals.lww.com/jorthotrauma/Fulltext/2005/01000/Differential_Effects_of_Nicotine_and_Smoke.4.aspx.

43. Sarin CL, Austin JC, Nickel WO. Effects of Smoking on Digital Blood-Flow Velocity. JAMA 1974;229(10): 1327–8.

44. Hess DE, Carstensen SE, Moore S, et al. Smoking Increases Postoperative Complications After Distal Radius Fracture Fixation: A Review of 417 Patients From a Level 1 Trauma Center. Hand (New York, N,Y) 2020;15(5):686–91.

45. Hall MJ, Ostergaard PJ, Dowlatshahi AS, et al. The Impact of Obesity and Smoking on Outcomes After Volar Plate Fixation of Distal Radius Fractures. J Hand Surg Am 2019;44(12):1037–49.

46. Galivanche AR, FitzPatrick S, Dussik C, et al. A Matched Comparison of Postoperative Complications Between Smokers and Nonsmokers Following Open Reduction Internal Fixation of Distal Radius Fractures. J Hand Surg Am 2021;46(1):1–9.e4.

47. Lee JJ, Patel R, Biermann JS, et al. The Musculoskeletal Effects of Cigarette Smoking. J Bone Joint Surg Am 2013;95(9). Available at: https://journals.lww.com/jbjsjournal/Fulltext/2013/05010/The_Musculoskeletal_Effects_of_Cigarette_Smoking.12.aspx.

48. Nåsell H, Adami J, Samnegård E, et al. Effect of Smoking Cessation Intervention on Results of Acute Fracture Surgery: A Randomized Controlled Trial. J Bone Joint Surg Am 2010;92(6). Available at: https://journals.lww.com/jbjsjournal/Fulltext/2010/06000/Effect_of_Smoking_Cessation_Intervention_on.1.aspx.

49. Kanis JA, Johnell O, Oden A, et al. Smoking and fracture risk: a meta-analysis. Osteoporos Int 2005; 16(2):155–62.

50. Shi Y, Warner DO. Surgery as a Teachable Moment for Smoking Cessation. Anesthesiology 2010; 112(1):102–7.

51. Boylan MR, Bosco JA, Slover JD. Cost-Effectiveness of Preoperative Smoking Cessation Interventions in Total Joint Arthroplasty. J Arthroplasty 2019;34(2): 215–20.

52. Zhuang T, Ku S, Shapiro LM, et al. A Cost-Effectiveness Analysis of Smoking-Cessation Interventions Prior to Posterolateral Lumbar Fusion. J Bone Joint Surg Am 2020;102(23):2032–42.

53. Truntzer J, Comer G, Kendra M, et al. Perioperative Smoking Cessation and Clinical Care Pathway for Orthopaedic Surgery. JBJS Rev 2017;5(8). Available at: https://journals.lww.com/jbjsreviews/Fulltext/2017/08000/Perioperative_Smoking_Cessation_and_Clinical_Care.11.aspx.

54. Zwar NA, Mendelsohn CP, Richmond RL. Supporting smoking cessation. BMJ 2014;348:f7535.

55. Stead L, Koilpillai P, Fanshawe T, et al. Combined pharmacotherapy and behavioural interventions for smoking cessation. Cochrane Database Syst Rev 2016;3. https://doi.org/10.1002/14651858.CD008286.pub3.

56. Dodds RA, Catterall A, Bitensky L, et al. Abnormalities in fracture healing induced by vitamin B6-deficiency in rats. Bone 1986;7(6):489–95.

57. Mohan S, Kapoor A, Singgih A, et al. Spontaneous Fractures in the Mouse Mutant sfx Are Caused by

Deletion of the Gulonolactone Oxidase Gene, Causing Vitamin C Deficiency. J Bone Miner Res 2005;20(9):1597–610.

58. Sarisözen B, Durak K, Dinçer G, et al. The Effects of Vitamins E and C on Fracture Healing in Rats. J Int Med Res 2002;30(3):309–13.

59. Alcantara-Martos T, Delgado-Martinez AD, Vega MV, et al. Effect of vitamin C on fracture healing in elderly Osteogenic Disorder Shionogi rats. Bone Joint Lett J 2007;89-B(3):402–7.

60. Day SM, DeHeer DH. Reversal of the Detrimental Effects of Chronic Protein Malnutrition on Long Bone Fracture Healing. J Orthop Trauma 2001;15(1). Available at: https://journals.lww.com/jorthotrauma/Fulltext/2001/01000/Reversal_of_the_Detrimental_Effects_of_Chronic.9.aspx.

61. Meesters DM, Wijnands KAP, Brink PRG, et al. Malnutrition and Fracture Healing: Are Specific Deficiencies in Amino Acids Important in Nonunion Development? Nutrients 2018;10(11). https://doi.org/10.3390/nu10111597.

62. Aldebeyan S, Nooh A, Aoude A, et al. Hypoalbuminaemia—a marker of malnutrition and predictor of postoperative complications and mortality after hip fractures. Injury 2017;48(2):436–40.

63. O'Daly BJ, Walsh JC, Quinlan JF, et al. Serum albumin and total lymphocyte count as predictors of outcome in hip fractures. Clin Nutr 2010;29(1):89–93.

64. Yuwen P, Chen W, Lv H, et al. Albumin and surgical site infection risk in orthopaedics: a meta-analysis. BMC Surg 2017;17(1):7.

65. Zhuang T, Shapiro LM, Fogel N, et al. Perioperative Laboratory Markers as Risk Factors for Surgical Site Infection After Elective Hand Surgery. J Hand Surg Am 2021;46(8):675–84.e10.

66. Wilson JM, Holzgrefe RE, Staley CA, et al. The Effect of Malnutrition on Postoperative Complications Following Surgery for Distal Radius Fractures. J Hand Surg Am 2019;44(9):742–50.

67. Nagai T, Tanimoto K, Tomizuka Y, et al. Nutrition status and functional prognosis among elderly patients with distal radius fracture: a retrospective cohort study. J Orthop Surg Res 2020;15(1):133.

68. Ernst A, Wilson JM, Ahn J, et al. Malnutrition and the Orthopaedic Trauma Patient: A Systematic Review of the Literature. J Orthop Trauma 2018;32(10). Available at: https://journals.lww.com/jorthotrauma/Fulltext/2018/10000/Malnutrition_and_the_Orthopaedic_Trauma_Patient__A.1.aspx.

69. Cross MB, Yi PH, Thomas CF, et al. Evaluation of Malnutrition in Orthopaedic Surgery. J Am Acad Orthop Surg 2014;22(3). Available at: https://journals.lww.com/jaaos/Fulltext/2014/03000/Evaluation_of_Malnutrition_in_Orthopaedic_Surgery.7.aspx.

70. Cong T, Hall AJ, Jia Z, et al. Conceptualizing Biological Aging and Frailty in Orthopaedics: A

Framework for Clinical Practice. J Bone Joint Surg Am 2022. Available at: https://journals.lww.com/jbjsjournal/Fulltext/9900/Conceptualizing_Biological_Aging_and_Frailty_in.482.aspx.

71. George EL, Hall DE, Youk A, et al. Association Between Patient Frailty and Postoperative Mortality Across Multiple Noncardiac Surgical Specialties. JAMA Surg 2021;156(1):e205152.

72. Shinall MC Jr, Youk A, Massarweh NN, et al. Association of Preoperative Frailty and Operative Stress With Mortality After Elective vs Emergency Surgery. JAMA Netw Open 2020;3(7):e2010358.

73. Shinall MC Jr, Arya S, Youk A, et al. Association of Preoperative Patient Frailty and Operative Stress With Postoperative Mortality. JAMA Surg 2020;155(1):e194620.

74. Rothenberg KA, Stern JR, George EL, et al. Association of Frailty and Postoperative Complications With Unplanned Readmissions After Elective Outpatient Surgery. JAMA Netw Open 2019;2(5):e194330.

75. Lemos JL, Welch JM, Xiao M, et al. Is Frailty Associated with Adverse Outcomes After Orthopaedic Surgery?: A Systematic Review and Assessment of Definitions. JBJS Rev 2021;9(12). Available at: https://journals.lww.com/jbjsreviews/Fulltext/2021/12000/Is_Frailty_Associated_with_Adverse_Outcomes_After.6.aspx.

76. Rege RM, Runner RP, Staley CA, et al. Frailty predicts mortality and complications in chronologically young patients with traumatic orthopaedic injuries. Injury 2018;49(12):2234–8.

77. Wilson JM, Holzgrefe RE, Staley CA, et al. Use of a 5-Item Modified Frailty Index for Risk Stratification in Patients Undergoing Surgical Management of Distal Radius Fractures. J Hand Surg Am 2018;43(8):701–9.

78. Congiusta D, Amer K, Merchant AM, et al. A simplified preoperative risk assessment tool as a predictor of complications in the surgical management of forearm fractures. J Clin Orthop Trauma 2021;14:121–6.

79. Saxton A, Velanovich V. Preoperative Frailty and Quality of Life as Predictors of Postoperative Complications. Ann Surg 2011;253(6). Available at: https://journals.lww.com/annalsofsurgery/Fulltext/2011/06000/Preoperative_Frailty_and_Quality_of_Life_as.26.aspx.

80. Kojima G, Iliffe S, Walters K. Frailty index as a predictor of mortality: a systematic review and meta-analysis. Age Ageing 2018;47(2):193–200.

81. Hall DE, Arya S, Schmid KK, et al. Development and Initial Validation of the Risk Analysis Index for Measuring Frailty in Surgical Populations. JAMA Surg 2017;152(2):175–82.

82. Kamal RN, Shapiro LM. American Academy of Orthopaedic Surgeons/American Society for Surgery of the Hand Clinical Practice Guideline Summary Management of Distal Radius Fractures. J Am Acad

Orthop Surg 2022;30(4). Available at: https://journals.lww.com/jaaos/Fulltext/2022/02150/American_Academy_of_Orthopaedic_Surgeons_American.7.aspx.

83. Gritsenko K, Helander E, Webb MPK, et al. Preoperative frailty assessment combined with prehabilitation and nutrition strategies: Emerging concepts and clinical outcomes. Best Pract Res Clin Anaesthesiol 2020;34(2):199–212.

84. Baimas-George M, Watson M, Elhage S, et al. Prehabilitation in Frail Surgical Patients: A Systematic Review. World J Surg 2020;44(11):3668–78.

85. Truntzer J, Vopat B, Feldstein M, et al. Smoking cessation and bone healing: optimal cessation timing. Eur J Orthop Surg Traumatol 2015;25(2):211–5.

86. Howard M, Curtis A, Everett S, et al. Does a delay in surgery for distal radial fractures affect patient outcome? J Hand Surg Eur 2021;46(1):69–74.

87. Aronson S, Murray S, Martin G, et al. Roadmap for transforming preoperative assessment to preoperative optimization. Anesth Analg 2020;130(4):811–9.

88. Williams DGA, Villalta E, Aronson S, et al. Tutorial: Development and Implementation of a Multidisciplinary Preoperative Nutrition Optimization Clinic. JPEN J Parenter Enteral Nutr 2020;44(7):1185–96.

89. Setji T, Hopkins TJ, Jimenez M, et al. Rationalization, Development, and Implementation of a Preoperative Diabetes Optimization Program Designed to Improve Perioperative Outcomes and Reduce Cost. Diabetes Spectr 2017;30(3):217–23.

Novel Tools to Approach and Measure Outcomes in Patients with Fractures

Edgar Garcia-Lopez, MD, MS[a], Ryan Halvorson, MD[a], Lauren Shapiro, MD[b],*

KEYWORDS

• PROM • Telemedicine • Wearables

KEY POINTS

- Telemedicine in hand and upper extremity surgery has the potential to increase productivity, reduce costs, and increase access to care. Identified limitations include the risk of misdiagnosis, required technologic literacy, equitable access.
- In the clinical setting PROMs be utilized to understand a patient's perception of their outcome, to forecast clinical outcomes, guide treatment decisions, and ultimately improve outcomes. Notably, however, investigation regarding the best use of PROMs is still underway (eg, how to utilize PROMs at point of care, how to utilize PROMs in linguistically and culturally diverse populations).
- The widespread commercial adoption of mobile phone technology and wearable devices has enabled the development of mobile health and sensor-based tools for orthopedic surgery outcome measures.

INTRODUCTION

Upper extremity fractures are prevalent and pose a great burden to patients and society. In the US alone, the annual incidence of upper extremity fractures is 67.6 fractures per 10,000 persons.[1] While the majority of patients with upper extremity fractures demonstrate satisfactory outcomes when treated appropriately (the details of which are discussed in prior articles), the importance of follow-up and outcome measurement cannot be understated. Outcome measurement allows for accountability and improvement in clinical outcomes and research. The purpose of this article is to describe recent advances in methods and tools for assessing clinical and research outcomes in hand and upper extremity care. Three specific advances that are broadly changing the landscape of follow-up care of our patients include: 1) telemedicine, 2) patient-reported outcome measurement, and 3) wearables/remote patient monitoring.

Telemedicine refers to the use of technology to remotely deliver clinical care.[2] Although its use has greatly expanded recently, telemedicine was used as early as the 19th century when the use of a telephone facilitated the first telemedicine visit.[2] More recently, advances in technology, as well as widespread access to videoconferencing, facilitated the expansion of telemedicine in the 21st century. In addition, the COVID-19 pandemic has hastened the process of shifting toward telemedicine. Patients and surgeons documented high levels of satisfaction with telehealth encounters during the novel coronavirus (COVID-19) pandemic.[3–6] Telemedicine in hand and upper extremity surgery has the potential to increase productivity, reduce costs, and increase access to care. Identified limitations include risk of misdiagnosis, required technologic literacy, and equitable access.[3] Telemedicine does not appear to be a replacement for all in-person clinic encounters, however

a Department of Orthopaedics, University of California San Francisco, 500 Parnassus Avenue, MU-320W, San Francisco, CA 94143-0728, USA; b Department of Orthopaedics, University of California San Francisco, 1500 Owens Street, San Francisco, CA 94158, USA
* Corresponding author.
E-mail address: Lauren.Shapiro@ucsf.edu

Hand Clin 39 (2023) 627–639
https://doi.org/10.1016/j.hcl.2023.06.005
0749-0712/23/© 2023 Elsevier Inc. All rights reserved.

when used in the appropriate context telemedicine demonstrates favorable results.

The shift in the healthcare landscape toward value-based and patient-centered health care has resulted in the growth of patient-reported outcome measures (PROMs). Although originally developed as research tools to measure a patient's report of their function and symptoms, PROMs have gained traction in the clinical setting. In the clinical setting, PROMs can not only be utilized to understand a patient's perception of their outcome, but PROMs can be utilized to forecast clinical outcomes, guide treatment decisions, and ultimately improve outcomes.[7–9] Notably, however, investigation regarding the best use of PROMs is still underway (eg, how to utilize PROMs at point of care, how to utilize PROMs in linguistically and culturally diverse populations). We will discuss how the expansion of PROM use in the clinical setting can provide great benefit, while acknowledging their limitations and opportunities for development.

Finally, the widespread commercial adoption of mobile phone technology and wearable devices has enabled the development of mobile health and sensor-based tools for orthopedic surgery. The low cost of these technologies compared to conventional tools has allowed for more widespread and remote data collection than was previously possible. These devices have demonstrated early impact in hand and upper extremity care, and eventually will expand capabilities for telemedicine and remote monitoring beyond the clinic.

Telemedicine

The World Health Organization defines telemedicine as, "The delivery of health care services, where distance is a critical factor, by all health care professionals using information and communication technologies for the exchange of valid information for diagnosis, treatment, and prevention of disease and injuries, research and evaluation, and for the continuing education of health care providers, all in the interests of advancing the health of individuals and their communities."[2,10] This definition was created in the Geneva 1997 conference, when the reach and capabilities of telemedicine were limited. The method of communication during telemedicine visits is most commonly videoconferencing which in 1997 would have been limited to a very select group of patients.[2] The Pew Research Center estimates that in the US, about three-quarters of the population owns a laptop, 97% of people own a cellphone, and 85% a smart cellphone, a dramatic increase of 245% during the last 10 years. Thus, the acceleration in technologic development has largely contributed to the accessibility of telemedicine for care by a larger population.

Advances in technology and accessibility have accelerated the use of telemedicine in orthopedic surgery. Furthermore, the utilization of telemedicine was further driven during the COVID-19 pandemic by accelerating adoption, lowering barriers to reimbursement, and reducing medicolegal concerns.[3–5] In orthopedics, telemedicine is being used for consultations services, post-operative care, telerehabilitation, and to reach rural and underserved areas.[2–5,11–15] Although fruitful, telemedicine has its limitations including the lack of in-person examinations, required technology literacy, and varying patient satisfaction and equitable access.[16–18]

Remote consultations

Remote consultation for the diagnosis of fractures has been implemented successfully on an outpatient basis in many countries and in rural areas for many years.[13,19–22] For instance, an early 1999 prospective study in Finland utilized telecommunication (via videoconferencing) to conduct orthopedic consultations on 29 patients who were an average if 150 miles away.[20] At that time, video quality was judged to be acceptable by physicians. Notably, none of the patients had used videoconferencing before yet 87% were satisfied and would participate in telecommunication again. Surgeons equally considered the videoconferencing system to be reliable and 69% of patients were given a diagnosis along with definitive treatment. Most importantly, this allowed for a previously secluded population to receive adequate care without traveling 150 miles for an in-person visit. As expected, the demand of telemedicine may exceed the availability of practicing providers. Thus, programs to help bridge this unmet need are under development. For example, more recently, The Arkansas Hand Trauma Telemedicine Program was created to meet the rising demand placed upon hand surgeons that care for mangled hand injuries in rural areas.[21,22] Through this program, remote Emergency Departments (ED) are able to videoconference with a hand surgeon to obtain management recommendations. They found that after the implementation of the program there was a significant decrease in the number of unnecessary transfers (from 73% to 45%) and transportation costs.[21,22] Telemedicine may be a cost-effective and option for orthopedic consultations particularly in rural areas.

Furthermore, in a randomized study of 389 patients from a remote northern region of Norway referred to an outpatient orthopedic center, Buvik and colleagues reported that video-assisted orthopedic consultations were not inferior to standard consultations.[19,23] In this study, radiographs were obtained immediately prior to 88% of the 199 remote consultations at the regional medical center and 89% of the 190 standard consultations at the University Hospital of North Norway.[23] For remote visits, a digitalized X-ray was shown to the patient if he or she wanted. No significant difference was found between groups in the number of patients who underwent a surgical procedure. Similarly, the mean visit duration was not significantly different. The orthopedic surgeons were pleased with the video consultations, rating 98% of the visits either "good" or "very good." From a patient perspective, the study demonstrated an annual savings of $18,161 euros per 300 consultants, primarily related to transportation costs and absenteeism from work, among others.

Post-operative care

Telemedicine has facilitated the evaluation of clinical outcomes in the post-operative setting including PROMs and range of motion (ROM).[2] Studies demonstrating this ability include those studying post-operative patients who have undergone elective surgeries (eg, arthroplasty) well as those undergoing surgeries for more traumatic injuries (eg, ankle, elbow, clavicle, humerus).[2,24–28] In these studies measured ROM through videoconferencing was comparable to clinical ROM measurements.[24–27] Ankle assessment by videoconference resulted in 93.3% similar agreement with face-to-face examination.[25] Elbow ROM by videoconferencing was comparable to in-person goniometry measurement.[27] In a prospective study of 87 post-operative upper extremity patients, Grandizio and colleagues, whose first post-op visit was through telemedicine and second post-op visit was in person, found that travel time and visit time was significantly decreased without change in patient satisfaction.[29] Notably, 90% of patients preferred telemedicine in subsequent encounters. Importantly, all patients had absorbable sutures, and during the visit, a wound check was performed and the patient was guided through a physical examination that involved ROM and sensation to light touch compared to the non-operative extremity. Patients who required radiographs obtained them at a location close to home and the imaging was available in electronic medical record as well as reviewed during the visit. Telemedicine for post-operative care has the potential to be reliable and efficient for a select group of post-op patients.

Telerehabilitation

Telerehabilitation is the delivery of comprehensive rehabilitation services at a distance using telecommunications technology as the delivery medium.[25] Telerehabilitation has been utilized previously by subspecialties such at orthopedics and neurology in the rehabilitation process of post-op arthroplasty and stroke patients, respectively.[25,30–32] In the subspecialty of arthroplasty, telemedicine has gained significant traction. Bini and colleagues in 51 post-op total knee arthroplasty patients found that clinical outcomes after telerehabilitation were not inferior to those receiving traditional physical therapy, and satisfaction was similar.[30] In another prospective study, 17 patients with non-surgically managed proximal humerus fractures were recruited into an 8-week telerehabilitation program.[33] Tousignant and colleagues reported that visual analog pain scale (VAS), shoulder range of motion, and upper limb function as measure by the Disability of the Arm, Shoulder, and Hand instrument all improved from pre to post 8-week telerehabilitation intervention. Additionally, patient satisfaction was high.[33] Although promising, there are limitations in not only evaluating and quantifying human movement remotely but also in providing rehabilitation not in person[25]

Telemedicine barriers

Multiple barriers challenge the continued expansion of telemedicine, including difficulty performing physical examinations, lack of perceived benefit of virtual care, concern for liability, and equitable access.[2,18,19,34] Numerous physical examination maneuvers including sensory examinations are difficult to perform through a virtual visit; however, standardized protocols of the virtual examination have been shown to be comparable to in person examinations.[18,35–40] In addition, telemedicine requires access to a device with a camera, Wi-Fi and a basic level of technological literacy that many socioeconomically disadvantaged patients may not have access to. There is also patient and provider concern of diagnostic accuracy and potential legal remefications.[18] Some of these challenges have been addressed with temporary state and federal mandates in response to the COVID-19 pandemic. However, continued research, technological advances, standardization of the telemedicine encounter, and focus on equitable access are needed to sustain widespread adoption by patients and providers.

There are concerns that the lack of being able to perform an in-person examination may limit the reach of telemedicine or worse, lead to misdiagnosis. There are maneuvers utilized in physical examination that are difficult to perform remotely. Some examples include motor testing to determine the strength of an extremity, passive motion, sensory examination (ie, 2-point discrimination), and palpation to determine sources of pain.[18,35–40] In a cross-sectional evaluation, Mehta and colleagues assessed wrist and knee ROM virtually and in person in 54 healthy patients and found a >90 interclass correlation coefficient between the virtual and in-person assessment of wrist and knee ROM.[37] In a prospective study of 32 patients evaluated either virtually or in person for carpal tunnel release, Grandizio and colleagues found generally good agreement in examination findings however noted that the sensory assessment had the lowest agreement (63%) between visit types.[40] Establishing consensus on how best to evaluate patients through telemedicine can help surgeons establish differential diagnoses and monitor patient outcomes and progress.

Telemedicine platforms circumvent barriers to access of care such as proximity or travel. However, it requires advanced technological requirements that may affect access to and use by populations such as those with limited English-language or technological proficiency and those that lack technological resources such as internet capabilities and teleconferencing devices. A study surveying the patient population of the greater Boston area from March to May of 2020, found that Hispanic and Asian patients were 41% and 27%, respectively, less likely to be seen by telemedicine when compared to white patients.[16] Similarly, non-English speakers and those with Medicaid were, 15% and 66% less likely to be seen via telemedicine visit when compared to English/Spanish speakers and those with private insurance, respectively.[16] Language and accessibility to interpreters has been and continues to be a barrier in access to the delivery of health care, that may be perpetuated by telemedicine. Similar, this patient cohort may not have access to the technology needed for videoconferencing and may not be able to work from home, as many fell under the designation of essential worker.[16,18,41] Implementation of telemedicine has the potential to worsen the already existing disparities in health care without ensuring the equitable distribution of resources necessary for its use.

Telemedicine future direction

A physical examination consisting of inspection, palpation, neurovascular and motor examination can be performed through videoconferencing with adequate preparation and standardization.[39] Van Nest and colleagues designed protocols and methods to standardize the virtual orthopedic hand examination.[39] In this study Van Nest and colleagues recommended that the camera should be centered at the shoulders and when a closer examination of the hands is necessary, the patient can be instructed to tilt the camera down to focus on the hands resting on table. A graphical depiction can be helpful for the patient to communicate effectively and for the surgeon to be able to guide the patient in the palpation of individual joints to assess pain (**Fig. 1**). For the sensory examination, the patient can compare sensation to light touch on regions of the affected extremity to the non-affected side.[29,39,40] To further evaluate numbness or paresthesias the patient can utilize a paper clip as the surgeon guides them through a sensory examination. Similarly, a diagram can be provided to the patient with specific sensory distributions. For the motor examination the patient can be guided though range of motion for each specific joint with visual demonstrations. This, however, does not evaluate strength to resistance. Another study suggested utilizing common household object as they go through range of motion exercises to better assess strength and can also be utilized for special provocative tests.[35] Some special tests that can be reliably performed include Phalen test, elbow flexion test, and modified versions of Finklestein, Froment, Cozen, and TFCC load test.[35,39] Other authors also have reported and validated the use of virtual tools, such as internet-based goniometer, to help doctors during a virtual examination.[13]

Technological advances and the COVID-19 pandemic have accelerated the use of telemedicine. Surveys suggest that telemedicine will continue well into the post-pandemic era given its utility in various facets of upper extremity management: consultations services, post-operative care, telerehabilitation, and ability to reach rural and underserved areas. Technological innovations in physical examination protocols and tools will continue to improve the effectiveness of virtual orthopedic visits. Recent technological advances that can be used in conjunction to the telemedicine visit will be reviewed in the sections later in discussion. As telemedicine continues to expand, it is important to consider and address systematic issues with accessibility and equitable care for all patient groups.

PATIENT REPORTED OUTCOME MEASURES

Outcome measurement in orthopedic and hand surgery classically involves objective measures, for example, range of motion and presence of infection. PROMs are designed to complement objective measures and provide a standardized assessment from a patient about their health

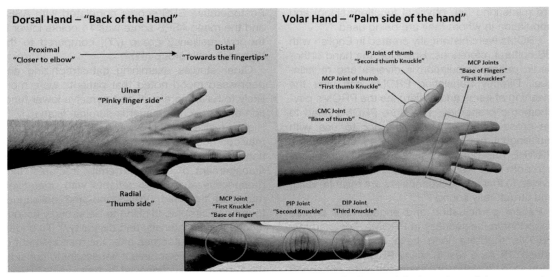

Fig. 1. Surface anatomy and anatomic orientation for patient review before and during telemedicine encounter. This identifies basic anatomic vocabulary and orientation with corresponding layman's terms in quotations marks. CMC, carpometacarpal; DIP, distal interphalangeal; IP, interphalangeal; MCP, metacarpophalangeal; PIP, proximal interphalangeal. (*From* Van Nest DS, Ilyas AM, Rivlin M. Telemedicine Evaluation and Techniques in Hand Surgery. J Hand Surg Glob Online. 2020;2(4):240–245; with permission.)

status (eg, ability to work or perform activities of daily living). PROMs can be utilized to gain a better understanding of the patient perspective and thus deliver more patient-centered care. While initially designed as research tools to measure outcomes, PROMs have been increasingly utilized in clinical settings not only to measure outcomes that matter to patients but also to predict outcomes, inform shared decision-making approaches, and guide treatment.[8,9,42,43]

There are multiple PROMs that are used to evaluate the upper extremity. Some common PROMs include the Australian/Canadian Osteoarthritis Hand Index (AUSCAN),[44–48] Patient-Rated Wrist-Hand Evaluation (PRWHE),[48–50] Disability of the Arm Shoulder and Hand (DASH),[50–53] the short form of the DASH (Quick-DASH), and the Patient-Reported Outcomes Measurement Information System Upper Extremity (PROMIS UE).

Patient-reported outcome measures at point of care

While traditionally utilized for research or retrospectively, the clinical benefits of PROM collection and use at the point of care in many specialties are being increasingly recognized. In the field of oncology, PROMs have demonstrated clinical benefits. Basch and colleagues demonstrate that the use of PROMs in monitoring symptoms during chemotherapy is associated with improved survival. In total joint arthroplasty, PROMs.[54] In

hand surgery, PROMs have the potential to be used for clinical decision making and to track longitudinal outcomes.[42,43] Less investigation has been conducted evaluating these clinical benefits to patients being seen by hand and upper extremity surgeons. In a prospective study of 227 workers with distal radius fractures (DRF), MacDermid et. al. found that patients' PRWE and DASH score were more closely associated with return to work than physical measures of impartment (ie, grip strength, wrist ROM, and dexterity) or radiographic measures.[8] The Hand Surgery Quality Consortium conducted an investigation to understand the literature and to create quality measures related to the routine collection and communication individualized PROMs to patients at point of care.[55–60] The group voted on measures that include collecting and communicating validated PROMs at every clinical visit for common conditions. Consensus was not achieved for any of the twelve measures developed. Notably, consensus was limited secondary to usability and evidence available. As such, additional investigation on the use of PROMs at point of care in hand surgery is needed as benefits of PROM use at point of care has demonstrated benefits in other fields.

Barriers to patient-reported outcome measures utilization

In order for PROMs to be utilized appropriately, they should be validated for the construct they are measuring (eg, physical function, sleep) and population in whom they are being used. ***

PROMs were historically created in English with US cultural references. However, the hand orthopedic patient population is diverse and multilingual. Directly translating PROMs can alter the meaning of items and undermine the PROMs psychometric properties. Therefore PROMs need to be cross-culturally validated prior to use with multilingual populations. For hand surgery, the PRWHE has been translated into 21 languages and both the PRWHE and DASH have high quality evidence that the questionnaires are reliable, valid, and structurally sound.[61–64]

Patient participation and engagement is also important in the success of PROMs. For example, PROMs that are long have lower completion rates.[65–68] As a result, many PROMS have been shortened, loosing precision but with enhanced responder compliance. Similarly, CAT questionaries have been developed, a model in which the instrument progressively adapts to the individual answering the questions and may be shorter based on the answers.[65,69–77] In a prospective study 744 patients with proximal humerus, elbow and distal radius fractures Jayakumar and colleagues found that patients who actively manage their health and demonstrate effective emotional and social functioning share a common underlying trait.[68,78,79] They have fewer limitations and greater satisfaction with care during recovery from upper limb fractures. It is important to consider patient engagement, starting by having PROMs that are user friendly, as well as identifying psychosocial factors and addressing them through patient education and coaching.[68,78,79]

Psychosocial factors and clinical outcomes

Outcomes in hand surgery are influenced by multiple factors. Historically a large emphasis was placed on surgical proficiency and outcomes related to the surgery. However, other factors beyond the surgeons' control, such as psychosocial factors, influence clinical outcomes. Recent studies have shown that psychological factors such as patient expectations, mental health (catastrophizing, depression, anxiety), pre-operative opioid use, and resiliency may be important predictors of patient outcomes for patients with proximal humerus fractures undergoing arthroplasty.[80–86] Resiliency is characterized as the ability to bounce back or return to healthy level of function after experiencing stress measured by the Brief Resiliency Scale (BRS). In a prospective study 77 patients that were 2 years post shoulder arthroplasty completed the BRS and ASES.[81,82]

Postoperative BRS scores correlated with ASES and the mean ASES score was 14 points lower in the low resiliency group (77), compared to the high resiliency group (91).

Other studies examining catastrophizing and depressed mood noted that patients were more likely to have more pain and perceive lower function after proximal humerus surgical fixation.[80–84] Higher resilience and lower pain catastrophizing may contribute to lower pain intensity, better function, and perception of greater normality after the management of upper extremity fractures. In a prospective study 152 patients with operatively managed fractures, Vranceanu and colleagues found catastrophic thinking to be strongly associated with pain intensity and disability.[87] To understand clinical outcomes after the management of upper extremity fractures it necessary to consider the impact of psychosocial factors.

Patient-reported outcome measures future direction

PROMs were developed as research tools with limited capabilities that have gained traction with the shift to patient-centered care and are now frequently used in the clinical setting. Efficiency in high volume hand clinics is important, as result utilizing PROMs that do not take away from valuable clinic time is important.[9] Various PROMs have now been transfer to electronic forms that the patient can fill out prior to their appointment or can be completed over a telephone visit. CAT questionaries have been developed, a model in which the instrument progressively adapts to the individual answering the questions and may be shorter based on the answers.[65,69,72,76] PROM data has the potential to provide signposts for when progress is stalled or important milestones are reached. In addition, PROM can be important predictors of clinical outcomes.[7–9] Expansion of the use of PROMs in the clinical setting can provide a large data base that can be used for research and continued improvement of patient care.

TRACKERS/WEARABLES/APPS

The extensive commercial adoption of mobile phone technology and wearable devices has enabled the development of mobile health and sensor-based tools for orthopedic surgery. Given the relatively low cost of these technologies compared to conventional tools, they allow for more widespread and remote data collection than was previously possible, which eventually will expand capabilities for telemedicine and remote monitoring beyond the clinic.

Modalities

Within orthopedic surgery, several key applications are being explored for clinical evaluation, rehabilitation, and postoperative monitoring. For example, quantifying muscular strength and joint range of motion has conventionally been limited by clinician subjectivity and expensive digital tools, which has limited the accuracy of evaluation in the clinic and prohibited evaluation remotely during telehealth visits. Several low-cost mechanical devices are being developed capable of accurately and reproducibly measuring muscular strength both in the clinic and at home for a variety of musculoskeletal applications.[88] Low-cost motion analysis systems (LCMAS) have also emerged as pragmatic tools for in clinic and at home assessment of range of motion as well as novel biomechanical biomarkers.[89,90]

Inertial measurement units (IMUs) are low-cost sensors capable of measuring linear and rotational acceleration, as well as gravitational forces. Various algorithms[91] have been developed to derive the joint range of motion (ROM) from these sensor data for a variety of musculoskeletal applications,[92] including the hand and upper extremity.[93–109] Because many modern mobile phones contain IMU's, several applications have been developed to measure hand and wrist ROM without the need for additional hardware.[110–114]

With the incorporation of sensor technologies or virtual reality environments telerehabilitation has been able to expand its reach.[12,25,31] Telerehabilitation utilizes sensors utilizes equipment such as tilt switches, accelerometers, and gyroscopes to measure movement through three-dimensional space.[25,93,109,115] These devices have been shown to be practical for home monitoring of patients creating opportunities for research and into improving post-operative clinical mobility. Virtual reality telerehabilitation utilizes computer-generated three-dimensional virtual environments that the patient is presented with eliciting specific movement to aid in motor learning that can be translated to the real world.[25,32] These capabilities have the ability to interface with live feed from the physical therapy team and measure ROM progression.

Use cases

Several notable applications of these technologies beyond conventional ROM measurement include the evaluation of wrist mobility in postoperative distal radius fracture patients,[116] monitoring of mobilization of geriatric fracture patients in the hospital setting,[117] and the incorporation of mobile games to encourage rehabilitation.[12,115,118] Digital health tools may improve adherence to postoperative therapy,[118] although data so far are mostly speculative. There is an ongoing clinical trial comparing 6 weeks of mobile serious game therapy, interactive computer application that incorporates gamification principles to achieve a predefined goal, versus conventional hand therapy following distal radius fractures.[115]

Like most early-stage clinical technologies, many of the aforementioned validation studies have occurred in healthy control samples or small clinical cohorts. Larger trials assessing the feasibility of widespread implementation and clinical efficacy of these technologies compared to the standard of care are required. While technologies developed around commercial sensors and mobile phones are more accessible than many conventional clinical technologies, access to a mobile device and the internet are still required, which may be prohibitive for certain patient populations. Finally, changes to physician and hospital reimbursement may be necessary to ensure providers and health care systems are compensated for the use of these technologies.

Future directions

Finally there are several emerging technologies that may have promise specifically for hand and upper extremity surgery, including "smart" graphene electronic tattoos capable of measuring electromyographic signals, skin stretch, temperature, and other physiologic metrics.[119] Stretchable carbon nanotubes have also been used to develop strain sensors which may have applications in the assessment of finger range of motion, which has previously been difficult to quantify.[120] Park and colleagues tested carbon nanotubes on the middle finger MTP joint of 12 healthy patients and reliably measured MCP ROM, as well as demonstrated the high durability of the sensor.

Mobile phone technology and wearable devices have enabled the development of mobile health and sensor-based tools for orthopedic surgery to help in the rehabilitation process. Ongoing research on validation and feasibility is necessary. Wearable technology is also being developed across orthopedic subspecialties including trauma,[121] sports medicine,[122,123] and spine surgery[124] highlighting the importance of collaboration across disciplines in the development of new technology.

SUMMARY

Recent advances in telemedicine, patient-reported outcome measurement, and wearables/remote patient monitoring are changing the landscape of follow-up care of clinical and research outcomes in hand and upper extremity patients. Telemedicine in hand and upper extremity surgery has the potential to increase productivity, reduce costs, and increase access to care. Telemedicine does not appear to be a replacement for all in-person clinic encounters, however, when used in the appropriate context demonstrates favorable results. PROMs have gained traction in the clinical setting to understand a patient's perception of their outcome, and to predict clinical outcomes, guide treatment decisions, and ultimately improve outcomes. Finally, the widespread commercial adoption of mobile phone technology and wearable devices has enabled the development of mobile health and sensor-based tools for orthopedic surgery to improve clinical outcomes. These devices have demonstrated early impact in hand and upper extremity care, and eventually will expand capabilities for telemedicine and remote monitoring beyond the clinic. In the continued development and expansion of these tools there should be continued focus on their potential limitations and provide equitable access to all patients.

CLINICS CARE POINTS

- In orthopedics, telemedicine is being used for consultations services, post-operative care, telerehabilitation, and to reach rural and underserved areas. Technological innovations in physical examination protocols and tools will continue to improve the effectiveness of virtual orthopedic visits. As telemedicine continues to expand, it is important to consider and address systematic issues with accessibility and equitable care for all patient groups.

- While initially designed as research tools to measure outcomes, PROMs have been increasingly utilized in clinical settings not only to measure outcomes that matter to patients but also to predict outcomes, inform shared decision-making approaches, and guide treatment. It is important to consider patient engagement, starting by having PROMs that are user friendly, as well as adapt PROMS to linguistically and culturally diverse populations

- In trackers/wereables/apps several key applications are being explored for clinical evaluation, rehabilitation, and postoperative monitoring. Digital health tools may improve adherence to postoperative therapy, although data so far are mostly speculative. Access to a mobile device and the internet are still required, which may be prohibitive for certain patient populations.

DISCLOSURE

The authors have nothing to disclose.

REFERENCES

1. Karl JW, Olson PR, Rosenwasser MP. The epidemiology of upper extremity fractures in the United States, 2009. J Orthop Trauma 2015;29(8):e242–4.
2. Fahey E, Elsheikh MFH, Davey MS, et al. Telemedicine in orthopedic surgery: a systematic review of current evidence. Telemed J E-Health Off J Am Telemed Assoc. 2022;28(5):613–35.
3. Moisan P, Barimani B, Antoniou J. Orthopedic surgery and telemedicine in times of COVID-19 and beyond: a review. Curr Rev Musculoskelet Med 2021;14(2):155–9.
4. Al-Kulabi A, Mansour MA, Thahir A. The orthopaedic experience of COVID-19: A literature review. J Perioper Pract 2021;31(3):102–7.
5. Rizzi AM, Polachek WS, Dulas M, et al. The new "normal": Rapid adoption of telemedicine in orthopaedics during the COVID-19 pandemic. Injury 2020;51(12):2816–21.
6. Henry TW, Fletcher D, Vaccaro AR, et al. Evaluating patient interest in orthopedic telehealth services beyond the COVID-19 pandemic. Cureus 2021; 13(7):e16523.
7. Dias J, Brealey S, Cook L, et al. Surgical fixation compared with cast immobilisation for adults with a bicortical fracture of the scaphoid waist: the SWIFFT RCT. Health Technol Assess Winch Engl 2020;24(52):1–234.
8. MacDermid JC, Roth JH, McMurtry R. Predictors of Time Lost from Work Following a Distal Radius Fracture. J Occup Rehabil 2007;17(1):47–62.
9. MacDermid JC. Patient-reported outcomes: state-of-the-art hand surgery and future applications. Hand Clin 2014;30(3):293–304.
10. WHO Group Consultation on Health Telematics (1997: Geneva S. A Health Telematics Policy in Support of WHO's Health-for-All Strategy for Global Health Development : Report of the WHO Group Consultation on Health Telematics, 11-16 December, Geneva, 1997. World Health Organization; 1998. Available at: https://apps.who.int/iris/handle/10665/63857. Accessed July 17, 2022.
11. Sandhu KS, Singh A, Singh A, et al. Telemedicine Versus In-Person Visits in Postoperative Care in Orthopedic Patients: Follow-Up Study From North India. Cureus 2021;13(9):e18399.
12. Berton A, Longo UG, Candela V, et al. Virtual Reality, Augmented Reality, Gamification, and Telerehabilitation: Psychological Impact on Orthopedic Patients' Rehabilitation. J Clin Med 2020;9(8):E2567.

13. Foni NO, Costa LAV, Velloso LMR, et al. Telemedicine: Is It a Tool for Orthopedics? Curr Rev Musculoskelet Med 2020;13(6):797–801.

14. Miller KL, Steffen MJ, McCoy KD, et al. Delivering fracture prevention services to rural US veterans through telemedicine: a process evaluation. Arch Osteoporos 2021;16(1):27.

15. Seron P, Oliveros MJ, Gutierrez-Arias R, et al. Effectiveness of Telerehabilitation in Physical Therapy: A Rapid Overview. Phys Ther 2021;101(6). pzab053.

16. Xiong G, Greene NE, Lightsey HMI, et al. Telemedicine Use in Orthopaedic Surgery Varies by Race, Ethnicity, Primary Language, and Insurance Status. Clin Orthop Relat Res 2021;479(7):1417–25.

17. Poeran J, Cho LD, Wilson L, et al. Pre-existing Disparities and Potential Implications for the Rapid Expansion of Telemedicine in Response to the Coronavirus Disease 2019 Pandemic. Med Care 2021;59(8):694–8.

18. Makhni MC, Riew GJ, Sumathipala MG. Telemedicine in Orthopaedic Surgery: Challenges and Opportunities. J Bone Joint Surg Am 2020;102(13):1109–15.

19. Buvik A, Bergmo TS, Bugge E, et al. Cost-Effectiveness of Telemedicine in Remote Orthopedic Consultations: Randomized Controlled Trial. J Med Internet Res 2019;21(2):e11330.

20. Aarnio P, Lamminen H, Lepistö J, et al. A prospective study of teleconferencing for orthopaedic consultations. J Telemed Telecare 1999;5(1):62–6.

21. Tripod M, Tait M, Bracey J, et al. The Use of Telemedicine Decreases Unnecessary Hand Trauma Transfers. Hand N Y N 2020;15(3):422–7.

22. Bracey JW, Tait MA, Hollenberg SB, et al. A Novel Telemedicine System for Care of Statewide Hand Trauma. Hand N Y N 2021;16(2):253–7.

23. Buvik A, Bugge E, Knutsen G, et al. Quality of care for remote orthopaedic consultations using telemedicine: a randomised controlled trial. BMC Health Serv Res 2016;16(1):483.

24. Moore MR, Galetta MS, Schwarzkopf R, et al, Force Writing Committee. Patient Satisfaction and Interest in Telemedicine Visits Following Total Knee and Hip Replacement Surgery. Telemed J E-Health Off J Am Telemed Assoc 2022. https://doi.org/10.1089/tmj.2021.0439.

25. Russell TG, Blumke R, Richardson B, et al. Telerehabilitation mediated physiotherapy assessment of ankle disorders. Physiother Res Int J Res Clin Phys Ther 2010;15(3):167–75.

26. Chande RD, Wayne JS. Neural Network Optimization of Ligament Stiffnesses for the Enhanced Predictive Ability of a Patient-Specific, Computational Foot/Ankle Model. J Biomech Eng 2017;139(9).

27. Dent PA, Wilke B, Terkonda S, et al. Validation of Teleconference-based Goniometry for Measuring Elbow Joint Range of Motion. Cureus 2020;12(2):e6925.

28. Tang P. Collateral ligament injuries of the thumb metacarpophalangeal joint. J Am Acad Orthop Surg 2011;19:287–96.

29. Grandizio LC, Mettler AW, Caselli ME, et al. Telemedicine After Upper Extremity Surgery: A Prospective Study of Program Implementation. J Hand Surg 2020;45(9):795–801.

30. Bini SA, Mahajan J. Clinical outcomes of remote asynchronous telerehabilitation are equivalent to traditional therapy following total knee arthroplasty: A randomized control study. J Telemed Telecare 2017;23(2):239–47.

31. Piron L, Turolla A, Agostini M, et al. Exercises for paretic upper limb after stroke: a combined virtual-reality and telemedicine approach. J Rehabil Med 2009;41(12):1016–102.

32. Holden MK. Virtual environments for motor rehabilitation: review. Cyberpsychology Behav Impact Internet Multimed Virtual Real Behav Soc 2005;8(3):187–211 [discussion 212-219].

33. Tousignant M, Giguère AM, Morin M, et al. In-home telerehabilitation for proximal humerus fractures: a pilot study. Int J Telerehabilitation 2014;6(2):31–7.

34. Chaudhry H, Nadeem S, Mundi R. How Satisfied Are Patients and Surgeons with Telemedicine in Orthopaedic Care During the COVID-19 Pandemic? A Systematic Review and Meta-analysis. Clin Orthop 2021;479(1):47–56.

35. Wahezi SE, Duarte RA, Yerra S, et al. Telemedicine During COVID-19 and Beyond: A Practical Guide and Best Practices Multidisciplinary Approach for the Orthopedic and Neurologic Pain Physical Examination. Pain Physician 2020;23(4S):S205–38.

36. Kumar S, Kumar A, Kumar M, et al. Feasibility of telemedicine in maintaining follow-up of orthopaedic patients and their satisfaction: A preliminary study. J Clin Orthop Trauma 2020;11:S704–10.

37. Mehta SP, Kendall KM, Reasor CM. Virtual assessments of knee and wrist joint range motion have comparable reliability with face-to-face assessments. Muscoskel Care 2021;19(2):208–16.

38. Wright-Chisem J, Trehan S. The Hand and Wrist Examination for Video Telehealth Encounters. HSS J Musculoskelet J Hosp Spec Surg 2021;17(1):70–4.

39. Van Nest DS, Ilyas AM, Rivlin M. Telemedicine Evaluation and Techniques in Hand Surgery. J Hand Surg Glob Online 2020;2(4):240–5.

40. Grandizio LC, Barreto Rocha DF, Foster BK, et al. Evaluation of a Comprehensive Telemedicine Pathway for Carpal Tunnel Syndrome: A Comparison of Virtual and In-Person Assessments. J Hand Surg 2022;47(2):111–9.

41. Rogers TN, Rogers CR, VanSant-Webb E, et al. Racial Disparities in COVID-19 Mortality Among Essential Workers in the United States. World Med Health Policy 2020;12(3):311–27.

42. Ingall EM, Bernstein DN, Shoji MM, et al. Using the QuickDASH to Model Clinical Recovery Trajectory After Operative Management of Distal Radius Fracture. J Hand Surg Glob Online 2021;3(1):1–6.

43. Lambert MJ, Whipple JL, Hawkins EJ, et al. Is It Time for Clinicians to Routinely Track Patient Outcome? A Meta-Analysis. Clin Psychol Sci Pract 2003;10(3):288–301.

44. MacDermid JC, Turgeon T, Richards RS, et al. Patient rating of wrist pain and disability: a reliable and valid measurement tool. J Orthop Trauma 1998;12(8):577–86.

45. Bellamy N, Campbell J, Haraoui B, et al. Dimensionality and clinical importance of pain and disability in hand osteoarthritis: Development of the Australian/Canadian (AUSCAN) Osteoarthritis Hand Index. Osteoarthr Cartil OARS Osteoarthr Res Soc 2002;10(11):855–62.

46. Bellamy N, Hochberg M, Tubach F, et al. Development of Multinational Definitions of Minimal Clinically Important Improvement and Patient Acceptable Symptomatic State in Osteoarthritis. Arthritis Care Res 2015;67(7):972–80.

47. Haugen IK, Slatkowsky-Christensen B, Bøyesen P, et al. Cross-sectional and longitudinal associations between radiographic features and measures of pain and physical function in hand osteoarthritis. Osteoarthr Cartil OARS Osteoarthr Res Soc 2013; 21(9):1191–8.

48. McQuillan TJ, Vora MM, Kenney DE, et al. The AUSCAN and PRWHE Demonstrate Comparable Internal Consistency and Validity in Patients With Early Thumb Carpometacarpal Osteoarthritis. Hand N Y N 2018;13(6):652–8.

49. MacDermid JC, Tottenham V. Responsiveness of the disability of the arm, shoulder, and hand (DASH) and patient-rated wrist/hand evaluation (PRWHE) in evaluating change after hand therapy. J Hand Ther 2004;17(1):18–23.

50. Phillips JLH, Warrender WJ, Lutsky KF, et al. Evaluation of the PROMIS Upper Extremity Computer Adaptive Test Against Validated Patient-Reported Outcomes in Patients With Basilar Thumb Arthritis. J Hand Surg 2019;44(7):564–9.

51. Gummesson C, Atroshi I, Ekdahl C. The disabilities of the arm, shoulder and hand (DASH) outcome questionnaire: longitudinal construct validity and measuring self-rated health change after surgery. BMC Musculoskelet Disord 2003;4:11.

52. Poole JL. Measures of hand function: Arthritis Hand Function Test (AHFT), Australian Canadian Osteoarthritis Hand Index (AUSCAN), Cochin Hand Function Scale, Functional Index for Hand Osteoarthritis (FIHOA), Grip Ability Test (GAT), Jebsen Hand Function Test (JHFT), and Michigan Hand Outcomes Questionnaire (MHQ). Arthritis Care Res 2011;63(Suppl 11):S189–99.

53. Hung M, Voss MW, Bounsanga J, et al. Examination of the PROMIS upper extremity item bank. J Hand Ther 2017;30(4):485–90.

54. Jayakumar P, Moore MG, Furlough KA, et al. Comparison of an Artificial Intelligence-Enabled Patient Decision Aid vs Educational Material on Decision Quality, Shared Decision-Making, Patient Experience, and Functional Outcomes in Adults With Knee Osteoarthritis: A Randomized Clinical Trial. JAMA Netw Open 2021;4(2):e2037107.

55. Shapiro LM, Ring D, Akelman E, et al. How Should We Use Patient-Reported Outcome Measures at the Point of Care in Hand Surgery? J Hand Surg 2021;46(12):1049–56.

56. Fogel N, Mertz K, Shapiro LM, et al. Outcome Metrics in the Treatment of Distal Radius Fractures in Patients Aged Above 50 Years: A Systematic Review. HAND 2021.

57. Velikova G, Booth L, Smith AB, et al. Measuring quality of life in routine oncology practice improves communication and patient well-being: a randomized controlled trial. J Clin Oncol Off J Am Soc Clin Oncol 2004;22(4):714–24.

58. Berry DL, Blumenstein BA, Halpenny B, et al. Enhancing patient-provider communication with the electronic self-report assessment for cancer: a randomized trial. J Clin Oncol Off J Am Soc Clin Oncol 2011;29(8):1029–35.

59. Detmar SB, Muller MJ, Wever LD, et al. The patient-physician relationship. Patient-physician communication during outpatient palliative treatment visits: an observational study. JAMA 2001;285(10):1351–7.

60. Wood SM, Kim YJ, Seyferth AV, et al. Quality Metrics in Hand Surgery: A Systematic Review. J Hand Surg 2021;46(11):972–9.e1.

61. Shafiee E, MacDermid J, Farzad M, et al. A systematic review and meta-analysis of Patient-Rated Wrist (and Hand) Evaluation (PRWE/PRWHE) measurement properties, translation, and/or cross-cultural adaptation. Disabil Rehabil 2021;1–15.

62. Rosales RS, García-Gutierrez R, Reboso-Morales L, et al. The Spanish version of the Patient-Rated Wrist Evaluation outcome measure: cross-cultural adaptation process, reliability, measurement error and construct validity. Health Qual Life Outcomes 2017;15(1):169.

63. Kim JK, Kang JS. Evaluation of the Korean version of the patient-rated wrist evaluation. J Hand Ther Off J Am Soc Hand Ther 2013;26(3):238–43 [quiz: 244].

64. Kennedy CA, Beaton DE, Smith P, et al. Measurement properties of the QuickDASH (disabilities of the arm, shoulder and hand) outcome measure and cross-cultural adaptations of the QuickDASH: a systematic review. Qual Life Res Int J Qual Life Asp Treat Care Rehabil 2013;22(9):2509–47.

65. Giladi AM, Chung KC. Measuring Outcomes in Hand Surgery. Clin Plast Surg 2008;35(2):239–50.

66. Rosenbaum S. The Patient Protection and Affordable Care Act: Implications for Public Health Policy and Practice. Public Health Rep 2011;126(1):130–5.

67. Kamal RN, Ring D, Akelman E, et al. Quality Measures in Upper Limb Surgery. J Bone Joint Surg Am 2016;98(6):505–10.

68. Jayakumar P, Teunis T, Vranceanu AM, et al. Relationship Between Magnitude of Limitations and Patient Experience During Recovery from Upper-Extremity Fracture. JB JS Open Access 2019;4(3):1–7. e0002.

69. Hung M, Tyser A, Saltzman C, et al. Establishing the Minimal Clinically Important Difference for the PROMIS and qDASH. J Hand Surg 2018;43:S22.

70. Constant CR, Murley AH. A clinical method of functional assessment of the shoulder. Clin Orthop 1987;214:160–4.

71. Richards RR, An KN, LU Bigliani, et al. A standardized method for the assessment of shoulder function. J Shoulder Elbow Surg 1994;3(6):347–52.

72. Beleckas CM, Padovano A, Guattery J, et al. Performance of Patient-Reported Outcomes Measurement Information System (PROMIS) Upper Extremity (UE) Versus Physical Function (PF) Computer Adaptive Tests (CATs) in Upper Extremity Clinics. J Hand Surg 2017;42(11):867–74.

73. Döring AC, Nota SPFT, Hageman MGJS, et al. Measurement of Upper Extremity Disability Using the Patient-Reported Outcomes Measurement Information System. J Hand Surg 2014;39(6):1160–5.

74. Jayakumar P, Teunis T, Vranceanu AM, et al. Construct Validity and Precision of Different Patient-reported Outcome Measures During Recovery After Upper Extremity Fractures. Clin Orthop 2019;477(11):2521–30.

75. Cella D, Riley W, Stone A, et al. The Patient-Reported Outcomes Measurement Information System (PROMIS) developed and tested its first wave of adult self-reported health outcome item banks: 2005-2008. J Clin Epidemiol 2010;63(11):1179–94.

76. Gausden EB, Levack AE, Sin DN, et al. Validating the Patient Reported Outcomes Measurement Information System (PROMIS) computerized adaptive tests for upper extremity fracture care. J Shoulder Elbow Surg 2018;27(7):1191–7.

77. Copay AG, Chung AS, Eyberg B, et al. Minimum Clinically Important Difference: Current Trends in the Orthopaedic Literature, Part I: Upper Extremity: A Systematic Review. JBJS Rev 2018;6(9):e1.

78. Jayakumar P, Teunis T, Vranceanu AM, et al. The impact of a patient's engagement in their health on the magnitude of limitations and experience following upper limb fractures. Bone Jt J 2020;102-B(1):42–7.

79. Schalet BD, Reise SP, Zulman DM, et al. Psychometric evaluation of a patient-reported item bank for healthcare engagement. Qual Life Res 2021;30(8):2363–74.

80. Vajapey SP, Cvetanovich GL, Bishop JY, et al. Psychosocial factors affecting outcomes after shoulder arthroplasty: a systematic review. J Shoulder Elbow Surg 2020;29(5):e175–84.

81. Tokish JM, Kissenberth MJ, Tolan SJ, et al. Resilience correlates with outcomes after total shoulder arthroplasty. J Shoulder Elbow Surg 2017;26(5):752–6.

82. Dombrowsky AR, Kirchner G, Isbell J, et al. Resilience correlates with patient reported outcomes after reverse total shoulder arthroplasty. Orthop Traumatol Surg Res OTSR 2021;107(1):102777.

83. Morris BJ, Sciascia AD, Jacobs CA, et al. Preoperative opioid use associated with worse outcomes after anatomic shoulder arthroplasty. J Shoulder Elbow Surg 2016;25(4):619–23.

84. Belayneh R, Lott A, Haglin J, et al. The role of patients' overall expectations of health on outcomes following proximal humerus fracture repair. Orthop Traumatol Surg Res 2021;107(8):103043.

85. Smith BW, Dalen J, Wiggins K, et al. The brief resilience scale: assessing the ability to bounce back. Int J Behav Med 2008;15(3):194–200.

86. Sheikhzadeh A, Wertli MM, Weiner SS, et al. Do psychological factors affect outcomes in musculoskeletal shoulder disorders? A systematic review. BMC Musculoskelet Disord 2021;22:560.

87. Vranceanu AM, Bachoura A, Weening A, et al. Psychological factors predict disability and pain intensity after skeletal trauma. J Bone Joint Surg Am 2014;96(3):e20.

88. Bechard L, Bell K, Lynch A. Preliminary validation of a mobile force Sensing device for clinical and telerehabilitation. J Biomech 2020;110:109973.

89. Halvorson RT, Castillo FT, Ahamed F, et al. Point-of-care motion capture and biomechanical assessment improve clinical utility of dynamic balance testing for lower extremity osteoarthritis. Awai C, ed. PLOS Digit Health. 2022;1(7):e0000068. doi: 10.1371/journal.pdig.0000068.

90. Ngan A, Xiao W, Curran PF, et al. Functional workspace and patient-reported outcomes improve after reverse and total shoulder arthroplasty. J Shoulder Elbow Surg 2019;28(11):2121–7.

91. Bravo-Illanes G, Halvorson R, Matthew R, et al. IMU Sensor Fusion Algorithm for Monitoring Knee Kinematics in ACL Reconstructed Patients. In: 2019 41st Annual International Conference of the IEEE Engineering in Medicine and Biology Society (EMBC), Berlin, Germany July 2019:5877-5881. https://doi.org/10.1109/EMBC.2019.8857431.

92. Rigoni M, Gill S, Babazadeh S, et al. Assessment of Shoulder Range of Motion Using a Wireless Inertial Motion Capture Device-A Validation Study. Sensors 2019;19(8):E1781.

93. Costa V, Ramírez Ó, Otero A, et al. Validity and reliability of inertial sensors for elbow and wrist range of motion assessment. PeerJ 2020;8:e9687.

94. Arora R, Gabl M, Gschwentner M, et al. A Comparative Study of Clinical and Radiologic Outcomes of Unstable Colles Type Distal Radius Fractures in Patients Older Than 70 Years: Nonoperative Treatment Versus Volar Locking Plating. J Orthop Trauma 2009;23(4):237–42.

95. Anzarut A, Johnson JA, Rowe BH, et al. Radiologic and patient-reported functional outcomes in an elderly cohort with conservatively treated distal radius fractures. J Hand Surg 2004;29(6):1121–7.

96. Choi WS, Hwang JS, Hur JS, et al. Correlation between patient-reported outcome measures and Single Assessment Numerical Evaluation score in patients treated with a volar locking plate for a distal radial fracture. Bone Jt J 2020;102-B(6):744–8.

97. Rangan A, Handoll H, Brealey S, et al. Surgical vs nonsurgical treatment of adults with displaced fractures of the proximal humerus: the PROFHER randomized clinical trial. JAMA 2015;313(10):1037–47.

98. Roberson TA, Granade CM, Hunt Q, et al. Nonoperative management versus reverse shoulder arthroplasty for treatment of 3- and 4-part proximal humeral fractures in older adults. J Shoulder Elbow Surg 2017;26(6):1017–22.

99. Bhashyam AR, Ochen Y, van der Vliet QMJ, et al. Association of Patient-reported Outcomes With Clinical Outcomes After Distal Humerus Fracture Treatment. J Am Acad Orthop Surg Glob Res Rev 2020;4(2):e19, 00122.

100. Van Lieshout EMM, Mahabier KC, Tuinebreijer WE, et al. HUMMER Investigators. Rasch analysis of the Disabilities of the Arm, Shoulder and Hand (DASH) instrument in patients with a humeral shaft fracture. J Shoulder Elbow Surg 2020;29(5):1040–9.

101. Hao KA, Kakalecik J, Delgado GA, et al. Current trends in patient-reported outcome measures for clavicle fractures: a focused systematic review of 11 influential orthopaedic journals. J Shoulder Elbow Surg 2022;31(2):e58–67.

102. Stirling PHC, Simpson CJ, Ring D, et al. Virtual management of clinically suspected scaphoid fractures. Bone Jt J 2022;104-B(6):709–14.

103. Kootstra TJM, Keizer J, Bhashyam A, et al. Patient-Reported Outcomes and Complications After Surgical Fixation of 143 Proximal Phalanx Fractures. J Hand Surg 2020;45(4):327–34.

104. Lee JK, Hong IT, Cho JW, et al. Outcomes Following Open Reduction and Internal Fixation in Proximal Phalangeal Fracture with Rotational Malalignment. J Hand Surg Asian-Pac 2020;25(2):219–25.

105. Wylie JD, Beckmann JT, Granger E, et al. Functional outcomes assessment in shoulder surgery. World J Orthop 2014;5(5):623–33.

106. Kleinlugtenbelt YV, Krol RG, Bhandari M, et al. Are the patient-rated wrist evaluation (PRWE) and the disabilities of the arm, shoulder and hand (DASH) questionnaire used in distal radial fractures truly valid and reliable? Bone Jt Res 2018;7(1):36–45.

107. Kleinlugtenbelt YV, Nienhuis RW, Bhandari M, et al. Are validated outcome measures used in distal radial fractures truly valid? A critical assessment using the COnsensus-based Standards for the selection of health Measurement INstruments (COSMIN) checklist. Bone Jt Res 2016;5(4):153–61.

108. Pourahmadi MR, Ebrahimi Takamjani I, Sarrafzadeh J, et al. Reliability and concurrent validity of a new iPhone® goniometric application for measuring active wrist range of motion: a cross-sectional study in asymptomatic subjects. J Anat 2017;230(3):484–95.

109. Santospagnuolo A, Bruno AA, Pagnoni A, et al. Validity and reliability of the GYKO inertial sensor system for the assessment of the elbow range of motion. J Sports Med Phys Fitness 2019;59(9):1466–71.

110. Engstrand F, Tesselaar E, Gestblom R, et al. Validation of a smartphone application and wearable sensor for measurements of wrist motions. J Hand Surg Eur 2021;46(10):1057–63.

111. Modest J, Clair B, DeMasi R, et al. Self-measured wrist range of motion by wrist-injured and wrist-healthy study participants using a built-in iPhone feature as compared with a universal goniometer. J Hand Ther Off J Am Soc Hand Ther 2019;32(4):507–14.

112. Alford SL. Remote self-measurement of wrist range of motion performed on normal wrists by a minimally trained individual using the iPhone level application only demonstrated good reliability in measuring wrist flexion and extension. J Hand Ther Off J Am Soc Hand Ther 2021;34(4):549–54.

113. Reid S, Egan B. The validity and reliability of DrGoniometer, a smartphone application, for measuring forearm supination. J Hand Ther Off J Am Soc Hand Ther 2019;32(1):110–7.

114. Wagner ER, Conti Mica M, Shin AY. Smartphone photography utilized to measure wrist range of motion. J Hand Surg Eur 2018;43(2):187–92.

115. Meijer HAW, Graafland M, Obdeijn MC, et al. Serious game versus standard care for rehabilitation after distal radius fractures: a protocol for a multicentre randomised controlled trial. BMJ Open 2021;11(3):e042629.

116. Zucchi B, Mangone M, Agostini F, et al. Movement Analysis with Inertial Measurement Unit Sensor After

Surgical Treatment for Distal Radius Fractures. Bio-Research Open Access 2020;9(1):151–61.

117. Keppler AM, Holzschuh J, Pfeufer D, et al. Postoperative physical activity in orthogeriatric patients - new insights with continuous monitoring. Injury 2020;51(3):628–32.

118. Meijer HA, Graafland M, Goslings JC, et al. Systematic Review on the Effects of Serious Games and Wearable Technology Used in Rehabilitation of Patients With Traumatic Bone and Soft Tissue Injuries. Arch Phys Med Rehabil 2018;99(9):1890–9.

119. Kabiri Ameri S, Ho R, Jang H, et al. Graphene Electronic Tattoo Sensors. ACS Nano 2017;11(8):7634–41.

120. Park JW, Kim T, Kim D, et al. Measurement of finger joint angle using stretchable carbon nanotube strain sensor. PLoS One 2019;14(11):e0225164.

121. Berwin JT, Macdonald H, Fleming T, et al. Using a Wearable Activity Monitor to Accurately Measure Mobility After Surgery for Hip Fractures (MASH)-A Feasibility Study Protocol. Geriatr Orthop Surg Rehabil 2020;11. 2151459320964086.

122. Li RT, Kling SR, Salata MJ, et al. Wearable Performance Devices in Sports Medicine. Sport Health 2016;8(1):74–8.

123. Burns D, Razmjou H, Shaw J, et al. Adherence Tracking With Smart Watches for Shoulder Physiotherapy in Rotator Cuff Pathology: Protocol for a Longitudinal Cohort Study. JMIR Res Protoc 2020; 9(7):e17841.

124. Lee TJ, Galetta MS, Nicholson KJ, et al. Wearable Technology in Spine Surgery. Clin Spine Surg 2020;33(6):218–21.

UNITED STATES POSTAL SERVICE

Statement of Ownership, Management, and Circulation
(All Periodicals Publications Except Requester Publications)

1. Publication Title	2. Publication Number	3. Filing Date
HAND CLINICS	000 – 709	9/18/2023

4. Issue Frequency	5. Number of Issues Published Annually	6. Annual Subscription Price
FEB, MAY, AUG, NOV	4	$444.00

7. Complete Mailing Address of Known Office of Publication (Not printer) (Street, city, county, state, and ZIP+4®)

ELSEVIER INC.
230 Park Avenue, Suite 800
New York, NY 10169

Contact Person
Malathi Samayan

Telephone (Include area code)
91-44-4299-4507

8. Complete Mailing Address of Headquarters or General Business Office of Publisher (Not printer)

ELSEVIER INC.
230 Park Avenue, Suite 800
New York, NY 10169

9. Full Names and Complete Mailing Addresses of Publisher, Editor, and Managing Editor (Do not leave blank)

Publisher (Name and complete mailing address)

Dolores Meloni, ELSEVIER INC.
1600 JOHN F KENNEDY BLVD. SUITE 1600
PHILADELPHIA, PA 19103-2899

Editor (Name and complete mailing address)

MEGAN ASHDOWN, ELSEVIER INC.
1600 JOHN F KENNEDY BLVD. SUITE 1600
PHILADELPHIA, PA 19103-2899

Managing Editor (Name and complete mailing address)

PATRICK MANLEY, ELSEVIER INC.
1600 JOHN F KENNEDY BLVD. SUITE 1600
PHILADELPHIA, PA 19103-2899

10. Owner (Do not leave blank. If the publication is owned by a corporation, give the name and address of the corporation immediately followed by the names and addresses of all stockholders owning or holding 1 percent or more of the total amount of stock. If not owned by a corporation, give the names and addresses of the individual owners. If owned by a partnership or other unincorporated firm, give its name and address as well as those of each individual owner. If the publication is published by a nonprofit organization, give its name and address.)

Full Name	Complete Mailing Address
WHOLLY OWNED SUBSIDIARY OF REED/ELSEVIER, US HOLDINGS	1600 JOHN F KENNEDY BLVD. SUITE 1600 PHILADELPHIA, PA 19103-2899

11. Known Bondholders, Mortgagees, and Other Security Holders Owning or Holding 1 Percent or More of Total Amount of Bonds, Mortgages, or Other Securities. If none, check box ► ☐ None

Full Name	Complete Mailing Address
N/A	

12. Tax Status (For completion by nonprofit organizations authorized to mail at nonprofit rates) (Check one)
The purpose, function, and nonprofit status of this organization and the exempt status for federal income tax purposes:
☒ Has Not Changed During Preceding 12 Months
☐ Has Changed During Preceding 12 Months (Publisher must submit explanation of change with this statement)

PS Form **3526**, July 2014 [Page 1 of 4 (see instructions page 4)] PSN: 7530-01-000-9931 PRIVACY NOTICE: See our privacy policy on www.usps.com

---

13. Publication Title	14. Issue Date for Circulation Data Below
HAND CLINICS	MAY 2023

15. Extent and Nature of Circulation			Average No. Copies Each Issue During Preceding 12 Months	No. Copies of Single Issue Published Nearest to Filing Date
a. Total Number of Copies (Net press run)			200	198
b. Paid Circulation (By Mail and Outside the Mail)	(1)	Mailed Outside-County Paid Subscriptions Stated on PS Form 3541 (Include paid distribution above nominal rate, advertiser's proof copies, and exchange copies)	124	113
	(2)	Mailed In-County Paid Subscriptions Stated on PS Form 3541 (Include paid distribution above nominal rate, advertiser's proof copies, and exchange copies)	0	0
	(3)	Paid Distribution Outside the Mails Including Sales Through Dealers and Carriers, Street Vendors, Counter Sales, and Other Paid Distribution Outside USPS®	60	68
	(4)	Paid Distribution by Other Classes of Mail Through the USPS (e.g., First-Class Mail®)	14	15
c. Total Paid Distribution (Sum of 15b (1), (2), (3), and (4))		►	198	196
d. Free or Nominal Rate Distribution (By Mail and Outside the Mail)	(1)	Free or Nominal Rate Outside-County Copies included on PS Form 3541	1	1
	(2)	Free or Nominal Rate In-County Copies Included on PS Form 3541	0	0
	(3)	Free or Nominal Rate Copies Mailed at Other Classes Through the USPS (e.g., First-Class Mail)	0	0
	(4)	Free or Nominal Rate Distribution Outside the Mail (Carriers or other means)	1	1
e. Total Free or Nominal Rate Distribution (Sum of 15d (1), (2), (3) and (4))		►	2	2
f. Total Distribution (Sum of 15c and 15e)		►	200	198
g. Copies not Distributed (See Instructions to Publishers #4 (page #3))		►	0	0
h. Total (Sum of 15f and g)		►	200	198
i. Percent Paid (15c divided by 15f times 100)			99%	98.99%

* If you are claiming electronic copies, go to line 16 on page 3. If you are not claiming electronic copies, skip to line 17 on page 3.

PS Form **3526**, July 2014 (Page 2 of 4)

16. Electronic Copy Circulation	Average No. Copies Each Issue During Preceding 12 Months	No. Copies of Single Issue Published Nearest to Filing Date
a. Paid Electronic Copies ►		
b. Total Paid Print Copies (Line 15c) + Paid Electronic Copies (Line 16a) ►		
c. Total Print Distribution (Line 15f) + Paid Electronic Copies (Line 16a) ►		
d. Percent Paid (Both Print & Electronic Copies) (16b divided by 16c × 100) ►		

☒ I certify that 50% of all my distributed copies (electronic and print) are paid above a nominal price.

17. Publication of Statement of Ownership

☒ If the publication is a general publication, publication of this statement is required. Will be printed ☐ Publication not required
in the **November 2023** issue of this publication.

18. Signature and Title of Editor, Publisher, Business Manager, or Owner

Malathi Samayan   Date 9/18/2023

Malathi Samayan - Distribution Controller

I certify that all information furnished on this form is true and complete. I understand that anyone who furnishes false or misleading information on this form or who omits material or information requested on the form may be subject to criminal sanctions (including fines and imprisonment) and/or civil sanctions (including civil penalties).

PS Form **3526**, July 2014 (Page 3 of 4) PRIVACY NOTICE: See our privacy policy on www.usps.com

Moving?

Make sure your subscription moves with you!

To notify us of your new address, find your **Clinics Account Number** (located on your mailing label above your name), and contact customer service at:

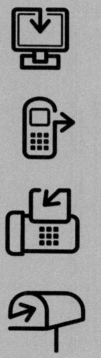

Email: journalscustomerservice-usa@elsevier.com

800-654-2452 (subscribers in the U.S. & Canada)
314-447-8871 (subscribers outside of the U.S. & Canada)

Fax number: 314-447-8029

Elsevier Health Sciences Division
Subscription Customer Service
3251 Riverport Lane
Maryland Heights, MO 63043

*To ensure uninterrupted delivery of your subscription, please notify us at least 4 weeks in advance of move.